# Community Organizing and Community Building for Health

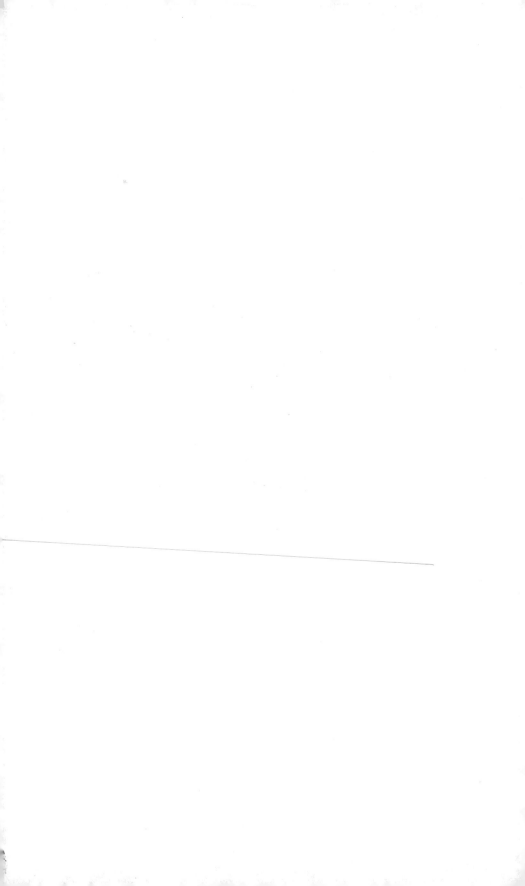

# Community Organizing and Community Building for Health

2nd edition

EDITED BY MEREDITH MINKLER

RUTGERS UNIVERSITY PRESS
New Brunswick, New Jersey, and London

Fourth paperback printing, 2008

**Library of Congress Cataloging-in-Publication data**

Community organizing and community building for health / edited by Meredith
Minkler. — 2nd ed.
  p.   cm.
  Includes bibliographical references and index.
  ISBN 0-8135-3473-9 (hardcover : alk. paper). — ISBN 0-8135-3474-7
(pbk : alk. paper)
    1. Health promotion.   2. Community health services—Citizen participation.
3. Community organization.   4. Community development.   I. Minkler,
Meredith.
RA427.8.C64   2005
362.1'2—dc22                                                    2004000307

**British Cataloging-in-Publication information is available from the British Library.**

Manufactured in the United States of America

# Contents

## Appendixes

# Acknowledgments

The second edition of a book like this one is in many respects a gift to the editor. It is a gift from many of the original authors, who cared enough to revisit, and often substantially revise and update, their earlier contributions; and it is a gift from new colleagues, who put other tasks aside to share their talents in this new collection. As in the previous volume, each of my fellow authors writes from the heart, and their combination of passion and professionalism has contributed greatly to the final product. This second edition also is a gift from the publisher, and I am indebted to Audra Wolfe, Marilyn Campbell, and the staff at Rutgers University Press for believing in this book enough to make a second edition a reality.

Many colleagues, practitioners, and community activists have shared with me and my fellow authors case studies and examples, ethical dilemmas faced in practice, and new ways of conceptualizing key aspects of community organizing and community building. Although too numerous to mention here by name, their contributions are cited throughout the book, and they deserve special thanks and recognition.

Like many of my co-authors, I have been blessed in the choice of a profession that places a strong emphasis on the centrality of empowerment and social justice for health and well-being. Numerous public health leaders and activists have inspired me in their unstinting efforts to live up to the profession's mission, but several in particular—Henrik Blum, E. Richard Brown, H. Jack Geiger, Joyce Lashof, Dorothy Nyswander, Victor Sidel and Ruth Sidel, and Rosalind Singer—have been special role models to whom I am deeply grateful.

My colleagues at the University of California, Berkeley's, School of Public Health have been a tremendous source of support and encouragement, and I acknowledge especially those current and former colleagues in community health education and health and social behavior who have contributed to my own thinking in the areas of community organizing and community building: Denise Herd, Len Duhl, Pat Morgan, Jeff Oxendine, Cheri Pies, Len Syme, and William Vega. My deepest thanks also go to my long-time faculty colleague and dear friend Lawrence Wallack, whose inspiration and help with so many things, including this project, are beyond measure. I am grateful as well to Dean Steve Shortell, whose emphasis on moving "from publication and public action" is consistent with much of the thinking behind this book and the theory-driven case studies shared in these pages.

I also owe a great debt to my colleagues at PolicyLink, especially Angela Glover Blackwell and Mildred Thompson, whose commitment to "lifting up what works"™ and using the lessons of community building on the ground to help inform and shape healthy public policy is a source of tremendous inspiration. My colleagues at the Youth Empowerment Strategies (YES!) Project, particularly Nance Wilson and Stefan Dasho, have also been a source of friendship and learning, which I hope is reflected in these pages.

Like the original book, this second edition owes its existence to my current and former gradate students at the University of California, Berkeley, and I owe them a great debt of gratitude for teaching me far more about community organizing and community building than I could ever have hoped to teach them. My other best teachers, however, have tended to be people on the front lines, and I wish to acknowledge especially some of my early teachers: the residents of San Francisco's Tenderloin District, whose tireless efforts with the Tenderloin Senior Organizing Project demonstrated over sixteen years what courage, power, and community are all about. The many staff members, board members, and volunteers involved in the project also deserve my deep thanks, particularly co-founders Sheryl Kramer and Robin Weschler, former directors Diana Miller and Lydia Ferrante, and project adviser Mike Miller. I am grateful as well to my colleagues in the Gray Panthers, the disability movement, and in the local and national communities of grandparents raising grandchildren, who have further deepened my understanding of what committed organizing and community building are all about.

Finally, while I have never had the privilege of working with them, I am indebted to the men and women of Concerned Citizens of Tillery, North Carolina, to their visionary leader Gary Grant, and to Steve Wing and their other academic partners at the University of North Carolina, who exemplify a standard of community organizing and true collaborative research to which I can only aspire. I also owe great thanks to the scholars, former scholars, staff members, and advisory board of the W. K. Kellogg Foundation's Community Health Scholars Program, from whom I also have learned a great deal about community-based participatory research and its deep roots in community building.

The second edition of this book, like the first, came to fruition thanks in part to the stimulation and support of my family and friends. My parents have been lifelong supporters and role models, providing encouragement and love beyond measure, even as their days grow more difficult. My siblings and extended family have, each in his or her own way, contributed to this project, as have close friends, including Diane Driver, Martha Holstein, Rena Pasick, Kathleen Roe, and

Rusty Springer. Finally, my friend and colleague Nina Wallerstein has again played a special role in this project, and her many contributions since its inception are, I hope, well reflected in these pages.

The sheer mechanics of a project like this one can be overwhelming, and I owe a special debt to my tireless research assistants, Alyssa Lafosse and Gena Anderson, without whose caring and commitment, organization skills, and unfailing sense of humor this project never could have been completed, much less done ahead of schedule. My copy editor, Dawn Potter, also made immense contributions, and her thoroughness and excellence are deeply appreciated.

Although I did the lion's share of the work on this book in the wee hours to avoid cutting into family time, I am grateful to SpongeBob SquarePants for buying me a couple of extra hours each Saturday morning. Above all, though, I am grateful to my husband, Jerry Peters, and our son, Jason, for their love and support. Together with my parents, siblings, and sibling-equivalent Kathy Roe, they have been a constant reminder that real "family values" are embedded, in large part, in the support and love that families, however they are defined, give to and receive from their members.

# Community Organizing and
# Community Building for Health

# Chapter 1

# Introduction to Community Organizing and Community Building

Civic engagement scholar Suzanne W. Morse (1997) is fond of describing two large signs that greet tourists at the airport customs area in a small Caribbean nation: "Belongers" and "Visitors." As health educators, social workers, and other professionals engaged in community building and community organizing, we sometimes are belongers, working within our own communities of geography or identity, helping to build a sense of connection and working collectively to bring about change. Others of us straddle two or more worlds, sharing a sense of community by virtue of race, ethnicity, or status as a breast cancer survivor or person with a disability yet remaining outsiders because of other factors, such as our education or professional credentials. Finally, many of us engage in work that requires us to stand in the visitors' line, where our effectiveness will depend in large part on our ability to demonstrate the cultural humility (Tervalon and Murray-Garcia 1998), authenticity, and respect for the belongers' strengths and wisdom that are central to successful community organizing and community building.

This book is designed for those visitors and belongers who also are professionals in fields, such as health education, which lie at the interface of health systems and communities. The book's diverse contributors share a common belief that community organizing and community building must occupy a central place in health education, health promotion, and related fields in the twenty-first century. With Lawrence Wallack and his colleagues (1993), we argue that "contemporary public health is as much about facilitating a process whereby communities use their voice to define and make their health concerns known as it is about providing prevention and treatment" (5). As professionals concerned with helping communities have their voices heard and their strengths realized and nurtured, health educators and their allies in fields such as health planning and social welfare have a critical role to play.

Playing this role and doing so effectively has seldom been more challenging. On the positive side, the importance of broadening our gaze beyond the individual to the community and broader systems levels is increasingly accepted. *Community-based, community empowerment, community participation,* and *community partnerships* are among a litany of terms used with increasing frequency among health agencies, outside funders, and policymakers. Although the reality of the accent on community has not begun to match the rhetoric (Green and Frankish 1997, Robertson and Minkler 1994), clear movement in this direction is evident on a number of fronts.

In the United States, a plethora of new community-based organizations and coalitions have sprung up in the past three decades. Through them, local communities have mobilized to fight environmental racism, domestic violence, HIV/AIDS, the targeting of youth and communities of color by the tobacco and alcohol industries, and cutbacks in health care for the uninsured. On a global scale, the Healthy Cities Movement counts among its members approximately 1,000 official community projects (http://www.healthycities.org), with estimates reaching 8,000 worldwide (Dr. Len Duhl, personal communication, July 2003). These projects are using intersectoral cooperation and high-level public participation to assess their health and mobilize their resources to create healthy cities and communities (Norris and Pittman 2000). The concepts of empowerment and community participation, defined as the "twin pillars" of the new health promotion movement (Robertson and Minkler 1994), are reflected in the World Health Organization's (WHO) (1986) definition of health promotion as "a process of enabling people to increase control over and to improve their health" (1). And that definition is replacing older conceptualizations of health promotion that focused on "individual responsibility for health" without attending to the equally important need for increasing individual and community "response-ability," in part through healthy environments and healthy public policies (Minkler 1994). The availability of powerful new organizing tools, such as media advocacy and online organizing, have further enhanced the prospects for effective community building and community organizing for health and welfare; and health education professionals have been in the forefront of developing, disseminating, and using these potent new resources (see chapters 18 and 23).

Such encouraging developments, however, have been accompanied by troubling ones. Economic inequalities in the United States have reached unprecedented levels: by the late 1990s, the top fifth of the population claimed 48.2 percent of national income and the bottom fifth had access to just 3.6 percent. In 1999, top executives were earning 531 times the wage of their average workers, up from a ratio of 42 to 1 in 1980 (Tobias 2003). Such disparities are likely to increase still further as a result of recent policy changes, including the historic ten-year $350 billion tax cut enacted in 2003, two-thirds of which will benefit the top 10 percent of the population, and a federal minimum wage, which at $5.15 an hour continues to keep a full-time working parent with one child at 12 percent below poverty line (Ryan 2003). Almost a decade ago, economist Lester Thurow (1996) asked, "How far can inequality rise before the system cracks?" (2). That question has taken on even greater urgency in the first years of the twenty-first century. Indeed, "the persistence of poverty and growing inequality in the midst of unprecedented affluence" has been called "the most urgent moral problem in contemporary America" (Putnam 2001, xv).

The health implications of these continuing inequities are profound. People who are disadvantaged by systems of inequality (Stoller and Gibson 2001) have more acute and more chronic health problems, and the continued disproportionate representation of people of color among the poor is a major reason why health disparities by race and ethnicity remain pronounced. Black babies continue to die at more than twice the rate of white babies (Moreno et al. 2000), and the life expectancy for African American men is 6.6 years less than that of white men (Arias 2002). Finally, and as discussed later in this chapter, the role of racism and differential treatment based on race or ethnicity is increasingly recognized as a major public health problem. A recent Institute of Medicine meta-analysis of more than one hundred studies of health care among insured Americans, for example, revealed stark disparities, with people of color significantly less likely to receive appropriate treatment for heart disease, HIV/AIDS, and a host of other conditions (Smedley et al. 2002).

Under former president Bill Clinton, an important step forward was taken with a bold new initiative to eliminate health disparities by 2010 (USDHHS 1998) and attempts to promote national dialogue about race. But the tragedy of September 11, an already slowing economy, the massive shift of funds to fight real and perceived terrorist threats, and the launch of a costly war against Iraq deflected attention from other important agendas, including the fight to end racial and ethnic inequalities in health. Individual and institutionalized racism and the undercurrent of racial and ethnic tensions in our society are constant reminders that the "problem of the color line," articulated by W.E.B. Du Bois more than one hundred years ago, remains very real today.

To the problems posed by continuing race, class, and gender inequities and tensions, Harvard University's Robert Putnam (1996) has added "the strange disappearance of civic America" (34). He laments the loss of our social capital—such "features of social life" as our norms, our networks, and our trust—and the loss of "civic engagement," defined as "people's connections with the life of their communities" (34). Putnam (2000) offers a stark picture of a nation in which television "privatizes our leisure time" (236) and supplants our connections with communities. His original analysis has been justifiably criticized as overly simplistic (Hawe and Shiell 2000, Wallerstein 2002; see also chapter 2), and he and others have been careful to argue that "social capital is not an alternative to providing greater financial resources and public services to poor communities (Warren et al. 2001, 2; Putnam 2000). Yet the heart of his message resonates with many who feel increasingly disconnected and disenfranchised in a land where ever-more sophisticated technology and an impoverished sense of individual and community embeddedness often lie side by side.

Finally, as this book goes to press, a conservative political climate, exacerbated by September 11 and its aftermath, is enabling even mainstream politicians in the United States to advocate openly for cutbacks in government commitments to health care and entitlements for the poor and other vulnerable groups. And while HIV/AIDS, violence, asthma, teen pregnancy, and a host of chronic illnesses and disabilities continue to affect large numbers of Americans and their families, the pool of available dollars for public health education and related functions falls further and further behind the need. Within such a climate, where is the place for community organizing and community building in our professional practice? And how relevant are these approaches in today's world?

The second edition of this book is premised on the belief that such approaches have never been more relevant or necessary. Like the original volume, it advocates for the adaptation and use of community organizing principles and methods in response to a host of public health issues, such as substance abuse, HIV/AIDS, and lead poisoning. But it also advocates for a purer approach to community organizing—that is, "a process through which communities are helped to identify common problems or goals, mobilize resources, and in other ways develop and implement strategies for reaching the goals they collectively have set" (chapter 2). In this latter process, the professional's role is to help create the conditions in which community groups, rather than outside experts, can determine and set the health agenda and then act effectively to help transform their lives and the life of their community (see chapters 14 and 15).

Although this second edition remains primarily concerned with community organizing, it also makes the case that health educators and other professionals should use their skills and resources to promote community building. As suggested in chapter 4, community building is an orientation to community that is strength-based rather than need-based and stresses the identification, nurture, and celebration of community assets. Broader macro-conceptualizations of community building have gained increasing currency in fields such as urban planning and community economic development (Walsh 1997) and are discussed and illustrated later in this book (see chapters 14, 22, and appendix 2). For the most part, however, the book takes a more modest perspective, focusing on community building as an orientation to practice.

Increased attention to community building, not merely community organizing around health issues, is well justified from a public health perspective. As Marc

Pilisuk and his colleagues argue in chapter 6, we confront daily the "fraying social fabric" of our postindustrial society, where individuals often lack secure embeddedness in a family, a workplace, a neighborhood, or a community of common interest. This lack of embeddedness represents not only a social hazard but also a public health hazard: alienation and lack of a sense of connection to others have long been associated with heart disease, depression, risky health behaviors, and a variety of other adverse health outcomes (Bloomberg et al. 1994; James et al. 2001). Professionals who draw on their resources to support community building can make a real contribution to improving the public's health and welfare.

## Social Change Professionals as Conscious Contrarians

Jacqueline Mondros and Scott Wilson (1994, 14–15) have described community organizers as conscious contrarians. They delineate three components of conscious contrarianism: a particular world view or set of beliefs and values about people and society, a power analysis that rejects the dominant ways of thinking about power and how power is distributed, and a deliberate selection of work (community organizing) that is consistent with the other two. I argue that community health educators, social workers, and other social change professionals may also be described as conscious contrarians along these three dimensions, but I add a forth and fifth dimension as well. Borrowed from the Lakota tribe's tradition of the Heyokas (sacred clowns), the fourth dimension involves the social change professional's role in doing things differently and, in the process, challenging traditional ways of thinking (Tilleras 1988). Finally, the fifth dimension involves the increasing willingness of community organizers to openly confront issues of racism and demonstrate cultural humility (Tervalon and Murray-Garcia 1998) as they engage with others in our increasingly diverse society and world.

### WORLD VIEW

Like professional organizers, health educators, social workers, and other social change professionals engaged in community organizing and community building tend to share a world view characterized by "a strong sense of what is just in and for the world" (Mondros and Wilson 1994, 15; Lippman 1937). Concerns with justice, fairness, the application of democratic principles, and a sense of collective responsibility thus can be seen to characterize the world view reflected in fields such as public health and social welfare. Indeed, as public health leader Dan Beauchamp (1976) argued almost thirty years ago, social justice is the very foundation of public health and is an ethic that contrasts sharply with the dominant American world view, which is characterized by a market-justice orientation. "Under the norms of market justice, people are entitled only to those valued ends such as status, income happiness, etc., that they have acquired . . . by their own individual efforts, actions or abilities. Market justice emphasizes individual responsibility, minimal collective action, and freedom from collective responsibility, except to respect other persons' fundamental rights" (4).

This market-justice ethic in turn underlies the strong American tendency to frame and view problems, including health problems and their solutions, in individual terms. As applied to health, the market-justice ethic is clearly reflected in the words of John K. Iglehart (1990), former editor of the journal *Health Affairs*: "Most illnesses and premature death are caused by human habits of living *that people choose for themselves*" (4, emphasis added).

The major role that individuals can play in improving their health through smoking cessation, diet and exercise, and other lifestyle modifications has, of course, been well demonstrated (McGinnis and Foege 1993, Rowe and Kahn 1998). And health educators and other health professionals often play an important role in helping to create programs through which individuals can be enabled to change unhealthy habits and in other ways improve their own and their families' health status. But without discounting the importance of such work, the world view of community health educators and other public health professionals recognizes its limitations. This alternative view sees health as intimately tied to social and environmental conditions and suggests that the primary focus of intervention be at the community and policy levels rather than at the level of the individual (Epp 1986, Freudenberg 2000, James et al. 2001, Schwab and Syme 1997).

The dimension of the public health and social change world view that sees health and social problems as deeply grounded in a broader social context is very much in keeping with a power analysis that departs from mainstream ways of thinking about how and why societal resources are allocated as they are. But another critical dimension of this viewpoint deserves mention as well: its embrace of diversity and multiculturalism not as a problem or obstacle to be dealt with but as a rich resource and opportunity to be seized. In a nation such as the United States, where politicians can make political hay through their promotion of border patrols and by clamping down on the rights of immigrants and of lesbian, gay, bisexual, and transgendered people, there is increasing need for professionals who can emphasize the many ways in which society benefits from its growing heterogeneity. The respect for diversity that health education leader Dorothy Nyswander (1967) argued for almost forty years ago as a central criterion against which to measure our professional work has only increased in significance in the intervening decades. Its importance, moreover, will reach new heights in the twenty-first century, whose halfway mark is projected to see a majority-minority nation in which African Americans, Hispanics, Asian/Pacific Islanders, and Native Americans together outnumber whites. The value of inclusion rather than exclusion and the embrace of diversity as a means of enriching the social fabric are central to the world view of practitioners in community health education, social work, and the other social change professions, who engage in what Angela Blackwell and her colleagues (2002) call in their title "searching for the uncommon common ground."

### POWER ANALYSIS

Closely intertwined with this world view is a power analysis that differs sharply from the dominant ideology. As Mondros and Wilson (1994) have pointed out, "Mainstream definitions of who benefits in society and why are questioned along class, racial, ethnic, gender and other lines" (15).

While typically not articulated as such, the power analysis of social change professionals often is rooted in political economy. This theoretical framework accepts Max Weber's (1978) classic definition of power as the probability that an individual or a group will have its will win out despite the resistance of others. A power analysis rooted in political economy argues that resources are allocated not on the basis of relative merit or efficiency but on the basis of power (Minkler et al. 1994–95, Navarro 1993). The unequal distribution of wealth, health, and life chances in a society is seen in this analysis as heavily determined by the interaction of political, economic, and sociocultural factors (Andersen and Collins 2003, Brenner 1995, Walton 1979, Stoller and Gibson 2001). The dynamics of race, class, and gender and the role of broad social influences in determining how health and social problems are defined and treated or ignored are among the central issues with which political economy is concerned, and each has a great deal to say about the nature of power in society (Brenner 1995).

As suggested in subsequent chapters, feminist perspectives on community organizing and community practice (Bradshaw et al. 1994, Hyde 1994, Weil 1995), together with community building perspectives (Himmelman 1992, McKnight 1987, Walsh 1997), often contain an alternative power analysis that stresses "power with" and "power to" (French 1986) rather than more traditional and hierarchical notions of "power over." Within such perspectives "the target of change, that is, the power structure, is not seen as the enemy but rather as a potential collaborator toward a win-win situation" (Bradshaw et al. 1994, 29).

Although the contributors to this book offer a number of perspectives on power, their power analyses have in common a rejection of the dominant notion that power accrues to individuals and groups on the basis of merit and deservingness (Katz 1995). Further, and whether visualized primarily in terms of power over or power to and power with, the role of factors such as race, class, gender, and sexual orientation in influencing power and access to societal resources is a critical component of contributors' power analyses.

Of equal importance, however, are the authors' conceptualizations of empowerment. As Nina Wallerstein (1992) has pointed out, "In the public health field, empowerment has traditionally been defined by its absence, as powerlessness" (198).

More recently, far more careful attention has been paid to this multilevel construct (Wallerstein 2002, Zimmerman 2000), which Julian Rappaport (1984) defines as an enabling process through which individuals and communities take control over their lives and their environment. In Wallerstein's (1992) words, empowerment is "a social-action process that promotes participation of people, organizations, and communities toward the goals of increased individual and community control, political efficacy, improved quality of community life, and social justice" (198).

Such a perspective figures prominently in the power analysis of many community organizers, health educators, social workers, and other social change professionals for whom facilitating individual and community empowerment is a central goal. Yet as discussed in subsequent chapters, a cautionary attitude toward the rhetoric of empowerment also is important. Particularly in these times of fiscal retrenchment, conservative policymakers frequently invoke the language of individual and community empowerment and self-reliance to justify cutbacks in entitlement programs and health and social services. Indeed, as Ronald Labonte (in Bernstein et al. 1994) points out, "Divorced of its historical contingency, empowerment is more a sop than a challenge to the status quo" (287). While embracing authentic notions of empowerment, then, part of the world view of health educators and other social change professionals involves a rejection of the argument that individual and community empowerment can take the place of a broader societal-level commitment to creating the conditions in which people and communities can be healthy.

### DELIBERATE CAREER CHOICE

The third component of Mondros and Wilson's (1994) conscious contrarianism involves the deliberate seeking out of jobs "that at least appear to contain the possibility to promote change" (16). As suggested previously, the promotion of change that organizers embrace is most heavily concentrated on the community and broader institutional and societal levels.

Fields such as public health bring little fame, glory, or money to those who select them. In Dan Callahan's (1995) words, disease prevention and health promotion "still remain the step-children of the American health care system: accepted but not well fed, praised but not always allowed in the living room, beloved unless they start making real financial demands" (2). For health educators, moreover, the goal of facilitating empowerment can be particularly hard to live up to when funding is not only grossly inadequate but also is often "from categorical sources requiring us . . . to reduce cholesterol levels among people who cannot find employment, or to develop smoking cessation methods for communities who are despairing over the drug wars being fought on their children's playgrounds" (Pasick 1987).

Yet the increasing emphasis being placed by funders, health departments, and policymakers on health promotion and on strategies such as community participation, partnerships, and coalition building offers unique opportunities to help broaden still further the scope of our professional contributions to improving the public's health. In the United States, the growing number of Americans without access to health insurance and the work many communities are now doing to fight the environmental and policy-related causes of asthma and other health problems (see chapter 22 and Wing 1998) offer fertile ground for an increased emphasis on community building as a vital and health-promoting part of the health educator's role. In short, and particularly at this critical juncture in our history, the choice of a career in fields such as community health education and social welfare can offer real opportunities for helping to create the conditions in which healthier communities and societies can emerge. As Barbara Kingsolver (1990) reminds us in her novel *Animal Dreams*, "The very least you can do with your life is to figure out what to hope for. And the most you can do is to live inside that hope. Not admire it from a distance but live right in it, under its roof." In choosing a career in community organizing, health education, or social welfare, we are in a real sense choosing to live inside the hope we share for a healthier society and a healthier world.

## DOING THINGS DIFFERENTLY

A fourth dimension of conscious contrarianism may be found in the Lakota tradition of the Heyokas—those people in the tribe who challenge people's thinking and shake them up. As Perry Tilleras (1988) explains, the historical function of the sacred clowns, also known as contraries, "was to keep people from getting stuck in rigid ways of thinking and living" (viii). And so these tribal members, who were often gay, "lived backward"—walking and dancing backward and doing everything contrary to the norm. According to Tilleras, the gay community's early response to HIV/AIDS kept pace with the Heyoka tradition: "When the normal response was to react with fear and panic, there were people dancing backwards, responding with love and confidence. . . . When the normal reaction to a diagnosis was isolation, the Heyoehkahs dragged us into community" (viii).

For organizers, community health educators, and other social change professionals, the Heyoka tradition of doing things differently is a familiar one. Whereas traditional medicine looks for pathogens and other agents of disease causation, health educators, for example, look for the strengths on which people and communities can build in achieving and maintaining health. And whereas in business and many other professions "getting ahead" means pushing oneself and one's achievements, the good community organizer, health educator, or social worker typically remains in the background so that achievements and victories are seen as accomplishments of and by people and communities rather than of and by outside professionals.

## CONFRONTING RACISM AND
## EMBRACING CULTURAL HUMILITY

To this list may be added a fifth dimension of conscious contrarianism: actively confronting and attempting to address racism in our personal and professional lives and our society. As Makani Themba (1999) points out, racism in the United States is like "the gorilla in the living room. It's running through the place making noises, and everyone is sitting politely trying to ignore it" (157). Ironically, the tendency to avoid dealing openly with racism has persisted even in the wake of Healthy People 2010's naming of the elimination of health disparities as one of its two overarching goals. Indeed, and with a few important exceptions (see, for example, the February 2003 issue of the *American Journal of Public Health*), the important new emphasis in public health practice and research on eliminating health disparities has not been accompanied by serious confrontation with the issues of racism and white privilege (McIntosh 1989), which are intimately interconnected with the existence and continuation of these disparities in the first place.

Angela Blackwell and her colleagues (2002) help explain this paradox, noting that because race is such a "difficult subject for Americans . . . there is growing currency to the idea that the nation has crossed into a post-racial era. The country's growing diversity is seen as having washed away the stark images of yesterday—the blocked schoolhouse doors and burning crosses. America's increasing diversity is seen as evidence of tolerance, and, by extension, justice" (47–48). For conscious contrarians in fields like public health and social welfare, the need to address rather than deny racial ethnic differences in our nation's opportunity structure and to confront racism head on in doing so is a paramount commitment. Race matters in our continued need to commit to the elimination of health disparities, and it matters in the way in which we approach our work. In the latter regard, as Melanie Tervalon and Jane Murray-Garcia (1998, 118) point out, it matters that we approach our work not with the goal of achieving "*cultural competence*" (a discrete end point), but rather with "*cultural humility*," defined as involving a "lifelong commitment to self evaluation and self-critique," to redress power imbalances and "develop and maintain mutually respectful and dynamic partnerships with communities" (see chapter 14). Finally, for professionals who are also Caucasian and working with communities of color, the vital need for recognizing and confronting the many sources of "white privilege" or "invisible systems conferring dominance" on the basis of one's skin color (McIntosh 1989, 12) is especially critical. As Tervalon and Murray-Garcia (1998) suggest, although we can never truly become competent in another's culture, we can demonstrate humility in our outsider status and an openness to learning and trying our best in cross-race or ethnic group interactions.

In these and other ways, community health educators and other social change professionals are indeed contrarians. As such, they play a role that is highly consistent with the philosophy and methods of community organizing and community building.

## Purposes and Organization of the Book

Although the second edition of this book expands on the first in several important ways (as described later in this section), it shares with the original the same three purposes. First, it attempts to put together in one place, for students of health education and other social change professions, much of the critical recent thinking in community organizing and community building theory and practice. These contributions address both long-valued aspects of organizing, such as issue selection and participation, and more recently applied perspectives, such as Brazilian educator Paulo Freire's (1973) education for critical consciousness (chapter 12) and the approaches to healthy community assessment (chapter 8), online community building and organizing (chapter 18), and media advocacy (chapter 23) that have emerged over the past two decades. It further builds on the first edition by adding new theoretical perspectives as well as new methods and approaches to community building and organizing. The inclusion of a gender analysis of community organizing models (chapter 11), a stronger accent on race-ethnicity, and the need for cultural humility in collaborative work with communities (chapter 14); the role of the arts in community building and organizing (chapter 19); and the use of community organizing as a potent approach to influencing policy (chapter 22) are among the additions to this second edition.

Second, the book attempts to demonstrate, through a series of case studies, the concrete application of many of the concepts and methods discussed in real-world organizing and community building settings. Most of these case studies demonstrate the adaptation and use of community organizing and community building strategies by health educators and other social change professionals as part of their efforts to address public health problems such as substance abuse, HIV/AIDS, and lead poisoning. In other case examples, however, the health educator engages in a purer approach to organizing, creating the conditions in which communities can identify and address their own health and social issues (see chapters 14, 15, and 19). The frequent use of such analytical case studies and illustrations is designed to help bridge the still sizable gap between theory and practice in community organizing and community building.

A third and final purpose of the book is to make explicit the kinds of hard questions and ethical challenges that should be reflected upon continually by those of us who engage in community organizing or community building as part of our professional practice. Questions regarding the appropriate role of people in positions of privilege vis-à-vis community empowerment; the problem of conflicting loyalties between one's agency or funder and the community; competing visions of "the community"; potential unanticipated consequences of an organizing intervention; issues of working across boundaries in terms of race, class, or other dividing lines; and questions of how to develop empowering rather than disempowering approaches to community health assessment and the evaluation of community health initiatives are among the questions with which we grapple. By raising these questions rather than providing pat answers, the book attempts to foster an approach to community organizing and community building that is, above all, self-critical, reflective, and respectful of the diverse communities with which health professionals are engaged.

As suggested, the second edition of this text includes many significantly revised and updated chapters that use new concepts (such as social capital, cultural humility, and partnership synergy [Lasker et al. 2001]) and new case studies to illustrate their applications in practice. It also includes several new chapters on topics not included in the first edition—for example, using the arts to promote community organizing and community building and using community organizing as a vehicle to promote healthier public policy. Finally, a substantially increased knowledge and practice base in areas such as the influence of the global economy on grassroots organizing, participatory evaluation, online community building and organizing, and new methods for fostering effective collaborations with community residents led to the inclusion of new or heavily revised chapters in these areas as well.

Before providing a chapter by chapter overview of what this second edition includes, however, I must state up front what it does not contain. First, the book does not provide a step-by-step approach to community organizing or community building. Excellent manuals are available elsewhere for this purpose (see Bobo et al. 2001, Homan 1999), and interested readers are encouraged to peruse several of them to get a sense of their differences in style and approach. Second, this volume is not intended to be a comprehensive casebook and consequently cannot begin to do justice to the myriad exciting community organizing and community building efforts taking place among and with different racial and ethnic communities in both urban and rural areas or in communities based on shared interests locally or internationally. Once again, the interested reader is directed to other volumes, such as Felix Rivera and John Erlich's (1995) *Community Organizing in a Diverse Society* and Robert Fisher and Joseph Kling's (1993) *Mobilizing the Community*, which provide useful collections of such case studies.

Third, as in the first edition, a distinction is made in this book between community-based interventions, such as the well-designed Community-Based Hypertension Control Project (CHIP) (Morisky et al. 2002) and true community organizing and community building efforts in which community empowerment is often *the* central feature of the project itself. Although interventions like CHIP make an important contribution and are discussed briefly in some of the chapters, they do not form a central focus of the book. Indeed, only one social planning effort (the Centers for Disease Control's HIV Prevention Planning Councils, which attempted to place a heavy emphasis on community empowerment) is discussed in detail (chapter 21).

Fourth, this volume does not attempt to cover the voluminous body of literature on social movements. Although more discussion is provided in this edition on the importance of linking community organizing efforts with broader social movement, particularly in the context of today's global economy (see chapters 3 and 6), such movements themselves are the topic of a number of comprehensive volumes. Again, the reader is directed to other sources, such as Steven Buechler and Frank Kurt Cylke, Jr.'s, (1996) *Social Movements,* for a fuller discussion of this subject.

In making these omissions, I in no way mean to downplay the importance of social movements in bringing about change or the role of social planning interventions in health education and related fields. Similarly, the inability of this book to address in detail the impressive community organizing efforts that are taking place in areas such as anti-tobacco organizing, breast cancer, disability rights, and homelessness as well as among many diverse racial, ethnic, and other communities reflects solely the practical matter of space. Given these limitations, I hope that this book enables the reader to think critically about community organizing and community building for health, asking hard questions and exploring their relevance in practice settings.

The next three chapters together provide several conceptual frameworks and models within which community organizing and community building for health can be understood. Meredith Minkler and Nina Wallerstein begin, in chapter 2, by providing an expanded theoretical and historical introduction to community organizing and community building and introducing several key themes (such as power and empowerment, community capacity, and participation) to set the stage for their more detailed examination in later chapters. The popular new concept of social capital also is introduced and critically examined in this chapter. In chapter 3, Robert Fisher provides a more in-depth look at grassroots social action as a distinct and widespread model of community organizing worldwide. The ideological and historical roots of social action organizing are discussed, as are issues such as culture and social identity and their implications for practice.

In chapter 4, Cheryl L. Walter shifts our focus from community organizing to community, arguing that in our preoccupation with "the community," we as social change professionals sometimes have lost sight of the broader concept of community and what it symbolizes. Viewing community as "an inclusive, complex, and dynamic system of which we are a part" rather than as an entity with which we as outsiders interact, Walter proposes a way of framing community practice that differs from that of many of the other contributors. Her conceptualization is consonant with a number of important skills for social change professionals, however, and is offered here as a means of stimulating fresh thinking and challenging us to reflect more critically about our roles in community.

In chapters 5 through 7, we turn our attention to the challenging and often difficult role of health educators and other social change professionals as community organizers. Ronald Labonte begins, in chapter 5, by questioning the prevailing wisdom about community and raising a number of cautions for health workers who engage in community development or community organizing with the goal of building authentic partnerships. Stressing the difference between *community-based* and true *community development/community organizing* approaches, he provides a number of criteria to be met if authentic partnerships between health agencies and communities are to be realized. In chapter 6, Marc Pilisuk and his colleagues examine the roles, functions, and dilemmas faced by today's community organizers within the context of the global economy. The importance of linking with larger social movements and the need for a broad infrastructure that connects diverse progressive causes and organizations are among the topics explored.

Several of the hard questions and issues raised in chapters 5 and 6 are examined in greater detail in chapter 7, as Meredith Minkler and Cheri Pies provide case examples of the ethical and practical challenges frequently faced by health educators and other professionals in their roles as community organizers. Problems such as conflicting loyalties and the potential for negative unanticipated consequences of our organizing efforts are considered. Questions are posed throughout for health educators and other social change professionals to ask themselves in an effort to make more explicit the difficult ethical terrain in which we operate.

One of the most important, and neglected, aspects of the health or social change professional's role as organizer involves his or her involvement in the process of community assessment. Chapters 8 and 9 are based on the premise that such assessments need to stress community strengths and assets rather than merely needs or perceived problems and that such assessments should truly be of, by, and for the community. In chapter 8, Trevor Hancock and Meredith Minkler introduce this perspective and challenge the reader to think not in terms of a *community health assessment* but in terms of a broader *healthy community assessment,* using tools such as community indicators to broaden the lens through which we view such processes. In chapter 9, this approach is translated into practice in the form of John L. McKnight and John P. Kretzmann's classic piece, "Mapping Community Capacity." The reader is provided with a simple yet effective tool that can help communities—and the professionals who work with or as part of them—find and map the building blocks or strengths and assets that can in turn be called upon in the building of healthier communities.

We conclude this part by turning our attention to the related area of issue selection with communities. In chapter 10, Lee Staples lays out the criteria for a good issue as well as the factors to be considered in cutting the issue as part of a strategic analysis. Frequently drawing on case examples, he helps illuminate the many ways in which outside professionals can ensure that the issue selected comes from the community and is cut in ways that help the community achieve its goals.

In part 4 we explore several alternative models of community organizing and community building, each of which has salience for health educators and other professionals engaged in social change. We begin, in chapter 11, with Susan Stall and Randy Stoecker's use of a gender analysis and the concept of liminal spaces—those border zones where cultures and other spheres cross over—to examine community organizing models. Saul Alinsky's (1972) classic approach to social action organizing is compared and contrasted with women-centered organizing, and the authors then discuss and illustrate the advantages of approaches that use the liminality of community to best advantage by combining elements of each. In chapter 12, Nina Wallerstein, Victoria Sanchez, and Lily Velarde build on a theme introduced in chapters 1 and 2, laying out in more detail Freire's (1973) philosophy and methods of empowerment education and demonstrating their application through a case study. The New Mexico–based Adolescent Social Action Program, which addressed substance abuse and related problems on multiple levels, is described and analyzed, as is its evaluation, a recent replication of the model, and implications for practitioners interested in adapting it for use in their own communities.

A major theme running through much of this book involves the role of community organizing and community building in and across diverse groups. In chapter 13, Lorraine M. Gutierrez and Edith A. Lewis describe their approach to organizing with women of color through the application of an empowerment framework stressing principles of education, participation, and capacity building. Arguing that existing models of community organizing fail to adequately address the strengths, needs, and concerns of women of color, they present a feminist perspective on organizing that specifically addresses problems and issues for organizing by and with this population.

In chapter 14, Galen El-Askari and Sheryl Walton return to the issue of bridging cultural divides in forging truly collaborative partnerships as they describe and analyze the Healthy Neighborhoods Project in a low-income community in Contra Costa County, California, and its replication in a neighboring city. The necessity of long-term commitment, high-level administrative support, systems change, and cultural humility each are illustrated in this case study.

In chapter 15, we conclude this part with Meredith Minkler's case study of the Tenderloin Senior Organizing Project, a sixteen-year effort to facilitate community building and community organizing among low-income elders. The project's evolution from an outreach to an organizing project is described, as is its theoretical grounding in social action organizing, community building, and

Freirian approaches. Project evaluation processes and outcomes, efforts to promote replication, problems with long-term sustainability, and implications for practice also are discussed.

Building and maintaining effective coalitions have increasingly been recognized as vital components of much effective community organizing and community building. In chapter 16, Abraham Wandersman, Robert M. Goodman, and Frances D. Butterfoss offer a new look at coalitions, their unique capabilities, and how they operate. Using as a conceptual framework an organizational systems model, this chapter examines coalition viability along several key dimensions and explores both the benefits and drawbacks of these popular organizing vehicles. In chapter 17, Susan Klitzman, Daniel Kass, and Nicholas Freudenberg draw on a number of Wandersman et al.'s observations to describe and analyze a twenty-year New York City–based effort at building and using a coalition to prevent childhood lead poisoning. Following a brief look at lead poisoning as a public health problem, the authors describe the formation and evolution of this citywide coalition, whose activities have included bringing a major lawsuit against the city and drafting state and local legislation. The victories achieved and barriers and dilemmas faced in this case study are examined, key among them the limitations of a litigation-driven approach. Issues concerning the coalition's structure and functioning also are critically analyzed, and lessons are drawn for health educators and other social change professionals.

Although community building and organizing often conjure up images of community meetings and door-to-door canvassing, many exciting new approaches to this work have come into play in recent years. In chapter 18, Sonja Herbert provides a provocative look at the power of the Internet for advocacy and organizing. Drawing on a diversity of case examples and web sites, she illustrates how the Internet has dramatically improved access to information and organizing tools, enabled the formation of new communities, and provided powerful new approaches to political activism. Yet she also posts a number of "hazard signs" along the way, including the persistence of a digital divide that results in unequal access to this powerful advocacy and organizing tool.

In chapter 19, Marian McDonald, Jennifer Sarché, and Caroline C. Wang explore the usefulness of a wide variety of art forms for community organizing around health issues. The theoretical bases for using the arts in organizing are explored, and examples including the AIDS memorial quilt, and an innovative arts project with youth in Louisiana are provided to illustrate the promise of such approaches. The chapter then explores the philosophy and method of photovoice, "a process by which people can identify, represent and enhance their community through a specific photographic technique" (Wang and Burris 1997, 369), and describes several diverse photovoice projects to demonstrate the potential of this method for community building, assessment, and policy advocacy.

A central dilemma faced by professionals as organizers is how to facilitate the evaluation of community organizing and community building efforts in ways that do not disempower communities in the process. In chapter 20, Chris M. Coombe describes how the process of evaluation can be used as a capacity-building tool in organizing as well as a source of knowledge for project improvement. Limitations of traditional approaches to evaluation are discussed, and the theoretical underpinnings of participatory evaluation are described, with special attention to the emancipatory or transformative tradition in such efforts (Cousins and Whitmore 1998). A practical framework then is offered for incorporating this approach at each step of the evaluation process. The utility of participatory approaches to evaluation is further demonstrated in chapter 21. Kathleen M. Roe and her colleagues describe and analyze one of the first efforts to evaluate the work of HIV Prevention Planning Councils, using as a framework a variant of David Fetterman et al.'s (1996) empowerment evaluation model. As noted previously, their analysis represents the only detailed look in this volume at a social planning, rather than social action or community building, approach to practice. It is included, however, both because of the importance of this decade-long national experiment and because the case study itself demonstrates many of the challenges, dilemmas, and rewards involved in a participatory approach to evaluation. Although the planning councils have moved away from the heavy accent on empowerment emblematic of their early years, this chapter is a powerful reminder of the important role outside evaluators can continue to play in stimulating community building and empowerment through their adoption of an emancipating and participatory evaluation approach.

In the final two chapters, we turn our attention to influencing policy through community organizing and community building. In chapter 22, Angela Glover Blackwell, Meredith Minkler, and Mildred Thompson offer an overview of the policy-making process and roles for advocates in that process and then use several case studies to illustrate how community organizing and community building "on the ground" have helped bring about changes in local, regional, and state policy. One of the techniques they introduce, media advocacy, is then explored in greater detail in chapter 23, as Lawrence Wallack discusses the strategic use of mass media to promote public policy initiatives (Wallack et al. 1993). Media advocacy is described in this chapter as a powerful community tool that is enabling community groups and professionals in fields like public health to get the media to reframe local and national problems and change the ways in which they are presented and viewed. An approach that seeks to enhance community groups' visibility, legitimacy, and power, media advocacy is seen as a critical tool for building healthier communities through advocacy for healthy public policy.

The volume ends with appendixes designed to provide the reader with concrete tools and applications that correspond to a number of the chapter themes and issues raised. Ranging from an action-oriented community assessment technique to principles for both advocacy campaigns and community-based research, the appendixes are designed to help practitioners put into practice some of the messages central to this volume and to community organizing and community building.

Although this book was written primarily for students and practitioners in fields such as community health education, health planning, and social welfare, it should be of interest as well to activists and others concerned with the many hard questions and realities that surround community building and community organizing in the early twenty-first century. As in the first edition, the contributors to this volume have attempted to write provocatively and critically, challenging the reader—and each other—to ask hard questions and rethink some of our most basic assumptions. We ask you, the reader, to join us in this process of critical questioning and dialogue as you seek to apply theory to practice and practice to the rethinking of theory, to the end of helping build healthier communities and more caring and humane societies.

## References

Alinsky, S. D. 1972. *Rules for Radicals*. New York: Random House.

Andersen, M. L., and P. Collins. 2003. *Race, Class and Gender: An Anthology*. 5th ed. Belmont, Calif.: Wadsworth.

Arias, E. 2002. "United States Life Tables, 2000." In *National Vital Statistics Reports*, vol. 51, no. 3. Washington, D.C.: U.S. Department of Health and Human Services, National Center for Health Statistics.

Beauchamp, D. 1976. "Public Health As Social Justice." *Inquiry* 12: 3–14.

Bernstein, E., N. Wallerstein, R. Braithwaite, et al. 1994. "Empowerment Forum: A Dialogue between Guest Editorial Board Members." *Health Education Quarterly* 21, no. 3: 281–94.

Blackwell, A. G., S. Kwoh, and M. Pastor. 2002. *Searching for the Uncommon Common Ground: New Dimensions on Race in America*. New York: Norton.

Bloomberg, L., J. Meyers, and M. T. Braverman. 1994. "The Importance of Social Interaction: A New Perspective on Social Epidemiology, Social Risk Factors, and Health." *Health Education Quarterly* 21, no. 4: 447–63.

Bobo, K., J. Kendall, and S. Max. 2001. *Organizing for Social Change*. 3d ed. Santa Ana, Calif.: Seven Locks.

Bradshaw, C., S. Soifer, and L. Gutierrez. 1994. "Toward a Hybrid Model for Effective Organizing in Communities of Color." *Journal of Community Practice* 1, no. 1: 25–41.

Brenner, M. H. (1995). "Political Economy and Health." In *Society and Health*, edited by B. Amick, S. Levine, A. Tarlov, and D. Walsh, 211–46. New York: Oxford University Press.

Buechler, S. M., and F. K. Cylke, Jr. 1996. *Social Movements: Perspectives and Issues*. Mountain View, Calif.: Mayfield.

Callahan, D. 1995. "Issues in Health Promotion and Disease Prevention." Unpublished paper. Hastings on the Hudson, N.Y.: Hastings Center.

Cousins, J. B., and E. Whitmore. 1998. "Framing Participatory Evaluation." Special issue. *New Directions for Evaluation* 80, no. 5.

Epp, J. 1986. "Achieving Health for All: A Framework for Health Promotion." *Canadian Journal of Public Health* 77, no. 6: 393–408.

Fetterman, D. M., S. J. Kaftarian, and A. Wandersman. 1996. *Empowerment Evaluation: Knowledge and Tools for Self-Assessment and Accountability.* Newbury Park, Calif.: Sage.

Fisher, R., and J. Kling. 1993. *Mobilizing the Community: Local Politics in a Global Era.* Newbury Park, Calif.: Sage.

Freire, P. 1973. *Education for Critical Consciousness.* New York: Seabury.

French, M. 1986. *Beyond Power: On Women, Men, and Morals.* London: Abacus.

Freudenberg, N. 2000. "Time for a National Agenda to Improve the Health of Urban Populations." *American Journal of Public Health* 90, no. 6: 837–40.

Green, L. W., and C. J. Frankish. 1997. "Implementing Nutritional Science for Population Health: Decentralized and Centralized Planning for Health Promotion and Disease Prevention." In *Beyond Nutritional Recommendations: Implementing Science for Healthier Populations,* edited by C. Garza, J. D. Haas, J. Habicht, and D. L. Pelletier. Ithaca, N.Y.: Cornell University and National Academy of Science.

Hawe, P., and A. Shiell. 2000. "Social Capital and Health Promotion: A Review." *Social Science and Medicine* 51: 871–85.

Himmelman, A. 1992. "Communities Working Collaboratively for a Change." Unpublished paper. Minneapolis: Himmelman Consulting Group.

Homan, M. S. 1999. *Promoting Community Change: Making It Happen in the Real World.* 2d ed. Pacific Grove, Calif.: Brooks/Cole.

Hyde, C. 1994. "Committed to Social Change: Voices from the Feminist Movement." *Journal of Community Practice* 1, no. 2: 45–64.

Iglehart, J. K. 1990. "From the Editor: Special Issue on Promoting Health." *Health Affairs* 9, no. 2: 4–5.

James, S. A., A. Schulz, and J. van Olphen. 2001. "Social Capital, Poverty, and Community Health: An Exploration of Linkages." In *Social Capital and Poor Communities,* edited by S. Saegert, J. P. Thompson, and M. R. Warren, 165–199. New York: Sage Foundation.

Katz, M. 1995. *Improving Poor People.* New York: Pantheon.

Kingsolver, B. 1990. *Animal Dreams.* New York: Perennial.

Lasker, R. D., E. S. Weiss, and R. Miller. 2001. "Partnership Synergy: A Practical Framework for Studying and Strengthening the Collaborative Advantage." *Milbank Quarterly* 79, no. 2: 179–205.

Lippman, W. 1937. *An Inquiry into the Principles of Good Society.* Boston: Little, Brown.

McGinnis, J. M., and W. H. Foege. 1993. "Actual Causes of Death in the United States." *Journal of the American Medical Association* 270, no. 18: 2207–12.

McIntosh, P. 1989. "White Privilege: Unpacking the Invisible Knapsack." *Peace and Freedom* (July-August): 10–12.

McKnight, J. 1987. "Regenerating Community." *Social Policy* 3 (winter): 54–58.

Minkler, M. 1994. "Ethical Challenges for Health Promotion in the 1990s." *American Journal of Health Promotion* 8, no. 6: 403–13.

Minkler, M., S. P. Wallace, and M. McDonald. 1994–95. "The Political Economy of Health: A Useful Theoretical Tool for Health Education Practice." *International Quarterly of Community Health Education* 15, no. 2: 111–25.

Mondros, J. B., and S. M. Wilson. 1994. *Organizing for Power and Empowerment.* New York: Columbia University Press.

Moreno L., B. Davaney, D. Chu, and M. Seeley. 2000. *Effects of Healthy Start on Infant Mortality and Birth Outcomes (Final Report Prepared for HRSA, DHHS).* Princeton, N.J.: Mathematica Policy Research.

Morisky, D. E., N. B. Lees, B. A. Sharif, K. Y. Liu, and H. J. Ward. 2002. "Reducing Disparities in Hypertension Control: A Community-Based Hypertension Control Project for an Ethnically Diverse Population." *Health Promotion Practice* 3, no. 2: 264–75.

Morse, S. 1997. "Plaza or Pyramid? Metaphors for Leadership." *Wingspread* 19, no. 4: 3–4.

Navarro, V. 1993. *Dangerous to Your Health: Capitalism in Health Care.* New York: Monthly Review Press.

Norris, T., and M. Pittman. 2000. "The Healthy Communities Movement and the Coalition for Healthier Cities and Communities." *Public Health Reports* 115: 118–24.

Nyswander, D. 1967. "The Open Society: Its Implications for Health Educators." *Health Education Monographs* 1, no. 1: 3–13.

Pasick, R. J. 1987. "Health Promotion for Minorities in California." Report to the East Bay Health Education Center. Berkeley: University of California, School of Public Health.

Putnam, R. 1996. "The Strange Disappearance of Civic America." *American Prospect* (winter): 24, 34–48.

———. 2000. *Bowling Alone: The Collapse and Revival of American Community.* New York: Simon and Schuster.

———. 2001. Foreword. In *Social Capital in Poor Communities*, edited by S. J. Saegert, J. P. Thompson, and M. R. Warren, xv–xvi. New York: Sage Foundation.

Rappaport, J. 1984. "Studies in Empowerment: Introduction to the Issue." *Prevention in Human Services* 32, no. 3: 1–7.

Rivera, F., and J. Erlich, eds. 1995. *Community Organizing in a Diverse Society.* 2d ed. Boston: Allyn and Bacon.

Robertson, A., and M. Minkler. 1994. "The New Health Promotion Movement: A Critical Examination." *Health Education Quarterly* 21, no. 3: 295–312.

Rowe, J. W., and J. L. Kahn. 1998. *Successful Aging: The MacArthur Foundation Study.* New York: Pantheon.

Ryan, J. 2003. "As Stimulating As a Tax Cut: A Living Wage." *San Francisco Chronicle,* July 11, p. A21

Schwab, M., and S. L. Syme. 1997. "On Paradigms, Community Participation, and the Future of Public Health." *American Journal of Public Health* 87: 2049–52.

Smedley, B. D., A. Y. Stith, and A. R. Nelson. 2002. *Unequal Treatment: Confronting Racial and Ethnic Disparities in Health Care.* Washington, D.C.: Institute of Medicine and the National Academy Press.

Stoller, E. P., and R. Gibson. 2001. *Worlds of Difference: Inequalities in the Aging Experience.* Thousand Oaks, Calif.: Pine Forge.

Tervalon, M., and J. Murray-Garcia. 1998. "Cultural Humility vs. Cultural Competence: A Critical Distinction in Defining Physician Training Outcomes in Medical Education." *Journal of Health Care for the Poor and Underserved* 9, no. 2: 117–25.

Themba, M. N. 1999. *Making Policy, Making Change: How Communities Are Taking Law into Their Own Hands.* Berkeley, Calif.: Chardon.

Thurow, L. 1996. *The Future of Capitalism.* New York: Morrow.

Tilleras, P. 1988. *The Color of Light: Meditations for All of Us Living with AIDS.* San Francisco: Harper and Row.

Tobias, A. 2003. "How Much Is Fair?" *Parade*, March 2, pp. 10–11.

U.S. Department of Health and Human Services (USDHHS). 1998. *Call to Action: Eliminating Racial and Ethnic Disparities in Health.* Washington, D.C.: U.S. Department of Health and Human Services and Grantmakers in Health.

Wallack, L., L. Dorfman, D. Jernigan, and M. Themba. 1993. *Media Advocacy and Public Health: Power for Prevention.* Newbury Park, Calif.: Sage.

Wallerstein, N. 1992. "Powerlessness, Empowerment, and Health: Implications for Health Promotion Programs." *American Journal of Health Promotion* 6, no. 3: 197–205.

———. 2002. "Empowerment to Reduce Health Disparities." *Scandinavian Journal of Public Health* 30, no. S59: 72–77.

Walsh, J. 1997. *Stories of Renewal: Community Building and the Future of Urban America.* New York: Rockefeller Foundation.

Walton, J. 1979. "Urban Political Economy: An Overview." *Comparative Urban Research* 7, no. 1: 5–17.

Wang, C. C., and M. Burris. 1997. "Photovoice: Concept, Methodology, and Use for Participatory Needs Assessment." *Health Education and Behavior* 24, no. 2: 369–87.

Warren, M. R., J. P. Thompson, and S. Saegert. 2001. "The Role of Social Capital in Combating Poverty." In *Social Capital and Poor Communities*, edited by S. Saegert, J. P. Thompson, and M. R. Warren, 1–28. New York: Sage Foundation.

Weber, M. 1978. *Economy and Society*. Berkeley: University of California Press.

Weil, M. 1995. "Women, Community, and Organizing." In *Tactics and Techniques of Community Intervention*, edited by J. E. Tropman, J. L. Erlich, and J. Rothman, 118–34. 3d ed. Itasca, Ill.: Peacock.

Wing, S. 1998. "Whose Epidemiology, Whose Health?" *International Journal of Health Services* 28, no. 2: 241–52.

Zimmerman, M. A. 2000. "Empowerment Theory: Psychological, Organizational, and Community Levels of Analysis." In *Handbook of Community Psychology*, edited by J. Rappaport and E. Seidman, 43–63. New York: Academic/Plenum.

# Part I

# Contextual Frameworks and Models

$A$T THE END of the twentieth century and the beginning of the twenty-first, we are faced with increasing concern about the erosion of civic engagement and sense of community in the United States. Books such as Robert Putnam's (2000) *Bowling Alone* have become best sellers, while terms like *social capital* have become topics of scholarly attention and debate. Some fifteen years ago, political scientist Richard Couto (1990) captured reasons for this fascination, pointing out that "because Americans have so little sense of community, we pay a great deal of attention to it" (144). He suggests that "our rose-tainted view of community and the processes we describe as empowerment, community development, and community organizing" have led to considerable conceptual confusion. That confusion in turn has enabled both political liberals and conservatives to claim these concepts and to use the term *grass roots* "as if it were herbal medicine for current public problems and to renew American social health."

The contributors to part 1 attempt to move us beyond our prevailing confusion by creating conceptual frameworks and models within which community, community organizing, and community building can be better understood. Although additional perspectives on these concepts are offered throughout the book, this opening section lays a foundation for their subsequent exploration.

In chapter 2, Meredith Minkler and Nina Wallerstein offer initial definitions of community organizing and community building and underscore the central notion of empowerment in both processes. Introducing a theme that appears throughout much of the book, they suggest that real community organizing must begin with a group's or community's identification of its issues and goals rather than with the goals or concerns of a health department, a social service organization, or an outside organizer or funder.

Following a brief historical overview, Minkler and Wallerstein introduce the best-known typology of community organization, Jack Rothman's (2001) locality development, social planning, and social action. Newer alternative and complementary models are also explored, including collaborative empowerment, community building, and approaches (such as Ronald Braithwaite and his colleagues' [1994] community organization and development [COD] model) that borrow from both community organizing and community building but accent culturally relevant practice.

The heart of this chapter is the discussion of several key concepts in community organizing and community building that are central to effecting change on the community level. Empowerment and critical consciousness, community capacity and social capital, the principles of participation and "starting where the people are," and issue selection are each examined briefly, as is the often neglected area of measurement and evaluation in community building and organizing. Although this chapter covers a wide terrain, it does so "once over lightly" as a prelude to the more in-depth discussions in subsequent chapters.

The following two chapters each look in more detail at one of the major approaches to community organizing and community building practice introduced in chapter 2. In chapter 3, Robert Fisher takes a closer look at the social action organizing approach most closely identified with Saul Alinsky, which continues to play a substantive role in both local organizing and the development of broader social movements in the early years of the twenty-first century. Fisher presents social action as a dynamic organizing model that uses both conflict and consensus strategies in the quest to redress power imbalances and promote social justice. Key characteristics of social action efforts worldwide are described, as are antecedents of present-day social action organizing such as the seminal work of Alinsky, the liberation struggles of people of color, the heavier accent on community participation of the 1960s and beyond, and the social movements born in the last half of the twentieth century.

Building on a wealth of experience and expertise in this field, Fisher presents a number of implications for practice. Prominent are the need for coalition building across diverse constituencies, the need to make government or the state the focus of organizing efforts, and the importance of combining postmodern demands for autonomy and identity with the older modern emphasis on social justice and connection among people.

In chapter 4, Cheryl L. Walter shifts our focus from community organizing to community, arguing that, in our attention to "the community," we as social change professionals sometimes lose sight of the broader concept of community and what it symbolizes. Walter envisions communities not as geographic or other units with which we, as outside professionals, interact but as inclusive and dynamic systems to which we belong. The various dimensions or attributes of community, including vertical and horizontal relationships to other units and the larger society or culture, give breadth and depth to our understanding of these communities.

Building on and refining her earlier work in this area (presented in the first edition of this book), Walter helps us explore the various dimensions of community building practice and again uses an AIDS walk to illustrate how such a practice orientation might guide health educators or other social change professionals involved in the creation and implementation of such an event.

Walter's approach to community building differs from that of a number of other contributors to this book in its emphasis on the professional as part of the community rather than as an outsider looking in and working with the community. As noted in chapter 1, her approach also differs in important ways from the macro-approach to community building captured in the principles laid out by Angela Glover Blackwell and Ray Colmenar in appendix 2. Yet the skills for community building practice that Walter elaborates, including awareness of the dynamic quality of community and an ability to articulate and foster a discussion of process, have great relevance for health educators and other social change professionals who work on the community level. Her conceptualization of community building presents an important new way of thinking about our roles in community and both complements and challenges more traditional approaches offered elsewhere in this book.

## References

Braithwaite, R. L., C. Bianchi, and S. E. Taylor. 1994. "Ethnographic Approach to Community Organization and Health Empowerment." *Health Education Quarterly* 21, no. 3: 407–16.

Couto, R. A. 1990. "Promoting Health at the Grass Roots." *Health Affairs* 9, no. 2: 144–51.

Putnam, R. (2000). Bowling Alone: The Collapse and Revival of American Community. New York: Simon and Schuster.

Rothman, J. 2001. "Approaches to Community Intervention." In *Strategies of Community Intervention*, edited by J. Rothman, J. L. Erlich, and J. E. Tropman, 27–64. 5th ed. Itasca, Ill.: Peacock.

MEREDITH MINKLER
NINA WALLERSTEIN

Improving Health
through Community
Organization and
*Chapter 2*      Community Building

*A Health Education Perspective*

ALTHOUGH HEALTH EDUCATION PROFESSIONALS have developed and adapted a number of new approaches and change strategies in recent years, the principles and methods loosely referred to as community organization remain a central method of practice. For the purposes of this chapter, *community organization* is defined as the process by which community groups are helped to identify common problems or goals, mobilize resources, and develop and implement strategies for reaching the goals they collectively have set. We see the newer and related concept of community building, as Cheryl L. Walter (chapter 4) and Angela Glover Blackwell and Raymond Colmenar (2000) suggest, not as a method so much as an orientation to how people who identify themselves as members of a shared community, and their allies in larger systems, engage together in the process of community change.

Implicit in both of these definitions is the concept of empowerment, viewed as an enabling process through which individuals or communities take control over their lives and their environment (Rappaport 1984). Indeed, we argue that community organization cannot not be said to have taken place unless community competence or problem-solving ability has been increased in the process.

Strict definitions of community organization also suggest that the needs or problems around which community groups are organized must of necessity be identified by the community itself, not by an outside organization or change agent. Thus, while a health education professional may borrow some principles and methods from community organization to help mount an organizing effort for obesity prevention in the community, he or she can't be said to be doing community organization in the pure sense unless the community itself has identified obesity as the problem area it wishes to address.

Community organization is important in health education because it reflects one of the field's most fundamental principles, that of "starting where the people are" (Nyswander 1956). The health education professional who begins with the community's felt needs rather than a personal or agency-dictated agenda will be far more likely to experience success in the change process and to foster real community ownership of programs and actions. Community organizing and community building are also important in light of the evidence that social involvement and participation can themselves be significant psychosocial factors in improving perceived control, individual coping capacity, health behaviors, and health status (James et al. 2002, Eng et al. 1990, Wandersman and Florin 2000). Finally, the "rediscovery" of community, and the heavy accent that government agencies, foundations and the like now place on community partnerships and community-based health initiatives, suggest a need to refine theory, methods, and measurement techniques in this area.

In this chapter, we examine key concepts and principles of community organization and community building as they relate to health education and related disciplines. Following a brief historical look at the field, the process of community organization, and the emergence of community building practice, we consider the concept of community and present several models of community organization and community building. We then explore key theoretical and conceptual bases of community organization and community building, topics that subsequent chapters will expand on.

## Community Organization and Community Building in Historical Perspective

The term *community organization* was coined by American social workers in the late 1800s in reference to their efforts to coordinate services for newly arrived immigrants and the poor. As Charles D. Garvin and Fred M. Cox (2001) have pointed out, although community organization is often seen as the offspring of the settlement house movement, several important milestones, which took place outside of social work, by rights should be included in any history of community organization practice. Prominent are (1) African American organizing efforts in the post-Reconstruction period to salvage newly won rights that were rapidly slipping away; (2) the Populist movement, which began as an agrarian revolution and became a multisectoral coalition and a major political force; and (3) the labor movement of the 1930s and 1940s, which taught participants the value of forming coalitions around issues, the importance of full-time professional organizers, and the use of conflict as a means of bringing about change (Garvin and Cox 2001).

Within the field of social work, early approaches to community organization stressed the use of consensus and cooperation as communities were helped to increase their problem-solving ability (Garvin and Cox 2001). By the 1950s, however, a new brand of community organization was gaining popularity, stressing confrontation and conflict strategies for social change. Most closely identified with Saul Alinsky (1969, 1972), social action organizing emphasized redressing power imbalances by creating dissatisfaction with the status quo among the disenfranchised, building community-wide identification, and helping members devise winnable goals and nonviolent conflict strategies as means to bring about change.

From the late 1950s onward, strategies and tactics of community organization were increasingly applied to the achievement of broader social change objectives, through the civil rights movement, followed by the women's movement, the gay rights movement, anti–Vietnam war organizing, and the disability rights movement (see chapter 3). The 1980s through the present have also witnessed the adaptation and development of new community organization tactics and strategies, in areas as diverse as the AIDS crisis and conservative Republican organizing to ban abortions and stem-cell research. The effective use of the Internet in community organizing and community building has increased dramatically, with groups across the political spectrum going on line to build community and to identify and organize supporters on a mass scale (see chapter 18).

In the health field, a major emphasis on community participation began in the 1970s and culminated in the World Health Organization's adoption in 1986 of a new approach to health promotion that stressed increasing people's control over the determinants of their health, high-level public participation, and intersectoral cooperation (WHO 1986). Reflecting this new approach, the WHO-initiated Healthy Cities/Healthy Communities movement emerged and grew to involve at its peak thousands of healthy cities and communities worldwide. It aims to create sustainable environments and processes through which governmental and nongovernmental sectors work in partnership to create healthy public policies, achieve high-level participation in community-driven projects, and, ultimately, reduce inequities and disparities among groups (Norris and Pittman 2000).

Alongside these developments has grown an appreciation for *community building*, conceptualized as a process that people in a community engage in themselves, rather than *community organizing*, viewed typically from the vantage point of the outside organizer (see chapter 6 and appendix 2). The community building orientation is reflected in efforts such as the National Black Women's Health Project, a twenty-five-year-old network of close to two dozen chapters with more than 10,000 members, which stresses empowerment through self-help and consciousness raising for social change (http://www.nationalblackwomenshealth-project.org). Community building projects are strength-based and grounded in feminist notions of "power to" and "power with" rather than the more masculine concept of "power over" frequently encountered in traditional organizing (French 1986). They also borrow from feminist organizing an accent on the process of practice (Hyde 1994) and the integration, through dialogue, of personal and political experiences (see chapters 11 and 13). Although theoretical work in the area of community building remains somewhat underdeveloped, community building practice has become an increasingly important complement to more traditional notions of community organization.

Finally, a growing interest in community-based participatory research (CBPR) in health and related fields has brought community organizing principles into the domain of research, challenging both positivist notions of knowledge and traditional top-down processes of academia (Minkler and Wallerstein 2003). Increasingly, academic-community partnerships are sought by funding agencies and by individual communities and researchers to support community-determined research agendas, mutual learning, and actions based on the research results to improve health.

## The Concept of Community

Integral to a discussion of community organization and community building practice is an examination of the concept of community. While typically seen in geographic terms, communities may be based instead on shared interests or characteristics such as ethnicity, sexual orientation, or occupation (Fellin 2001). Communities have been defined as (1) functional spatial units that meet basic needs for sustenance, (2) units of patterned social interaction, and (3) symbolic units of collective identity (Hunter 1975). Eng and Parker (1994) add a fourth political definition of community: people coming together to act politically to make changes.

Two sets of theories are relevant for understanding the concept of community. The first, the ecological system perspective, is particularly useful in the study of autonomous geographic communities, including population characteristics of size, density, and heterogeneity; the physical environment; the social organization or structure of the community; and the technological forces that affect it. In contrast, the social systems perspective focuses primarily on the formal organizations, exploring interactions of community subsystems (economic, political, and so on) both horizontally within the community and vertically as they relate to systems outside the community (Fellin 2001). Warren's (1963) classic approach to community clearly fits within the latter perspective, envisioning communities as entities that change their structure and function to accommodate various social, political, and economic developments. Similarly, Alinsky's (1972) view of communities as reflecting the social problems and processes of an urban society provides a good example of a social systems perspective (see also chapters 3 and 11).

Clearly, a person's perspective on community influences his or her view of the appropriate domains and functions of the community organization process.

Community development specialists (for example, agricultural extension workers and Peace Corps volunteers) have thus tended to focus on helping people identify with and bring about changes in their own geographic community (Rothman 2001). By contrast, proponents of a broader social action approach have encouraged organizing around issues such as public housing and unemployment, recognizing the tremendous impact of larger socioeconomic issues on local communities. Similarly, though communities are rich in diversity, with multiple interacting subcommunities, one's view of the community as more or less heterogeneous will determine the strategies employed and the types of organizing goals.

Finally, as Ronald Braithwaite et al. (2000), Felix Rivera and John Erlich (1995, 2000), and Lorraine M. Gutierrez and Edith A. Lewis (chapter 13) have suggested, an appreciation of the unique characteristics of communities of color should be a major consideration in thinking about organizing within such communities. As regards African American communities, for example, Cornel West (1993) argues that market exploitation has shattered the religious and civic organizations that have historically buffered these communities from hopelessness and nihilism. He calls for community change by re-creating a sense of agency and political resistance based on "subversive memory—the best of one's past without romantic nostalgia" (19). A view of community that incorporates such a perspective would support building on preexisting social networks and structures and emphasize self-determination and empowerment. The different models described in this chapter illustrate how alternative assumptions about the nature of community strongly shape the ways in which community organization and community building are conceptualized and practiced.

## Models of Community Organization

While community organization is frequently treated as if it were a singular model of practice, several typologies and change models of community organization have been developed. The best known of these typologies is Jack Rothman's (2001) three distinct models of practice: locality development, social planning, and social action. Briefly, *locality development* is defined as heavily process-oriented, stressing consensus and cooperation and aimed at building group identity and a sense of community. By contrast, *social planning* is heavily task oriented, focused on rational-empirical problem solving, usually by an outside expert. Finally, the *social action model* is both task- and process-oriented. It is concerned with increasing the community's problem-solving ability and achieving concrete changes to redress imbalances of power and privilege between an oppressed or disadvantaged group and the larger society.

Originally arguing that most community organizing efforts tend to fall in one or the other of these categories, Rothman (2001) more recently has suggested that many professionals use a mix of two or more of the models. Feminist organizing, for example, may combine the goals and assumptions of social action organizing with methods that often are consistent with locality development (Hyde 1994, Rothman 2001). Similarly, the heart health community trials and Planned Community Action toward Health (PATCH) interventions mix social planning with elements of locality development (Farquhar et al. 1994, Bracht et al. 1999), while many organizers in the Alinsky tradition have mixed social action and locality development in their community efforts (Marquez 1990, Homan 1999; see also chapter 15).

For more than three decades, Rothman's typology has remained the dominant framework within which community organization has been examined and understood and thus has had a significant impact on practice (see chapter 4). Despite its widespread application, however, the typology and its underlying assumptions have a number of important limitations. First, use of the term *locality development*, for example, may be unnecessarily restrictive, discouraging a consideration of organizing along nongeographic lines. Second, inclusion of a social planning model, which often relies heavily on outside technical experts and does not necessarily increase the community's problem-solving ability, appears to contradict one of the most basic criteria of effective organizing. Finally, as Walter argues in chapter 4, the fact that this typology is problem-based and organizer-centered rather than strength-based and community-centered constitutes a philosophical and practical limitation that may be particularly problematic when organizing occurs in multicultural contexts.

Partly in reaction to the perceived limitations of the Rothman typology, Walter (chapter 4) and others (Kaye and Wolff 1995, Gardner 1991, Himmelman 1992, Labonte 1994, Wallerstein and Sanchez-Merki 1994) have suggested newer models of collaborative empowerment and community building practice that provide important alternative approaches. Although these models are partial descendants of community development in their emphases on self-help and collaboration, they extend beyond the tradition of external origination, which may implicitly accept the status quo. They take their parentage from community-driven development, where community concerns direct the organizing in a process that creates healthy and more equal power relations (Labonte 1994, Purdey et al. 1994; see figure 2.1).

The newer community building model emphasizes community strengths, not as nostalgia for the good old days but as a diversity of groups and systems that can identify shared values and nurture the development of shared goals (Gardner 1991), including Arthur Himmelman's (1992) collaborative empowerment model and John McKnight's (1995, 161) notion of regenerating, which seeks to recognize people's "gifts" as community resources.

Along similar lines, Walter (chapter 4) describes the community building practice approach not as a method but as "a way of orienting oneself in the

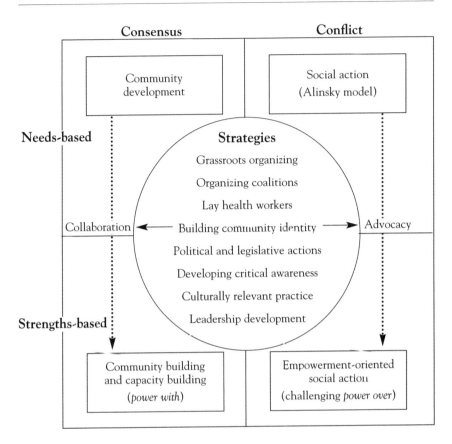

*Figure 2.1.* Community organization and community-building typology.

community" that places community "at the center of practice." Her concept of community building attempts to balance and blend elements of community such as historicity, identity, and autonomy with community development, community planning, community action, community consciousness, and "the commons." While placing a similarly strong emphasis on identifying and promoting community strengths and capacity, a macro-conceptualization of community building also emphasizes regional economic development and federal and state policy-level reinvestment in local communities as critical parts of the community building process (Blackwell and Colmenar 2000, Walsh 1997; see appendix 2). As such, community building approaches contrast significantly with more traditional notions of community practice that are community placed but not necessarily of and by the community (Kaye and Wolff 1995; see chapter 5).

Midway between older models of community organizing and newer conceptualizations of community building are models that incorporate some elements of each while accenting culturally relevant practice. Among the best known of these approaches in the health field is Braithwaite and colleagues' (1994, 2000) community organization and development (COD) model for health promotion in communities of color. Although written from the perspective of the outside organizer, the central thrust of the COD model involves facilitating the development and effective functioning of a community-dominated and -controlled coalition board. The latter undertakes its own community assessment, sets policy, facilitates leadership development, and, on the basis of bottom-up planning and community problem solving, designs culturally relevant interventions. The COD model moves from initial reliance on traditional community organizing to incorporating many of the principles of community building practice, while stressing throughout the cultural context of the practice.

Finally, coalition building is alternately defined as a model of community organization practice and a strategy used across models. Coalitions are increasingly popular in the health field in areas as diverse as chronic disease, drugs and alcohol, violence prevention, immunizations, and environmental justice (Goodman et al. 1993, Kaye and Wolff 1995, Sofaer 2002, Butterfoss 1998; see also chapters 16 and 17), and their particular relevance for organizing within communities of color also has been demonstrated (Braithwaite et al. 2000). Coalitions have attracted heavy public- and private-sector funding as well as increased scholarly attention (see Kreuter et al. 2000, Fawcett et al. 1997, Roussos and Fawcett 2000, Lasker et al. 2001).

In sum, several models of community organizing and community building have surfaced within the past decade to complement a long history of earlier organizing approaches. In figure 2.1, we integrate new perspectives with the older models, presenting a typology that incorporates both needs- and strengths-based approaches. Along the needs-based axis, community development, as primarily a consensus model, is contrasted with Alinsky's social action, conflict-based model. The newer strengths-based models contrast a capacity building approach with an empowerment-oriented, social action approach. When we look at primary strategies, we see that consensus approaches, whether needs- or strengths-based, primarily use collaboration strategies, whereas conflict approaches use advocacy strategies and ally building to support advocacy efforts.

Community organizing and community building are fluid endeavors. While some organizing efforts primarily focus in one quadrant, most incorporate multiple tendencies, possibly starting from a specific need or a crisis and moving to a strengths-based community capacity approach. Different organizing models, such as coalitions, lay health worker programs, political action groups, leadership development, or grassroots organizing, may incorporate needs- or strengths-based approaches at different times, depending on the starting place and the ever-changing social dynamic. It is important, however, that organizing efforts clarify their assumptions and make decisions about primary strategies based on skills of group members, history of the group, willingness to take risks, or comfort level with different approaches.

## Concepts in Community Organization and Community Building Practice

While no single unified model of community organization or community building exists, some key concepts are central to effecting and measuring change on the community level. In this section, we introduce several of these concepts and principles: empowerment and critical consciousness, community capacity and social capital, issue selection, and measurement and evaluation issues. They are summarized in table 2.1.

### EMPOWERMENT AND CRITICAL CONSCIOUSNESS

While the term *empowerment* has been justifiably criticized as a catch-all phrase in social science (Rappaport 1984), it nevertheless represents a central tenet of community organization and community building practice. Within public health, empowerment or community empowerment has been variously defined, from communities' achievement of equity or the capacity to identify problems and solutions (Cotrell 1976) to participatory self-competence in the political life of the community (Wandersman and Florin 2000).

Although many limit their definition to a narrow individual focus, similar to self-esteem or self-confidence, empowerment is a multilevel construct involving "participation, control and critical awareness," whether one focuses on the individual, organizational, or broader community level (Zimmerman 2000, 58). A broader definition is most useful—one that views empowerment as a social action process by which individuals, communities, and organizations gain mastery over their lives in the context of changing their social and political environment to improve equity and quality of life (Rappaport 1984, Wallerstein 1992).

Such a definition highlights issues of power or the ability to create change on a personal, interpersonal, and political level (see chapter 12). Ronald Labonte (1990) addresses power as a social relationship with contradictory elements (Bernstein et al. 1994). "Power from within" and "power with others" are moral, spiritual, and skill-based sources of power that can constantly expand as people empower themselves. "Power over" has a material and psychological base of domination through force or ideological hegemony. Although repressive power can be exercised directly or indirectly by controlling people's access to jobs, education, and living conditions, Michel Foucault (1977) argues that repressive power is not monolithic. He conceptualizes power as productive and relational; people produce their power through a web of complex practices and debates exercised within institutions and

Table 2.1
Key Concepts in Community Organization and Community Building

| Concept | Definition | Application |
|---|---|---|
| Empowerment | Social action process for people to gain mastery over their lives and the lives of their communities | Community members assume greater power or expand their power from within to create desired changes. |
| Critical consciousness | A consciousness based on continuous cycles of reflection and action in making change | People engage in dialogue that links root causes and community actions. |
| Community capacity | Community characteristics affecting its ability to identify, mobilize, and address problems | Community members participate actively in the life of their community through leadership, social networks, and access to power. |
| Social capital | Relationships and structures within a community that promote cooperation for mutual benefit | Community building efforts increase trust, reciprocity, and civic engagement and, ideally, makes connections to external resources. |
| Issue selection | Identifying winnable and specific targets of change that unify and build community strength | Issues are identified through community participation; targets are part of a larger strategy. |
| Participation and relevance | Community organizing that "starts where the people are" and engages community members as equals | Community members create their own agenda based on felt needs, shared power, and awareness of resources. |

communities. These power relationships are inherently unstable and therefore open to challenge by historically disenfranchised groups. Empowerment embraces both the challenge against power (resisting power structures through community organizing and advocacy) and community building efforts that expand power by strengthening community relationships.

For health educators, these contradictory elements raise issues about their own practice. Many professionals have higher-status positions than community members do. Can people in positions of dominance or privilege, in terms of either culture, gender, race, or class, empower others? Or must people empower themselves? If empowerment includes the dimension of transferring power to others, professionals may need to let go of their power, to make it more available to others. In Labonte's words, "Empowerment . . . is a fascinating dynamic of power given and taken all at once, a dialectical dance between consensus and conflict, professional expertise and lay wisdom, hierarchic institutions and community circles" (Bernstein et al. 1994, 285).

As a theory and a methodology, community empowerment is multilayered, representing both processes and outcomes of change for individuals, the organizations of which they are a part, and the community social structure itself (Zimmerman 2000). At the level of the individual, psychological empowerment extends beyond intrapsychic self-esteem to include people's perceived control in their lives, their critical awareness of their social context, and their political efficacy and participation in change (Zimmerman 1990, 2000). Empowerment challenges the perceived or real powerlessness that comes from the health injuries of poverty, chronic stressors, lack of control, and few resources—what epidemiologist S. Leonard Syme (2004) calls a lack of "control over destiny."

Organizational empowerment incorporates both the processes of organizations (for example, whether they are acting to influence societal change) and the outcomes, such as their effectiveness in gaining new resources (Zimmerman 2000). At the community level, as individuals engage in community organizing efforts, community empowerment outcomes can include an increased sense of community; greater community participation; and actual changes in policies, transformed conditions, or increased resources that may reduce inequities. As communities become empowered and better able to engage in collective problem solving, key health and social indicators may reflect this shift, perhaps in declining rates of alcoholism, depression, suicide, and other social problems. Moreover, the empowered community that works effectively for change can help bring about changes in some of the very conditions that contributed to its ill health in the first place (Israel 1985, James et al. 2002).

The link between psychological, organizational, and community level empowerment is strengthened through critical consciousness, or conscientization, a concept from Brazilian educator Paulo Freire (1970, 1973). Freire developed a method for teaching illiterate peasants to read by teaching them to "read" their political and social reality. Over the past four decades, his work has been a catalyst worldwide for programs in adult education, health, and community development (Carroll and Minkler 2000, Hope and Timmel 1984, Wallerstein and Bernstein 1994, Wallerstein and Weinger 1992, Arnold et al. 1995).

Freire's central premise is that the purpose of education should be liberating, transforming the status quo in the classroom and in people's lives. He questions whether education reinforces powerlessness (by treating people as objects who receive knowledge) or whether it enables people to challenge the conditions that keep them powerless. Freire proposes a dialogical problem-posing process, with equality and mutual respect between learner-teachers and teacher-learners. Problem posing contains a cycle of listening-dialogue-action that enables all participants to engage in continuous reflection and action. Through structured dialogue, group participants listen for the issues contained in their own experiences, discuss common problems, look for root causes and the connections among the "problems behind the problem-as-symptom," and devise strategies to help transform their reality (Freire 1970, 1973).

*Conscientization* is the consciousness that comes through the social analysis of conditions and people's role in changing those conditions. This awareness enables community groups to analyze moments and open spaces to enact change or to understand those limit-situations that may deter change (Barndt 1989). Conscientization is a key ingredient to maintaining a broader vision and sustaining community organizing efforts over time and, as such, is one of the most important links between psychological and community empowerment.

## COMMUNITY CAPACITY AND SOCIAL CAPITAL

Closely related to the concept of empowerment is the notion of *community capacity*, defined as "the characteristics of communities that affect their ability to identify, mobilize, and address social and public health problems" (Goodman et al. 1999, 259). Community capacity has multiple dimensions: active participation, leadership, rich support networks, skills and resources, critical reflection, a sense of community, an understanding of history, the articulation of values, and access to power (Goodman et al. 1999). Definitions of community capacity have drawn from other related concepts, such as community competence and social capital. *Community competence* was originally defined by community psychologist Leonard Cottrell (1976) as the community's ability "to collaborate effectively on identifying [its] problems and needs . . . ; to achieve a working consensus on goals and priorities; to agree on ways and means to implement the agreed upon goals; to collaborate effectively in the required actions" (403). Important refinements in community competence have accompanied lay health worker programs that focus on these workers as community activists in addition to their role of working with clients (Eng and Parker 2002, Ovrebo et al. 1994).

Social capital has more recently captured imaginations in the field of public health. A term that originated in political science and sociology, *social capital* is defined as the structures and relationships within social organization that facilitate coordination and cooperation for mutual benefit (Putnam 1996, Coleman 1988). "Social capital is a collective asset, a feature of communities rather than the property of individuals. As such, individuals both contribute to it and use it, but they cannot own it" (Warren et al. 2001, 1).

Within epidemiology, social capital has been seen predominantly as a horizontal or bonding relationship between neighbors or community members, with variables such as trust, reciprocity, and civic engagement operating in venues such as voluntary organizations, soccer leagues, and parent-teacher organizations (Kawachi et al. 1997; Kreuter et al. 1997). Lack of social capital has been correlated with poor health status, such as increased homicide rates, all-cause mortality, and other morbidities, and may mediate the relationship between income inequality and health (Kawachi et al. 1997, Sampson et al. 1997).

Despite social capital's correlational associations with health outcomes, the ascendance of the construct remains problematic. First, there is little evidence that lack of social capital causes poor health outcomes that are independent from the material conditions that inform day-to-day experience (Lynch et al. 2000). Second, an epidemiological focus on horizontal relationships ignores the issues of power between communities and the outside world (Hawe and Shiell 2000, Warren et al. 2001). More promising is the newer concept of *bridging social capital*—the connection that communities have with local government and external resources (Gitell and Vidal 1998, Harpham et al. 2002), an idea partly based on Pierre Bourdieu's depiction in the early 1980s of the economic benefits of a durable social network (Portes 1998). Robert J. Sampson's novel reconfiguration of social capital as collective efficacy, or the belief of community members that they have the capacity to create change, is an important recognition of bridging social capital (Sampson and Morenoff 2000). The tendency of many social capital advocates, however, to deemphasize issues of power and relationships beyond the local community level remains disconcerting (Hawe and Shiell 2000, Saegert et al. 2001). For as Mark Warren and his colleagues (2001) point out, "Social capital is not an alternative to providing greater financial resources and public services to poor communities. Rather, it constitutes an essential means to increase such resources and to make more effective use of them" (2). A related concern is the potential victim-blaming mentality: communities would be healthier if they just got it together themselves. Such an attitude, as Warren et al. (2001, 2) suggest, can have the effect of replacing "the moral deficit argument" (for example, that poor people lack a work ethic and an adequate sense of responsibility for their children) with an equally troubling "social deficit" perspective that implicitly holds up the middle-class community as the standard for comparison.

Finally, the major concern for health educators and organizers is that social capital is not an intervention construct, as are community capacity development, community organizing, and community empowerment. Unlike these other constructs, social capital does not provide theories of change, tools, or time lines for change; nor does it necessarily guarantee improved health outcomes if social capital is improved. As Bob Edwards and Michael Foley (1997) have suggested, it remains unclear whether and to what extent the concept of social capital has an analytic payoff distinct from that of these other well-known constructs in the field of public health.

Returning to community capacity building and community empowerment theories of change, let's look at tools that may be helpful in organizing. *Social networks* (the web of relationships in which people are embedded) and *social support* (the tangible and intangible resources they give and receive through these networks [Cohen and Syme 1985]), for example, provide ways in which we can map individuals' social ties, identify natural helpers or leaders within a community, help these natural leaders in turn identify their own networks, identify high-risk groups in the community, and involve network members in undertaking their own community assessment and actions necessary to strengthen their networks. A number of network assessment tools are available for mapping personal and community networks and other community assets (Sharpe et al. 2000).

Leadership development represents a key aspect of fostering community capacity and effectiveness, encouraging leadership roles as *animator* (stimulating people to think critically and identify problems and new solutions) and *facilitator* (providing a process through which the group can discuss its own content in the most productive possible way) (Hope and Timmel 1984). As Gutierrez and Lewis suggest in chapter 13, an emphasis on leadership development may be especially important in communities of color, where "a unidirectional outreach approach" is often taken, meaning that such communities are "targets of change rather than active participants and collaborators." By involving people of color in leadership roles from the outset and nurturing the development of new leaders, health education professionals can make important contributions to capacity building that reflect feminist notions of strength through diversity.

### ISSUE SELECTION

One of the most important steps in community organization practice involves the effective differentiation between *problems* (things that are troubling) and *issues* (problems the community feels strongly about). As Mike Miller (1986) suggests, a good issue must meet several important criteria. (1) It must be winnable, ensuring that working on the campaign doesn't simply reinforce fatalistic attitudes and beliefs. (2) It must be simple and specific so that any member of the group can explain it clearly in a sentence or two. (3) It must unite members of the group and must involve them in a meaningful way in achieving problem resolution. (4) It should affect many people and build up the community or organization (giving leadership experience, increased visibility, and so on). (5) Finally, it should be part of a larger plan or strategy. Focus groups, nominal group processes, and other popular education approaches can provide mechanisms to select and identify the priority issue for organizing (see chapter 8).

Even if organizers genuinely attempt to start where the people are, they may lack access to the hidden discourse in a community and misinterpret apparent community apathy because of their own lack of cultural competence, lack of access to key stakeholders or cultural translators, or lack of reflection about the problematic nature of power dynamics between themselves and community members (Scott 1990). As Vivian Chavez and her colleagues (2003) suggest with respect to community-based participatory research, community partners of color "may express defiance, make jokes, and express tensions not safe to bring up in the presence of their white counterparts from university or professional settings" (87). In other instances, the outside organizer, particularly if he or she is racially or in other ways a part of the group in which he or she is organizing, may have access to community discourse yet find community resistance and organizing strategies that challenge his or her own level of comfort. The person may have a working relationship with community leaders yet find that the group has chosen issues that are too broad to be winnable. In the case of issue selection, the organizer has the responsibility to pose questions to refocus the group onto specific targets.

Further, as Labonte (1994) has suggested, the community's selection of an issue may reflect racism, sexism, homophobia, or other discriminatory attitudes (as when communities in California, Oregon, and Colorado organized to put anti-gay-rights ballot initiatives on their state or local ballots). In such cases, the health education practitioner's commitment to starting where the people are and to community self-determination must be tempered by concern about the paramount principle of social justice in the larger community, whose interests would not be served by the parochial and prejudicial concerns and actions of one subgroup (Minkler 1994).

Freire's (1970, 1973) dialogical problem-posing method has proven to be especially helpful in overcoming some of these difficulties in issue selection. Community development approaches worldwide have adopted his educational strategies to identify the core themes that generate social and emotional commitment for starting organizing efforts (Arnold et al. 1995, Carroll and Minkler 2000, Hope and Timmel 1984).

Community organizers in the United States also have adopted organizational development strategic action plans to prioritize issues by available resources, appropriate time lines, and barriers to reaching goals (French and Bell 1990). Politically minded organizers have analyzed the power brokers, allies, and resisters in choosing an issue that may be feasible to win (Homan 1999; see also chapter 10).

As we have suggested, issue selection processes, undertaken thoughtfully, can contribute to community empowerment and serve as a positive force for social change. On the other hand, there have been increasing calls for "a new process of community organizing—one relying less on issue based mobilization and more on community education, leadership development and support, and building local sustainable organizations" (Traynor 1993). Community building practice is becoming less concerned with community issue selection and more with the identification, nurture, and celebration of community strengths and the creation of a context, by people in the community, for sharing those strengths (see chapters 4 and 9). Among the useful new approaches to combining issue selection with this positive emphasis on community strengths and assets is Caroline Wang's (Wang et al. 2000) photovoice method (Wang and Burris 1994; see also chapter 19). Health education professionals provide community residents with cameras and skills training, and the residents then use the cameras to convey their own images of their community problems and strengths. Together, participants select the pictures that best capture their collective wisdom and use them to tell their stories and to stimulate change through local organizing. Whether with homeless people in Detroit or rural women in China, this approach has been used with considerable success and offers new and innovative models for "integrating community capacity, health concerns and the visual image" (Wang and Burris 1994, 177; Wang et al. 2000).

## MEASUREMENT AND EVALUATION ISSUES

To date, a major limitation of most community organizing and community building efforts has been the failure to address evaluation processes and outcomes adequately. This failure typically stems from several sources, among them severe funding constraints and lack of knowledge about how to build a meaningful evaluation component into the organizing effort. The evolving nature of community organizing initiatives, complex and dynamic contexts, and the fact that these projects often seek change on multiple levels make many traditional evaluative approaches inappropriate or ill-suited to such organizing endeavors (Goodman 2000, Connell et al. 1995, Wallerstein et al. 2002). Similarly, many standard evaluation approaches focus on long-term change in health and social indicators and thus may miss the short-term, system-level effects with which community organizing is heavily concerned, such as improvements in organizational collaboration, participation, leadership, and healthier public policies or environmental conditions.

This lack of formal evaluation, coupled with the failure of many of those engaged in community organizing projects to write up and publish their results, have made it difficult to amass a literature of successful and unsuccessful organizing efforts and the hallmarks of each. Fortunately, since the late 1980s, we have witnessed important gains in the evaluation of community organizing and related areas. Key was the convening of a round-table meeting on community initiatives for children and families and the group's development of *New Approaches to Evaluating Community Initiatives* (Connell et al. 1995). This edited volume explores dilemmas commonly faced in the design, measurement, and interpretation of community initiatives as well as a variety of options and strategies for evaluators working with such projects. A special issue of the journal *Health Education Research* on community coalitions included several articles that addressed measurement and evaluation issues (Goodman et al. 1993). Much research has focused on internal dynamics and other characteristics that may influence a coalition's effectiveness, including shared vision, strong leadership, and an accent on process (Connell et al. 1995, Goodman et al. 1996, Butterfoss 1998, Kegler et al. 1998, Helitzer 2000). Determinants of effective partnership synergy identified for further research include the ability to bring in resources, level of involvement and heterogeneity of partners, trust and power relationships, and governance (Lasker et al. 2001).

Evaluation and measurement of community empowerment was brought to the fore in a two-part issue of *Health Education Quarterly* (1994) titled "Community Empowerment, Participatory Education, and Health," which included both tools and case studies. Measurement of community empowerment, capacity, and social capital has proceeded slowly. But measures do exist for community competence (Eng and Parker 1994); community collaboration (Backer 2003); multilevel perceived control (appendix 9); social cohesion and social influence (Speer et al. 2001); social capital (Lochner et al. 1999, Kreuter et al. 1997, Kawachi et al. 1997); collective efficacy and social norm control (Sampson et al. 1997, Bandura 1995); psychological empowerment beliefs of perceived control, critical understanding of one's social environment, and participation in social action (Zimmerman 2000); and perceived neighborhood control and neighborhood participation (Parker et al. 2001). A recent multisite Centers for Disease Control (CDC) study of social capital–community capacity in ethnic-minority communities is identifying new understandings and measures particular to grassroots organizing, coalition building, and community identity.

Equally important is whether or not new capacities lead to health and health behavior outcomes, a process that may be both direct and indirect. Direct health outcomes may result from coalition or neighborhood activity to prevent the siting of a toxic waste facility or to pass a clean air ordinance that leads to reduced tobacco use. Indirectly, participation may lead to empowerment (Speer et al. 2001), less social isolation, greater self-efficacy to change health behaviors, increased access to care, and other intermediate outcomes that may lead to improved health (Abatena 1997, Eng et al. 1990, Minkler et al. 2002).

Despite the advances in measurement for capturing these kinds of changes, however, there are limits to any tool or set of scales. Self-report measures of individuals cannot capture the full organizational and community-level processes over a period of time. Qualitative approaches are therefore needed to enhance understanding of the context; dynamics of change; and the range of intermediate outcomes such as new policies, levels of participation, political voice, and changed conditions, which in turn may lead to improved health.

Just as important to the development of validated scales, however, may be the process by which communities develop their own sets of capacity and empowerment indicators. Some community groups have already developed indicators of capacity and sustainability (Norris 1997, Aspen 1996, Bauer 2003, Wallerstein et al. 2002). A useful resource for communities that wish to engage in a participatory process to develop their own indicators can be found in the self-reflection workbook developed in New Mexico to evaluate system and population health changes from community organizing and community building in the context of creating healthier communities (Maltrud et al. 1997). The workbook focuses on changes in community processes (such as grassroots participation) and changes in short-term, system-level outcomes (such as the development of new programs) as a result of the organizing experience. These midlevel outcomes, rather than long-term changes in self-rated health and other health and social indicators, are often most important in documenting community capacity and empowerment.

A major contribution to the literature in this area was the publication of David Fetterman et al.'s (1996) comprehensive *Empowerment Evaluation*, defined as "an interactive and iterative process by which the community, in collaboration with the support team, identifies its own health issues, decides how to address them, monitors progress toward its goals and uses the information to adapt and sustain the initiative" (Fawcett et al. 1996, 169). Although some of the evaluation approaches described in this book (such as the "empowering evaluation" of HIV prevention community planning in chapter 21) fit better into a social planning rather than a true organizing approach to practice, most have immediate relevance for health education professionals concerned with the evaluation of community organizing efforts.

Recent work by Stephen B. Fawcett and his colleagues (1997, 2001) in the Work Group on Health Promotion and Community Development at the University of Kansas has helped tailor empowerment evaluation methods more directly to the evaluation of community coalitions for health. Stressing both processes (such as community mobilization to address substance abuse) and outcomes (such as changes in youth self-reports of substance abuse and community-level effects attributed to coalition efforts), this approach uses qualitative and quantitative measurement instruments and actively involves community members in the evaluation. A web site created by the work group (http://ctb.lsi.ukans.edu) was developed to help other groups use a "community tool box" to better document and evaluate their own community organizing and community building efforts in health promotion (Fawcett et al. 2000).

The availability of new theoretical contributions and practical tools that lend themselves to evaluation of community organizing fails, of course, to solve the problem of insufficient funding or commitment to carrying out high-quality evaluative research. Yet the increased attention of both foundation and government funders to evaluation and measurement issues in community organizing and community-based initiatives is encouraging. If translated into increased funding, this attention, together with the availability of new measurement tools and processes, should spur major advances in the evaluation and documentation of community organizing and community building.

## Conclusion

The continued pivotal role of community organization in health education practice reflects not only its time-tested efficacy but also its close philosophical fit with the most fundamental principles of effective community health education. Community organization stresses the principle of relevance, or starting where the people are; the principle of participation; and the importance of creating environments in which individuals and communities can become empowered as they increase their community problem-solving ability.

Newer conceptualizations of community building stress many of the same principles within an overall approach that focuses on community growth and change from the inside through increased group identification; discovery, nurture, and mapping of community assets; and creation of critical consciousness. Both community organizing and community building also stress the role of the larger systems in which communities are embedded in enabling them to grow and thrive by building relationships with external resource institutions and breaking down the social isolation of local communities (Blackwell and Colmenar 2000).

Professionals in health education and related fields sometimes have the opportunity to engage in pure community organizing in which the community, rather than a health department, an outside agency, or a funder, fully determines the issues to be addressed, the strategies and tactics employed and so forth. Yet even professionals who are helping to mobilize a community around a predetermined health or social problem, such as reducing rates of HIV, youth violence, or asthma, can effectively apply many of the core principles and approaches of community organization and community building practice. They can thus elicit high-level community participation or involvement and strive to build leadership skills and increase community capacity and social capital as integral parts of the overall health education project. Further, as demonstrated in several of the case studies in this volume, while the overall problem area (such as alcohol and substance abuse) may initially have been identified by an outside group or agency, the health education professional, using community organizing and community building skills and approaches, can help communities identify, within this broader framework, those specific issues they feel are most relevant.

Most important, professionals can challenge themselves to examine their own dynamic of power with their professional colleagues and members of the community, learning to understand the complexities of working in partnership toward community ownership of the projects undertaken and increased empowerment and community competence (Wallerstein 1999). In sum, both community organization and newer conceptions of community building practice have essential messages for health education professionals in a wide variety of settings and may hold particular relevance in the changing sociopolitical climate of the twenty-first century.

### Acknowledgments

Portions of this chapter are based on M. Minkler and N. Wallerstein, 2002, "Improving Health through Community Organizing and Community Building," in *Health Behavior*

## References

Abatena, H. 1997. "The Significance of Planned Community Participation in Problem Solving and Developing a Viable Community Capability." *Journal of Community Practice* 4, no. 2: 13–34.

Alinsky, S. D. 1969. *Reveille for Radicals.* Chicago: University of Chicago Press.

———. 1972. *Rules for Radicals.* New York: Random House.

Arnold, R., B. Burke, C. James, D. A. Martin, and B. Thomas. 1995. *Educating for a Change.* Toronto: Between the Lines and Doris Marshall Institute for Education and Action.

Backer, T. E. 2003. *Evaluating Community Collaborations.* New York: Springer.

Bandura, A. 1995. "Exercise of Personal and Collective Efficacy." In *Self-Efficacy in Changing Societies,* edited by A. Bandura, 1–45. New York: Cambridge University Press.

Barndt, D. 1989. *Naming the Moment: Political Analysis for Action.* Toronto: Jesuit Center for Social Faith and Justice.

Bauer, G. 2003. "Sample Community Health Indicators on the Neighborhood Level." In *Community-Based Participatory Research for Health,* edited by M. Minkler and N. Wallerstein. San Francisco: Jossey-Bass.

Bernstein, E., N. Wallerstein, R. Braithwaite, L. Gutierrez, R. Labonte, and M. Zimmerman. 1994. "Empowerment Forum: A Dialogue between Guest Editorial Board Members." *Health Education Quarterly* 21, no. 3: 281–94.

Blackwell, A. G., and R. Colmenar. 2000. "Community Building: From Local Wisdom to Public Policy." *Public Health Reports* 113, nos. 2 and 3: 167–73.

Bracht, N., L. Kingsbury, and C. Rissel. 1999. "A Five-Stage Community Organization Model for Health Promotion: Empowerment and Partnership Strategies." In *Health Promotion at the Community Level,* edited by N. Bracht, 83–104. Thousand Oaks, Calif.: Sage.

Braithwaite, R. L., C. Bianchi, and S. E. Taylor. 1994. Ethnographic approach to community organization and health empowerment. *Health Education Quarterly* 21, no. 3: 407–19.

Braithwaite, R. L., S. E. Taylor, and J. N. Austin. 2000. *Building Health Coalitions in the Black Community.* Thousand Oaks, Calif.: Sage.

Butterfoss, F. D. 1998. *Coalition Effectiveness Inventory Self-Assessment Tool.* Columbia: South Carolina Center for Pediatric Research, Center for Health Promotion.

Carroll, J., and M. Minkler. 2000. "Freire's Message for Social Workers: Looking Back and Looking Ahead." *Journal of Community Practice* 8, no. 1: 21–36.

Chavez, V., B. Duran, Q. E. Baker, M. M. Avila, and N. Wallerstein. 2003. "The Dance of Race and Privilege in Community-Based Participatory Research." In *Community-Based Participatory Research for Health,* edited by M. Minkler and N. Wallerstein, 81–97. San Francisco: Jossey-Bass.

Cohen, S., and S. L. Syme, eds. 1985. *Social Support and Health.* New York: Academic Press.

Coleman, J. S. 1988. "Social Capital in the Creation of Human Capital." *American Journal of Sociology* 94, supp.: S95–S121.

Connell, J. P., A. C. Kubisch, L. B. Schorr, and C. H. Weiss, eds. 1995. *New Approaches to Evaluating Community Initiatives: Concepts, Methods, and Contexts.* Washington, D.C.: Aspen Institute.

Cotrell, L. S., Jr. 1976. "The Competent Community." In *Further Explorations in Social Psychiatry,* edited by B. H. Kaplan and R. N. Wilson. New York: Basic Books.

———. 1983. "The Competent Community." In *New Perspectives on the American Community,* edited by R. Warren and L. Lyon, 398–432. Homewood, Ill.: Dorsey.

Edwards, B., and M. Foley. 1997. "Escape from Politics? Social Theory and the Social Capital Debate." *American Behavioral Scientist* 40, no. 5: 549–60.

Eng, E., J. Briscoe, and A. Cunningham. 1990. "The Effect of Participation in Water Projects on Immunization." *Social Science and Medicine* 30, no. 12: 1349–58.

Eng, E., and E. Parker. 1994. "Measuring Community Competence in the Mississippi Delta: The Interface between Program Evaluation and Empowerment." *Health Education Quarterly* 21, no. 2: 199–220.

———. 2002. "Natural Helper Models to Enhance a Community's Health and Competence." In *Emerging Theories in Health Promotion Practice and Research: Strategies for Improving Public Health*, edited by R. J. DiClemente, R. A. Crosby, and M. C. Kegler, 126–56. San Francisco: Jossey-Bass.

Farquhar, J., S. P. Fortmann, N. Maccoby, P. D. Wood, W. L. Haskell, C. B. Taylor, J. A. Flora, D. S. Solomon, T. Rogers, E. Adler, P. Breitrose, and L. Weiner. 1984. "The Stanford Five City Project: An Overview." In *Behavioral Health: A Handbook of Health Enhancement and Disease Prevention*, edited by J. D. Matarazzo, N. E. Miller, S. M. Weiss, and J. A. Herd, 1154–65. Silver Spring, Md.: Wiley.

Fawcett, S. B., V. T. Francisco, J. A. Schultz, B. Berkowitz, T. J. Wolff, and G. Nagy. 2000. "The Community Tool Box: A Web-Based Resource for Building Healthier Communities." *Public Health* 113, nos. 2 and 3: 274–78.

Fawcett, S. B., R. K. Lewis, A. Paine-Andrews, V. T. Francisco, K. P. Richter, E. L. Williams, and B. Copple. 1997. "Evaluating Community Coalitions for Prevention of Substance Abuse: The Case of Project Freedom." *Health Education and Behavior* 24, no. 6: 812–28.

Fawcett, S. B., A. Paine-Andrews, V. Francisco, J. Schultz, K. P. Richter, R. K. Lewis, K. J. Harris, E. J. Williams, J. Y. Berkley, C. M. Lopez, and J. L. Fisher. 1996. "Empowering Community Health Initiatives through Evaluation." In *Empowerment Evaluation*, edited by D. Fetterman, S. Kaftarian, and A. Wandersman, 161–87. Thousand Oaks, Calif.: Sage.

Fawcett, S., A. Paine-Andrews, V. T. Francisco, J. Schultz, K. P. Richter, J. Berkley-Patton, and J. L. Fisher. 2001. "Evaluating Community Initiatives for Health and Development." In *Evaluation in Health Promotion Approaches*, edited by I. Rootman, D. McQueen, L. Potvin, J. Springett, and E. Ziglio, 241–70. Copenhagen: World Health Organization, European Series, No. 92.

Fellin, P. 2001. "Understanding American Communities." In *Strategies of Community Intervention*, edited by J. Rothman, J. Erlich, and J. Tropman, 118–33. 5th ed. Itasca, Ill.: Peacock.

Fetterman, D., S. Kaftarian, and A. Wandersman, eds. 1996. *Empowerment Evaluation*. Thousand Oaks, Calif.: Sage.

Foucault, M. 1977. *Power/Knowledge: Selected Interviews and Other Writings*, edited by C. Gordon. New York: Pantheon.

Freire, P. 1970. *Pedagogy of the Oppressed*, translated by M. B. Ramos. New York: Seabury.

———. 1973. *Education for Critical Consciousness*. New York: Seabury.

French, M. 1986. *Beyond Power: On Women, Men, and Morals*. London: Abacus.

French, W., and C. Bell. 1990. *Organization Development: Behavioral Science Interventions for Organization Improvement*. 2d ed. Englewood Cliffs, N.J.: Prentice Hall.

Gardner, J. 1991. *Building Community*. Washington, D.C.: Independent Sector Leadership Studies Program.

Garvin, C. D., and F. M. Cox. 2001. "A History of Community Organizing Since the Civil War with Special Reference to Oppressed Communities." In *Strategies of Community Intervention*, edited by J. Rothman, J. L. Erlich, and J. E. Tropman, 65–100. 5th ed. Itasca, Ill.: Peacock.

Gitell, R., and A. Vidal. 1998. *Community Organizing: Building Social Capital As a Development Strategy*. Newbury Park, Calif.: Sage.

Goodman, R. M. 2000. *Evaluation of Community-Based Health Programs: An Alternate Perspective in Integrating Behavioral and Social Sciences with Public Health,* edited by N. Schneiderman, M. A. Speers, J. M. Silva, H. Tomes, and J. H. Gentry. Washington, D.C.: American Psychological Association Press.

Goodman, R. M., J. Burdine, E. Meehan, and K. McLeroy. 1993. "Coalitions." *Health Education Research* 8, no. 3: 313–14.

Goodman, R. M., M. A. Speers, K. McLeroy, S. Fawcett, M. Kegler, E. Parker, S. R. Smith, T. D. Sterling, and N. Wallerstein. 1999. "Identifying and Defining the Dimensions of Community Capacity to Provide a Basis for Measurement." *Health Education and Behavior* 25, no. 3: 258–78.

Goodman, R. M., A. Wandersman, M. Chinman, P. Imm, and E. Morrissey. 1996. "An Ecological Assessment of Community-Based Interventions for Prevention and Health Promotion: Approaches to Measuring Community Coalitions." *American Journal of Community Psychology* 24, no. 1: 33–61.

Harpham, T., E. Grant, and E. Thomas. 2002. "Measuring Social Capital within Health Surveys: Key Issues." *Health Policy and Planning* 17, no. 1: 106–11.

Hawe, P., and A. Shiell. 2000. "Social Capital and Health Promotion: A Review." *Social Science and Medicine* 51: 871–85.

Helitzer, D. 2000. *Coalition Member Survey.* Albuquerque: University of New Mexico, Office of Evaluation.

Himmelman, A. 1992. "Communities Working Collaboratively for a Change." Unpublished paper. July.

Homan, M. 1999. *Promoting Community Change: Making It Happen in the Real World.* Pacific Grove, Calif.: Books/Cole.

Hope, A., and S. Timmel. 1984. *Training for Transformation: A Handbook for Community Workers.* Gweru, Zimbabwe: Mambo.

Hunter, A. 1975. "The Loss of Community: An Empirical Test through Replication." *American Sociology Review* 40, no. 5: 537–52.

Hyde, C. 1994. "Committed to Social Change: Voices from the Feminist Movement." *Journal of Community Practice* 1, no. 2: 45–64.

Israel, B. A. 1985. "Social Networks and Social Support: Implications for Natural Helper and Community Level Interventions." *Health Education Quarterly* 12, no. 1: 65–80.

James, S. A., A. Schulz, and J. van Olphen. 2001. "Social Capital, Poverty, and Community Health: An Exploration of Linkages." In *Social Capital and Poor Communities,* edited by S. Saegert, J. P. Thompson, and M. R. Warren, 165–99. New York: Sage Foundation.

Kawachi, I., B. P. Kennedy, K. Lochner, and D. Prothrow-Stith. 1997. "Social Capital, Income Equality, and Mortality." *American Journal of Public Health* 87, no. 9: 1491–97.

Kaye, G., and T. Wolff. 1995. *From the Ground Up: A Workbook on Coalition Building and Community Development.* Amherst, Mass.: AHEC/Community Partners.

Kegler, M., A. Steckler, K. McLeroy, and S. Malek. 1998. "Factors That Contribute to Effective Community Health Promotion Coalitions: A Study of 10 Project ASSIST Coalitions in North Carolina." *Health Education and Behavior* 25, no. 3: 338–53.

Kreuter, M. W., N. A. Lezin, and A. N. Koplan. 1997. *Social Capital: Evaluation Implications for Community Health Promotion.* Atlanta: World Health Organization.

Kreuter, M. W., N. A. Lezin, and L. A. Young. 2000. "Evaluating Community Based Collaborative Mechanisms: Implications for Practitioners." *Health Promotion Practice* 1, no. 1: 49–63.

Labonte, R. 1990. "Empowerment: Notes on Professional and Community Dimensions." *Canadian Review of Social Policy* 26: 1–12.

———. 1994. "Health Promotion and Empowerment: Reflections on Professional Practice." *Health Education Quarterly* 21, no. 2: 253–68.

Lasker, R. D., E. S. Weiss, and R. Miller. 2001. "Partnership Synergy: A Practical Framework for Studying and Strengthening the Collaborative Advantage." *Milbank Quarterly* 79, no. 2: 179–205.

Lochner, K., I. Kawachi, and B. P. Kennedy. 1999. "Social Capital: A Guide to Its Measurement." *Health and Place* 5: 259–70.

Lynch, J., G. D. Smith, G. A. Kaplan, and J. S. House. 2000. "Income Inequality and Mortality: Importance to Health of Individual Income, Psychosocial Environment, or Material Conditions." *British Medical Journal* 320, no. 7243: 320.

Maltrud, K., M. Polacsek, and N. Wallerstein. 1997. *Participatory Evaluation Workbook for Community Initiatives.* Albuquerque: University of New Mexico, Masters in Public Health Program.

Marquez, B. 1990. "Organizing the Mexican American Community in Texas: The Legacy of Saul Alinsky." *Policy Studies Review* (winter): 355–73.

McKnight, J. 1995. "Regenerating Community." In *The Careless Society: Community and Its Counterfeits,* edited by J. McKnight, 161–72. New York: Basic Books.

Miller, M. 1986. "Turning Problems into Actionable Issues." Unpublished paper. San Francisco: Organize Training Center.

Minkler, M. 1994. "Ten Commitments for Community Health Education." *Health Education Research* 9, no. 4: 527–34.

Minkler, M., M. Thompson, J. Bell, K. Rose, and D. Redman. 2002. "Using Community Involvement Strategies in the Fight against Infant Mortality: Lessons from a Multisite Study of the National Healthy Start Experience." *Health Promotion Practice* 3, no. 2: 176–87.

Minkler, M., and N. Wallerstein. 2003. "Introduction to Community Based Participatory Research." In *Community Based Participatory Research,* edited by M. Minkler and N. Wallerstein, 3–26. San Francisco: Jossey-Bass.

Norris, T. 1997. *The Community Indicators Handbook: Redefining Progress.* Denver: Tyler Norris Associates.

Norris, T., and M. Pittman. 2000. "The Healthy Communities Movement and the Coalition for Healthier Cities and Communities." *Public Health Reports* 113, nos. 2 and 3: 118–24.

Nyswander, D. B. 1956. "Education for Health: Some Principles and Their Application." *Health Education Monographs* 14: 65–70.

Ovrebo, B., M. Ryan, K. Jackson, and K. Hutchinson. 1994. "The Homeless Prenatal Program: A Model for Empowering Homeless Pregnant Women." *Health Education Quarterly* 21, no. 2: 187–98.

Parker, E. A., R. L. Lichtenstein, A. J. Schultz, B. A. Israel, M. Schork, K. J. Steinman, and S. A. James. 2001. "Disentangling Measures of Individual Perceptions of Community Social Dynamics: Results of a Community Survey." *Health Education and Behavior* 28, no. 4: 462–86.

Portes, A. 1998. "Social Capital: Its Origins and Applications in Modern Sociology." *Annual Review of Sociology* 24: 1–24.

Purdey, A., G. Adhikari, S. Robinson, and P. Cox. 1994. "Participatory Health Development in Rural Nepal: Clarifying the Process of Community Empowerment." *Health Education Quarterly* 21, no. 3: 329–44.

Putnam, R. D. 1996. "The Strange Disappearance of Civic America." *American Prospect* 24: 34–48.

Rappaport, J. 1984. "Studies in Empowerment: Introduction to the Issue." *Prevention in Human Services* 3, nos. 2 and 3: 1–7.

Rivera, F., and J. Erlich. 1995. *Community Organizing in a Diverse Society.* Boston: Allyn and Bacon.

———. 2000. "An Option Assessment Framework for Organizing in Emerging Minority Communities." In *Tactics and Techniques of Community Intervention,* edited by J. Tropman, J. Erlich, and J. Rothman, 94–102. Chicago: Peacock.

Rothman, J. 2001. "Approaches to Community Intervention." In *Strategies of Community Intervention*, edited by J. Rothman, J. L. Erlich, and J. E. Tropman, 27–64. Itasca, Ill.: Peacock.

Roussos, S. T., and S. B. Fawcett. 2000. "A Review of Collaborative Partnerships As a Strategy for Improving Community Health." *Annual Review of Public Health* 21: 369–402.

Saegert, S., J. P. Thompson, and M. R. Warren. 2001. *Social Capital and Poor Communities*. New York: Sage Foundation.

Sampson, R. J., and J. D. Morenoff. 2000. "Public Health and Safety in Context: Lessons from Community-Level Theory on Social Capital." In *Promoting Health Intervention Strategies from Social and Behavioral Research*, edited by B. D. Smedley and S. L. Syme. Washington, D.C.: National Academy Press.

Sampson, R. J., S. W. Raudenbush, and F. Earls. 1997. "Neighborhoods and Violent Crime: A Multilevel Study of Collective Efficacy." *Science* 277: 918–24.

Scott, J. 1990. *Domination and the Arts of Resistance: Hidden Transcripts*. New Haven, Conn.: Yale University Press.

Sharpe, P. A., M. L. Greaney, P. R. Lee, and S. W. Royce. 2000. "Assets-Oriented Community Assessment." *Public Health Reports* 113, nos. 2 and 3: 205–11.

Sofaer, S. 2001. *Working Together, Moving Ahead: A Manual to Support Effective Community Health Coalitions*. New York: Baruch College, School of Public Affairs.

Speer, P. W., C. B. Jackson, and N. A. Peterson. 2001. "The Relationship between Social Cohesion and Empowerment: Support and New Implications for Theory." *Health Education and Behavior* 28, no. 6: 716–32.

Syme, S. L. 2004. "Social Determinants of Health: The Community As an Equal Partner." Retrieved January 5, 2004. http://www.cdc.gov/pcd/issues/2004/jan/syme.htm.

Traynor, B. 1993. "Community Development and Community Organizing." *Shelterforce* (March–April): 4–7.

Wallerstein, N. 1992. "Powerlessness, Empowerment, and Health: Implications for Health Promotion Programs." *American Journal of Health Promotion* 6: 197–205.

———. 1999. "Power between Evaluator and Community: Research Relationships within New Mexico's Healthier Communities." *Social Science and Medicine* 49: 39–53.

Wallerstein, N., and E. Bernstein, eds. 1994. "Community Empowerment Participatory Education and Health." *Health Education Quarterly* 21, nos. 2 and 3: 141–48.

Wallerstein, N., M. Polascek, and K. Maltrud. 2002. "Participatory Evaluation Model for Coalitions: The Development of Systems Indicators." *Health Promotion Practice* 3, no. 3: 361–73.

Wallerstein, N., and V. Sanchez-Merki. 1994. "Freirian Praxis in Health Education: Research Results from an Adolescent Prevention Program." *Health Education Research* 9, no. 1: 105–18.

Wallerstein, N., and M. Weinger, eds. 1992. *American Journal of Industrial Medicine* 22, no. 5.

Walsh, J. 1997. *Stories of Renewal: Community Building and the Future of Urban America*. New York: Rockefeller Foundation.

Wandersman, A., and P. Florin. 2000. "Citizen Participation and Community Organizing." In *Handbook of Community Psychology*, edited by J. Rappaport and E. Seidman. New York: Kluwer Academic/Plenum.

Wang, C., and Burris, M. A. 1997. "Photovoice: Concept, Methodology, and Use for Participatory Assessment." *Health Education and Behavior* 3, no. 24: 369–87.

Wang, C., J. Cash, and L. Powers. 2000. "Who Knows the Streets As Well As the Homeless? Promoting Personal and Community Action through Photovoice." *Health Promotion Practice* 1, no. 1: 81–89.

Warren, M. R. 1963. *The Community in America*. Chicago: Rand McNally.

Warren, M. R., J. P. Thompson, and S. Saegert. 2001. "The Role of Social Capital in Combating Poverty." In *Social Capital and Poor Communities*, edited by S. Saegert, J. P. Thompson, and M. R. Warren, 1–28. New York: Sage Foundation.

West, C. 1993. *Race Matters*. Boston: Beacon.

World Health Organization (WHO). 1986. "Ottawa Charter for Health Promotion." *Health Promotion* 1, no. 1: iii–v.

Zimmerman, M. 1990. "Taking Aim on Empowerment Research: On the Distinction between Individual and Psychological Conceptions." *American Journal of Community Psychology* 18: 169–77.

———. 2000. "Empowerment Theory: Psychological, Organizational, and Community Levels of Analysis. In *Handbook of Community Psychology*, edited by J. Rappaport and E. Seidman, 43–63. New York: Kluwer Academic/Plenum.

| | Social Action |
|---|---|
| Chapter 3 | Community Organizing |

*Proliferation, Persistence,*
*Roots, and Prospects*

SOCIAL ACTION is a distinctive type of community organization practice (Burghardt 1987). As articulated by Rothman (1968), in a seminal essay that provides the framework for much work in the field, it is different in a number of critical respects from other forms of community intervention, such as community locality development and community social planning. The "classic" social action effort is grassroots based, conflict oriented, with a focus on direct action, and geared to organizing the disadvantaged or aggrieved to take action on their own behalf. It has a long and important history, including, for example, such practitioners and efforts as Saul Alinsky and the numerous Industrial Areas Foundation projects associated with the "Alinsky method" since the late 1930s; Communist Party community organizing in the 1930s and 1940s; civil rights efforts in the 1950s and 1960s; the work of Cesar Chávez and the United Farm Workers; Community Action Programs and the confrontational organizing of SDS, SNCC, the Black Panthers, the Brown Berets, and La Raza Unida in the 1960s; and the wave of community-based social action since the 1970s organized around identity groups based on gender, sexual orientation, ethnicity, race, or neighborhood (Fisher 1994, Fisher and Kling 1993). Unlike community development and social planning efforts, social action focuses on power, pursues conflict strategies, and challenges the structures that oppress and disempower constituents. It is the type of community intervention that most lives up to the social justice and social change mission of social work, and yet, because of its oppositional politics, tends to be the least practiced within social work institutions and social service agencies.

Community-based social action, however, is not a static phenomenon. Social action is always changing in response to the conditions and opportunity structures in which it operates. In the 1980s, for example, one hallmark of community-based social action, as practiced by Alinsky groups and many others, was its withdrawal from a singular emphasis on conflict theory and confrontational politics. Involved in developing housing projects, organizing community development projects, and handling job training grants, these efforts, the heirs to classic social action community organization, now look more like a blending of social action with community development and social planning (Fisher 1994).

This essay seeks to contribute to the expanding knowledge of community-based social action by making four essential points. First, because community-based social action is an evolving and ever-changing phenomenon, we must now view it beyond our national borders, as a global phenomenon. The community development literature has done this for more than a generation. Moreover, unlike in the past, when social action efforts were said to last no more than six years, current efforts persist much longer and often become important community institutions. Second, these social action community organizations share common characteristics, reflective of what some observers call the new social movements. Third, new social theory and histories of social action efforts have reconceptualized contemporary community-based social action as primarily a product of post-1945 social movement organizing. These movement roots help further distinguish community-based social action from other forms of community organization and help explain why Rothman's model of social action continues to have salience for the study of grassroots oppositional movement efforts. Fourth, like all eras, but perhaps even more so for the current one, our contemporary context poses both significant opportunities and immense barriers to effective community-based social action and practice. It is these changing conditions and the responses of organizers and organizations to them that are significantly expanding and altering our knowledge and understanding of social action.

## Proliferation and Persistence

Two things are certain about contemporary community-based social action organizing. It is both a widespread and a long-term phenomenon. Once thought of as confined to narrow geographic areas (like New York City or Chicago) or to a specific historical era (like the late 1960s and early 1970s), proliferation and persistence, not provincialism and short-term existence, are the hallmarks of contemporary efforts. Without doubt, community-based social action has a long history in both social work practice and social work education (Burghardt 1987, Fisher 1994). Most social action, however, occurs outside of social work. That has always been the case. Since the 1960s, when the social work profession first began to take a very strong interest in social action approaches to community organization, grassroots organizing has become the dominant form of popular resistance and social change worldwide. Instead of not "enjoy[ing] the currency it once had" (Rothman with Tropman 1987, 7), these efforts have proliferated widely outside the social work profession, and within as well as outside of the United States.

Jeff Drumtra (1991–92) provided sketches of citizen action in thirty-eight countries. His research emphasized how political reform in twenty-five countries in Asia, Africa, and Latin America allowed for wide voter participation in free elections with multiple candidates. Durning (1989, 5) goes further. In a comparable comparative study he argues that people are coming together "in villages, neighborhoods, and shantytowns around the world," in response to the forces which endanger their communities and planet. More than a decade ago, Paget (1990) estimated two million grassroots social action groups in the United States alone. Lowe (1986) sees a similar upsurge of activity in the United Kingdom. The same is true for most of Western Europe. Grassroots social action organizing and urban protest have been key elements of politics in the West since the late 1960s. But community-based social action is not limited to Western industrial states. What happened in the West is only part of a widespread escalation of urban resistance throughout the world. The picture shows "an expanding latticework covering the globe," Durning (1989, 6–7) continues. Community organizing efforts, with hundreds of millions of members, have proliferated worldwide in the past thirty years, extending from nations in the West to those in the South, and, with extraordinary results, to those in the East.

Similarly, the persistence of grassroots social action, as well as their proliferation, is another hallmark of our contemporary era. Many efforts have come and gone in the past decade. But the old rule of thumb that social action community organizing, like that pioneered by Saul Alinsky, lasts no more than six years, is no longer valid. ACORN celebrated its twentieth anniversary in 1990, National People's Action (NPA) did so two years later, and COPS soon thereafter. Citizen Action, TMO in Houston, the New Jersey Tenants Union (NJTU), and many others recently passed the ten-year mark, with no signs of declining despite having to organize in very adverse conditions. Grassroots efforts tied to national issues, such as pro-choice, gay rights, and the environmental movement, not only persist but continue to grow.

## The Nature of Contemporary Social Action

But what is the nature of contemporary, community-based, social action organizing? Are these community-based social action efforts all of the same piece? Do prior models (Rothman, 1968, 2001; Fisher 1994) capture the complexity of current efforts? If a global proliferation exists, what are the shared, essential characteristics of contemporary, community-based, social action organizing? Building on the insights from new social movement theory (Epstein 1990, Melucci 1989), contemporary social organizing worldwide shares the following characteristics.

First, the efforts are community based, that is, organized around communities of interest or geography, not at the site of production (the factory) or against the principal owners of capital as was the case of most pre-1960s organizing (Offe 1987).

Second, the organizations are transclass groupings of constituencies and cultural identities such as blacks, ethnics, women, gay men, neighborhood residents, students, ecologists, and peace activists. Labor becomes one, not the, constituency group. Class becomes part of, not the, identity (Brecher and Costello 1990, Fisher 1992).

Third, the ideological glue is a neopopulist vision of democracy. The groups reject authoritarianism: in the state, leadership, party, organization, and relationships (Amin et al. 1990). Their organizational form is most often sufficiently small, loose, and open to be able to "tap local knowledge and resources, to respond to problems rapidly and creatively, and to maintain the flexibility needed in changing circumstances" (Durning 1989, 6–7). Some see contemporary social action as "nonideological," because the organizations dismiss the old ideologies of capitalism, communism, and nationalism and because they tend to be without a clear critique of the dominant system. But others argue that ideological congruence is their essence. Their "neopopulist" principles and beliefs are what make them so important and filled with potential (Dalton and Kuechler 1990, Offe 1987, Boyte and Riessman 1986, Fisher and Kling 1988, Boyte et al. 1986).

Fourth, struggle over culture and social identity play a greater role in these community-based efforts, especially when compared to the workplace-based organizing of the past, which focused more on economic and political issues. "After the great working class parties surrendered their remaining sense of radical political purpose with the onset of the cold war," Bronner (1990, 161) writes, "new social movements emerged to reformulate the spirit of resistance in broader cultural terms." Feminism. Black Power. Sexual identity. Ethnic nationalism. Victim's rights. Of course, culture and identity—grounded in historical experience, values, social networks, and collective solidarity—have always been central to citizen social action (Gutman 1977). And, of course, identity and constituency efforts include economic and political issues. But as class becomes increasingly fragmented in the postindustrial city and as the locus of workplace organizing declines in significance, resistances that emerge increasingly do so at the community level around cultural issues and identity bases (Touraine 1985, Fisher and Kling 1991).

Fifth, strategies include elements of locality development self-help and empowerment. An aim is building community capacity, especially in an era hostile to social change efforts and unwilling to support them. Some of the more effective efforts go beyond community capacity building to target and make claims against the public sector. They see the future of community-based social action as interdependent with political and economic changes outside their communities. They understand that the state is the entity potentially most responsible and vulnerable to social action claims and constituencies (Piven and Cloward 1982, Fisher 1992). But most contemporary community-based organizing seeks independence from the state rather than state power. As Midgley (1986, 4) points out, central to the rationale of community participation "is a reaction against the centralization, bureaucratization, rigidity, and remoteness of the state. The ideology of community participation is sustained by the belief that the power of the state has extended too far, diminishing the freedoms of ordinary people and their rights to control their own affairs." Community capacity building becomes a natural focus, reflecting antistatist strategies and decentralization trends of the postindustrial political economy.

## Historical Antecedents:
## The Roots of Ideologies and Strategies

One of the key causes for this common form of social action organization is the common heritage of citizen resistance since the end of World War II. It is this common heritage that continues to structure and inform contemporary efforts. For our purposes I emphasize five major historical roots: the (1) community-based resistance of Saul Alinsky, (2) liberation struggles of people of color, (3) urban decentralization and citizen participation programs, (4) New Left movement, and (5) new social movements. Of course, this is not to suggest that the heritage of community resistance does not include efforts prior to 1945 (Fisher 1992). Nor is it to suggest that all contemporary community mobilization efforts build on each of these antecedents or that these are the only sources. Admittedly, roots are more numerous and entangled than here suggested, but the following five are essential to contemporary community-based social action.

### COMMUNITY-BASED RESISTANCE OF SAUL ALINSKY
While the organizing projects of Saul Alinsky during his lifetime never amounted to much in terms of material victories and while his projects only took off when the southern civil rights movement shifted to northern cities in the 1960s, the community-based, constituency-oriented, urban populist, confrontational politics developed by Alinsky in the United States provides one of the earliest models of the community-based social action form (Fisher and Kling 1988). Beginning just before World War II, Alinsky's work in Chicago built on the older, union-based models of social action, such as the Congress of Industrial Organizations and Communist Party United States of America (Horwitt 1989, Fisher 1984). From these

it drew its labor organizing style, conflict strategies, direct-action politics, and the idea of grounding organizing in the everyday lives and traditions of working people. But Alinsky's model added something new: a kind of labor organizing in the social factory (Boyte 1981). The community organizer was the catalyst for change. The task was to build democratic, community-based organizations. The goal was to empower neighborhood residents by teaching them basic political and organizing skills and getting them or their representatives to the urban bargaining table (Fisher 1994, Boyte 1981). Both the site of production (supporting labor demands) and the public sector (making City Hall more accountable) served as the primary targets of Alinsky organizing.

This was an insurgent consciousness of "urban populism," based in neighborhood "people's organizations," oriented to building community power, discovering indigenous leaders, providing training in democratic participation, and proving that ordinary people could challenge and beat City Hall (Boyte et al. 1986, Swanstrom 1985, Horwitt 1989). At their weakest, Alinsky efforts sought to replace the political program and ideology of the old social action efforts with the skills of democratic grassroots participation, the abilities of professionally trained organizers, a faith in the democratic tendencies of working people to guide organizations toward progressive ends, and a reformist vision of grassroots pluralistic politics. At their best, however, Alinsky efforts continue to empower lower- and working-class, black and Latino community residents to demand expanded public sector accountability and public participation in an increasingly privatized political context (Fisher 1994, Horwitt 1989, Rogers 1990, Delgado 1986, Kahn 1970). Alinsky may not be the "father of community organizing," but, especially in the United States, his work and the work of his successors have been seminal to social action community organizing (Boyte 1981).

## LIBERATION STRUGGLES OF PEOPLE OF COLOR
Much more significant in terms of impact are the liberation struggles of people of color throughout the world since the 1950s. The civil rights movement in the United States and the national liberation struggles in the southern hemisphere served as important models for a community-based, ethnic/nationalist politics oriented to self-determination and sharing the political liberties and material affluence of the societies that exploited people of color. As a model for grassroots direct action and insurgent consciousness, the southern civil rights movement spawned most of what was to follow in the United States and established important precedents for others throughout the world (Branch 1988, Morris 1984, Reagon 1979). The liberation struggles in Africa, Asia, Latin America, and the Middle East, as well as specifically early efforts in Ghana, Vietnam, Iran, Guatemala, and Cuba, not only provided models for people worldwide, including activists in the civil rights movement in the United States, but symbolized the mobilization of a world-

wide liberation struggle for people of color. The demand for national self-determination for all people (not just those of European descent), the opposition to policies of racism and imperialism, and the plea of the civil rights movement for "beloved community" helped pierce the consensus politics of the 1950s and early 1960s. More recent liberation struggles in Nicaragua, El Salvador, and South Africa, to name but a few, continued to challenge conservative, racist, and imperialist paradigms in the 1980s and 1990s.

The continuous liberation struggles of people of color emphasize three lessons critical to the insurgent consciousness of contemporary community activism. First, citizen insurgency is not a political aberration. It is a legitimate and important, informal part of the political process to which all those without access to power can turn. Second, if oppressed people—often illiterate, rural peasants with few resources—could mobilize, take risks, and make history, then people of other oppressed or threatened constituencies can, with sufficient organization and leadership, do the same. Third, strategy must include both community self-help and constituency empowerment, on the one hand, and the struggle for state power, or at least the targeting of the public sector as the site of grievances and as a potential source of support, on the other. This dual quality of building community capacity and targeting the state, though not always in equal balance and often in tension, as exemplified in struggles between the Southern Christian Leadership Conference (SCLC) and the Student Nonviolent Coordinating Committee (SNCC), was as true for the civil rights movement in the United States as it was for the liberation struggles in the Third World (Carson 1982).

### URBAN DECENTRALIZATION AND CITIZEN PARTICIPATION

The struggles of people in the southern hemisphere dramatized the exploitative nature of the imperial postwar political economy at the very moment in the 1960s that some progressive capitalists, political leaders, and planners in both the public and voluntary sectors found themselves unable to address mounting urban problems at home. From 1960 onward, as liberal leaders such as presidents Kennedy and Johnson in the United States advocated for modest social reforms and a more democratized public sector, pressure mounted for urban decentralization and citizen participation. The Community Action Program of the 1960s in the United States and the Urban Programme of the late 1960s in Britain were among the most noted of public projects seeking "maximum feasible participation" at the grassroots level. But such programs proliferated widely, making state-sponsored municipal decentralization and community participation an international phenomenon (Kjellberg 1979, Blair 1983, Midgley 1986, Chekki 1979).

Of course, such postwar programs differ dramatically from Alinsky and liberation movement efforts in their origins and problem analysis. They are initiated largely by reformers in the public and voluntary sectors—professionals such as urban planners and social workers who either seek modest structural change or find themselves too constrained on the job to do much more in their agencies than deliver needed services at the grassroots level. As such, these initiatives represent a more institutionalized, more formalized wing of the community-based social action phenomenon. They tend, as well, to implement decentralized structure and democratic participation into public agencies without a sense for the contradictions inherent in doing so, but with a knowledge of the importance of linking the state and grassroots activism. The state becomes not the target of democratic insurgency but the employer and supporter of citizen initiatives (Merkl 1985). At their worst, these measures defuse and co-opt insurgency. At their best, contemporary organizing draws from this legacy a commitment to serving the people, to advocacy, and to citizen participation: (a) Deliver services at a grassroots level where people will have better access. (b) Include more people, even lay people, in the decision-making process at a more decentralized level. (c) Make sure they have real power to make decisions and control resources. (d) Struggle from within the state bureaucracies and agencies to achieve economic and participatory democracy for the greatest number of urban dwellers.

## THE NEW LEFT MOVEMENT

Despite the efforts noted so far, urban problems and tensions continued to escalate in the late 1960s. In response, direct-action movements mounted, especially in the United States. Early SDS (Students for a Democratic Society) and SNCC (Student Nonviolent Coordinating Committee) community organizing projects focused on "participatory democracy" and "letting the people decide," seeking not only to pressure local and national policy but to create "prefigurative," that is, alternative, social groups (Breines 1982, Evans 1979). They also developed a critique of American policy abroad and the liberal consensus at home. They built a movement in opposition to the politics of both corporate capital and the old social movement. After 1965, organizing adopted more nationalist and Marxist perspectives; Black Power efforts, for example, were less concerned with participatory democracy and more interested in challenging imperialism abroad and at home, winning "community control," and building black identity (Jennings 1990).

Such efforts in the United States were part of an insurgent trend in the West. Massive peace protests in the United Kingdom registered strong disapproval of Cold War policies, directly challenging social democratic regimes. These early efforts, among others, initiated a widespread "New Left" movement throughout the West, one which was soon to expand beyond university sites and student constituencies to develop, according to Ceccarelli (1982, 263), into "an unprecedented outburst of urban movements": Paris and West German cities in the spring of 1968; Prague, Chicago, and Monterrey, Mexico, during that summer; in Italy the "hot autumn" of 1969 and the urban conflicts of the early 1970s; squatters in Portuguese cities after the April Revolution; and urban social movements in Madrid and other Spanish cities after Franco. All testify to a massive grassroots mobilization which developed rapidly, and perhaps even unprecedentedly, throughout Europe, the United States, and parts of the Third World (Ceccarelli 1982, Teodori 1969).

Concern for and experimentation with participatory democracy, nonhierarchical decision making, prefigurative cultural politics, linking the personal with the political, direct-action tactics, and constituency-based organizing (students, the poor, etc.) characterized New Left insurgent consciousness (Jacobs and Landau 1966, Breines 1982). Unlike the new social movement resistances to follow, the New Left emphasized the formation of coalitions or political parties tied to national revolutionary/emancipatory struggles. There was a sense in the late 1960s, in cities as disparate as Paris, Berlin, Berkeley, and Monterrey, that "successful and autonomous urban movements are not a real alternative outside the context of a revolutionary national movement" (Walton 1979, 12). The struggle over state power, over who should make public policy, fueled local organizing efforts. Grassroots efforts were for most activists a democratic means to larger objectives which transcended the local community. This strategy persists, in a more reformist form, in certain notable national efforts since then, such as the Green parties in Europe, the Workers Party in Brazil, and the Rainbow Coalition idea in the United States (Spretnak and Capra 1985, Alvarez 1993, Collins 1986).

Community-based social action efforts which followed tended to borrow more heavily from the "newer" side of the New Left. These activists saw community organizing, alternative groupings, and grassroots efforts as at least the primary focus, if not the sole end. They emphasized democratic organizational structure, the politics of identity and culture, existential values of personal freedom and authenticity, and the development of "free spaces" where people could learn the theory and practice of political insurgency while engaging in it. So did much of the New Left, but the other, more Marxist segments, closer in style and politics to the old labor-based social action, adhered strongly to older concerns with public policy and winning state power (Evans 1979, Evans and Boyte 1986, Carson 1982).

## New Social Movements

Despite a marked backlash worldwide against the radical activism of the late 1960s, the 1970s and 1980s witnessed not the end of community-based activism but the proliferation of grassroots activism and insurgency into highly diversified, single-issue or identity-oriented, community-based efforts. These efforts, the subject of this essay, include women's shelters and feminist organizations; efforts in defense of the rights and the communities of oppressed people of color; struggles around housing, ecology, and peace issues; gay and lesbian rights and identity groups; and thousands of neighborhood and issue-based citizen initiatives, complete with organizer training centers. While these organizing efforts vary from one national and local context to another, they share a common form and movement heritage. Based in geographic communities or communities of interest, decentralized according to constituencies and identity groups, democratic in process and goals, and funded most often by voluntary sources, they serve as the archetype for contemporary social action.

The roots of their insurgent consciousness, while not always direct, can be found in the ideals discussed thus far: (1) that ordinary and previously oppressed people should have a voice and can make history; (2) that citizen and community participation, which gives "voice" to people previously silent in public discourse, is needed to improve decision making, address a wide range of problems, and democratize society; (3) that "by any means necessary" covers the gamut of strategies and tactics from revolutionary to interest-group politics; (4) that culture, whether found in a traditional ethnic neighborhood, battered women's shelter, counterculture collective, or gay men's organization, must be blended with the quest for "empowerment" into an identity- or constituency-oriented politics; and (5) that "the personal is political," articulated first by radical feminists in the late 1960s, guides people to organize around aspects of daily life most central to them, while keeping in mind that struggles over personal issues and relationships—personal choice, autonomy, commitment, and fulfillment—are inextricably tied to collective ones of the constituency group and the larger society.

Most commentators tend to see the focus on democracy as the essence of new social movement insurgent consciousness and the source of its potential. As Frank and Fuentes (1990, 142) put it, the new social movements "are the most important agents of social transformation in that their praxis promotes participatory democracy in civil society." Pitkin and Shumer (1982, 43) go further, declaring that "of all the dangerous thoughts and explosive ideas abroad in the world today, by far the most subversive is that of democracy. . . . [It] is the cutting edge of radical criticism, the best inspiration for change toward a more humane world, the revolutionary idea of our time." And these democratic projects have had profound impact: empowering participants, teaching democratic skills, transforming notions of political life, expanding political boundaries, returning politics to civic self-activity, strengthening a sense of public activism, raising new social and political issues, struggling against new forms of subordination and oppression, and even advancing agendas of the middle class to which formal, institutional politics remain closed (Roth 1991, Slater 1985).

But while the emphasis on democracy unites these efforts, it also helps detach them in the Western industrialized nations from the material needs of the poor, and it contributes to their fragmentation into a plethora of diverse, decentralized community organizations. The pursuit of democracy, without sufficient concern for equality, has resulted in the failure of the new social movements to address the material needs of the most disadvantaged. Moreover, the new social movement origins in culturally oriented, identity-based efforts tend to fragment social change efforts in general (Fisher and Kling 1993). For example, the diversity and flexibility that theorists of postmodernity attribute to contemporary society are nowhere more evident than in the variety of these new social movement efforts. A commitment to diversity embodies their emphasis on democratic politics. It encourages each constituency or identity group to name its own struggles, develop its own voice, and engage in its own empowerment. This may be the future of politics, a "postmodernization of public life," with its "proliferation of multiple publics [and] breaking down of rigid barriers between political and private life" (Kaufmann 1990, 10). But the central challenges to these efforts require more immediate and realistic strategies. How do they encourage diversity and counteract fragmentation? How do they influence or get power at levels—the city, state, and nation—beyond their own limited universes and at the same time build community capacity? How do we organize grassroots social action efforts and at the same time build a larger social change movement or political party, the size of which can only accomplish the needed, large structural changes?

## Practice Implications

Without question, the fragmentation of contemporary social action weakens the possibility for coherently imagined challenges to current problems. To address this problem of contemporary organizing, the historical dialectic of domination and resistance must be understood and fashioned in terms of the interplay between class, community, and the search for new cultural orientations. In this regard Kling and I have offered elsewhere the following sets of strategies (Fisher and Kling 1991).

First, mobilization in the fragmented metropolis demands that broad coalitions be sought between various constituency groups, and that community politics be more cohesively integrated with electoral activity. Single community-based efforts are not large enough to challenge the enormous power of corporate capital or centralized government. Because community problems almost always originate beyond local borders, the ability to affect change depends to a great extend upon coalition building. The success of coalition building, however, ultimately will be based upon whether specific ways can be found to break down the racial and cultural barriers that are so entrenched in the United States and growing again in Western Europe.

Pressure group politics, even through powerful coalitions, is not enough; movements must also struggle to win and hold power, not simply to influence it. The electoral arena must become a prime target for social movement mobilizing while, at some later point, political parties serve the critical role of formalizing and structuring relationships between loosely formed coalitions and constituency-based groups (Boyte et al. 1986,. Delgado 1986, Spretnak and Capra 1985). We offer such advice knowing how coalition and electoral efforts draw already scarce resources away from the fundamental task of grassroots organizing. But the local and the global are equally necessary, and numerous models of such dually focused practice have emerged over time. The experience of leading organizing efforts in the United States, such as IAF, ACORN and Citizen Action, and in Western Europe, such as the Green parties, illustrates how, while still focusing on the grassroots, they recognized the importance of coalition building and electoral activity.

Second, as others argue (Evans et al. 1985), we need to bring back in, and use legislative policy to challenge the ideology of privatization and free enterprise that meets so well the needs of international capital. The state, of course, is not inherently an ally of low- and moderate-income people. But in the late twentieth century, where private sector targets disappear in the electronic global economy, and where, in a new social movement context, the community replaces the workplace as the locus of organizing, a legitimized and expanded public sector becomes a critical ingredient for continued citizen action. Without it public life cannot even begin to be restored; without it grassroots mobilization devolves into self-help strategies which further fragmentation and perpetuate the use of private, voluntary solutions to massive, public problems (Fisher 1993).

For example, take the worldwide push for privatization (Barnekov et al. 1989). By undermining government legitimacy and responsibility, it results not only in a declining public life and fewer public services, but also in loss of access to a potentially accountable and responsible public sector, the major victory of pre-1945 social movements and a crucial target of some of the earlier antecedents to current social action efforts (Fisher 1988, 1992; Piven and Cloward 1982). Increasingly, in our current context, as the public sector declines as a source of grievances or solutions, citizen action is undercut. Contemporary resistance focuses its attention on community-based self-help and empowerment partly because the state—one of the primary arenas and targets for antecedents such as Alinsky, the civil rights movement, national liberation efforts, and the New Left—has been delegitimized. But contemporary social action community organization requires a public-sector arena and target because, unlike union organizing, which had some power at the site of production, in our current era of high-velocity global capital and declining labor activism, where it is much more difficult for workers and citizens to affect the private sector, community-based social action efforts have the state as the entity most responsible and vulnerable to their constituencies (Fisher 1992; Piven and Cloward 1982).

Third, we must move to a more consciously ideological politics. We must seek new, centering narratives, or, at least, more common programs that can draw the decentered narratives of our time toward a focal point. New formations and groupings will make mobilization on local levels more potent, perhaps, but they will not resolve the fundamental divisions that plague the effort to challenge broad, culturally entrenched structures of domination, prejudice, and exploitation.

Organizers must continue to teach the techniques of organization—the knowledge of how to bring people together to identify common grievances; to get them to communicate with each other across differing and even conflicting agendas; to enable them to run effective meetings; and to empower them to recognize what sorts of strategies are most suitable for particular contexts, and identify those points in the political regime most vulnerable to the pressures of collective action. But among the organizer's most valuable skills remains the ability to challenge the accepted vision of things and to develop ideological congruence with other oppositional efforts. Good organizational leadership—and good community practice—lies with understanding what is involved in moving people beyond their received notions of how they are related to other cultural and identity-based groups. An authentic commitment to "human solidarity, mutual responsibility, and social justice" demands that people engage in a profound reexamination of the values on which their society and way of life are based. Such transformations of consciousness do not emerge without intervention and engagement.

An organizing ideology for our times needs to combine the new postmodern demands for autonomy and identity with older, modernist ones for social justice, production for human needs, rather than profit, and the spirit of connectedness and solidarity among people, rather than competition. Day-to-day organizing, if it is to move beyond fragmented values and cultures, still needs to be informed by this sort of centering, oppositional ideology. To continue to open activists and constituencies to broader conceptions of social action and social change remains the primary responsibility of the organizer in the early twenty-first century.

### Acknowledgments

From *Strategies of Community Intervention: Macro Practice*, ed. J. Rothman, J. L. Erlich, and J. E. Tropman, 6th ed. (Itasca, Ill.: F. E. Peacock, Inc.). © 2001. Reprinted with permission of Wadsworth, a division of Thomson Learning: www.thomsonrights.com. Fax (800) 730-2215. Parts of the chapter appeared earlier as "Community Organizing Worldwide," in *Mobilizing the Community*, ed. R. Fisher and J. Kling (Newbury Park, Calif.: Sage, 1993).

### References

Alvarez, S. 1993. "Deepening Democracy: Social Movement Networks, Constitutional Reform, and Radical Urban Regimes in Contemporary Brazil." In *Mobilizing the Community: Local Politics in a Global Era*, edited by R. Fisher and J. Kling, 191–219. Newbury Park, Calif.: Sage.

Amin, S., G. Arrighi, A. G. Frank, and I. Wallerstein. 1990. *Transforming the Revolution.* New York: Monthly Review Press.

Barnekov, T., R. Boyle, and D. Rich. 1989. *Privatism and Urban Policy in Britain and the United States.* Oxford: Oxford University Press.

Blair, H. W. 1983. "Comparing Development Programs." *Journal of Community Action* 1.

Boyte, H. 1981. *The Backyard Revolution.* Philadelphia: Temple University Press.

Boyte, H., H. Booth, and S. Max. 1986. *Citizen Action and the New American Populism*. Philadelphia: Temple University Press.

Boyte, H., and F. Riessman. 1986. *The New Populism*. Philadelphia: Temple University Press.

Branch, T. 1988. *Parting the Waters: America in the King Years, 1954–1963*. New York: Simon and Schuster.

Brecher, J., and T. Costello. 1990. *Building Bridges: The Emerging Grassroots Coalition of Labor and Community*. New York: Monthly Review Press.

Breines, W. 1982. *Community and Organization in the New Left, 1962–1968: The Great Refusal*. New York: Praeger.

Bronner, S. E. 1990. *Socialism Unbound*. New York: Routledge.

Burghardt, S. 1987. "Community-Based Social Action." In *Encyclopedia of Social Work*, 18th ed. New York: National Association of Social Work.

Carson, C., Jr. 1982. *In Struggle: SNCC and the Black Awakening of the 1960s*. Cambridge, Mass.: Harvard University Press.

Ceccarelli, P. 1982. "Politics, Parties, and Urban Movements: Western Europe." In *Urban Policy under Capitalism*, edited by N. Fainstein and S. Fainstein. Beverly Hills, Calif.: Sage.

Chekki, D. 1979. *Community Development: Theory and Method of Planned Change*. New Delhi: Vikas.

Collins, S. 1986. *The Rainbow Challenge*. New York: Monthly Review Press.

Dalton, R., and M. Kuechler, eds. 1990. *Challenging the Political Order: New Social and Political Movements in Western Democracies*. New York: Oxford University Press.

Delgado, G. 1986. *Organizing the Movement: The Roots and Growth of ACORN*. Philadelphia: Temple University Press.

Diumtra, J. 1991–92. "Power to the People." *World View* 4 (winter): 8–13.

Durning, A. B. 1989. "Action at the Grassroots: Fighting Poverty and Environmental Decline." *Worldwatch Paper* 88 (January): 1–70.

Epstein, B. 1990. "Rethinking Social Movement Theory." *Socialist Review* 90 (January–March): 35–65

Evans, P., D. Rueschemeyer, and T. Skocpol, eds. 1985. *Bringing the State Back In*. New York: Cambridge University Press.

Evans, S. 1979. *Personal Politics: The Roots of Women's Liberation in the Civil Rights Movements and the New Left*. New York: Vintage.

Evans, S., and H. Boyte. 1986. *Free Spaces: The Sources of Democratic Change in America*. New York: Harper and Row.

Fisher, R. 1988. "Where Seldom Is Heard a Discouraging Word: The Political Economy of Houston, Texas." *Amerika-studien* 33 (winter): 73–91.

———. 1992. "Organizing in the Modern Metropolis." *Journal of Urban History* 18: 222–37.

———. 1993. "Grassroots Organizing Worldwide." In *Mobilizing the Community: Local Politics in a Global Era*, edited by R. Fisher and J. Kling, 3–27. Newbury Park, Calif.: Sage.

———. 1994. *Let the People Decide: Neighborhood Organizing in America*. Revised edition. Boston: Twayne.

Fisher, R., and J. Kling. 1988. "Leading the People: Two Approaches to the Role of Ideology in Community Organizing." *Radical America* 21, no. 1: 31–46.

———. 1991. "Popular Mobilization in the 1990s: Prospects for the New Social Movements." *New Politics* 3: 71–84.

———, eds. 1993. *Mobilizing the Community: Local Politics in a Global Era*. Newbury Park, Calif.: Sage.

Frank, A. G., and M. Fuentes. 1990. "Civil Democracy: Social Movements in Recent World History." In *Transforming the Revolution: Social Movements and the World-System*, edited by S. Amin, G. Arrighi, A. G. Frank, and I. Wallerstein. New York: Monthly Review Press.

Gutman, H. G. 1977. *Work, Culture, and Society in Industrializing America.* New York: Vintage.

Horwitt, S. 1989. *Let Them Call Me Rebel: Saul Alinsky, His Life and Legacy.* New York: Knopf.

Jacobs, P., and S. Landau. 1966. *The New Radicals: A Report with Documents.* New York: Vintage.

Jennings, J. 1990. "The Politics of Black Empowerment in Urban America: Reflections on Race, Class, and Community." In *Mobilizing the Community: Local Politics in a Global Era,* edited by R. Fisher and J. Kling. Newbury Park, Calif.: Sage.

Kahn, S. 1970. *How People Get Power: Organizing Oppressed Communities for Action.* New York: McGraw-Hill.

Kaufmann, L. A. 1990. "Democracy in a Postmodern World." In *Social Policy* (fall): 6–11.

Kjellberg, F. 1979. "A Comparative View of Municipal Decentralization: Neighborhood Democracy in Oslo and Bologna." In *Decentralist Trends in Western Democracies,* edited by L. J. Sharpe. London: Sage.

Lowe, S. 1986. *Urban Social Movements: The City after Castells.* London: Macmillan.

Merkl, P. 1985. *New Local Centers in Centralized States.* Berkeley, Calif.: University Press of America.

Melucci, A. 1989. *Nomads of the Present: Social Movements and Individual Needs in Contemporary Society.* Philadelphia: Temple University Press.

Midgley, J. 1986. *Community Participation, Social Development, and the State.* London: Methuen.

Morris, A. 1984. *The Origins of the Civil Rights Movement: Black Communities Organizing for Change.* New York: Free Press.

Offe, C. 1987. "Challenging the Boundaries of Institutional Politics: Social Movements Since the 1960s." In *Changing Boundaries of the Political: Essays on the Evolving Balance between the State and Society, Public and Private in Europe,* edited by C. Maier, 63–106. Cambridge: Cambridge University Press.

Paget, K. 1990. "Citizen Organizing: Many Movements, No Majority." *American Prospect* 1 (summer): 115–28.

Piven, F., and R. Cloward. 1982. *The New Class War: Reagan's Attack on the Welfare State and Its Consequences.* New York: Pantheon.

Pitkin, H., and S. Shumer. 1982. "On Participation." *Democracy* 2 (fall): 43–54.

Reagon, B. 1979. "The Borning Struggle: The Civil Rights Movement." In *They Should Have Served That Cup of Coffee,* edited by D. Cutler. Boston: South End.

Rogers, M. B. 1990. *Cold Anger: A Story of Faith and Power Politics.* Denton: University of North Texas Press.

Roth, R. 1991. "Local Green Politics in West German Cities." *International Journal of Urban and Regional Research* 15: 75–89.

Rothman, J. 1968. "Three Models of Community Organization Practice." In *National Conference on Social Welfare, Social Work Practice 1968.* New York: Columbia University Press.

Rothman, J., with J. Tropman. 1987. "Models of Community Organization and Macro Practice Perspectives: Their Mixing and Phasing." In *Strategies of Community Organization,* edited by F. Cox, J. L. Erlich, J. Rothman, and J. E. Tropman, 3–26. 4th ed. Itasca, Ill.: Peacock.

Slater, D., ed. 1985. *Social Movements and the State in Latin America.* Amsterdam: Foris.

Spretnak, C., and F. Capra. 1985. *Green Politics.* London: Grafton.

Swanstrom, T. 1985. *The Crisis of Growth Politics: Cleveland, Kucinich, and the Challenge of Urban Populism.* Philadelphia: Temple University Press.

Teodori, M. 1969. *The New Left: A Documentary History.* New York: Bobbs-Merrill.

Touraine, A. 1985. "An Introduction to the Study of Social Movements." *Social Research* 52 (winter): 749–87.

Walton, J. 1979. "Urban Political Movements and Revolutionary Change in the Third World." *Urban Affairs Quarterly* 15 (September): 3–22.

CHERYL L. WALTER

|  | Community |
| --- | --- |
| *Chapter 4* | Building Practice |

*A Conceptual Framework*

How we conceptualize community powerfully influences what we see and do in community practice. We draw upon theories of community and the models of community practice rooted in those theories to orient ourselves, assess what is going on, and help us make decisions about what to do, why, and how.

As suggested in chapter 2, community practice has been defined and categorized primarily according to various strategies and methods of practice, such as Jack Rothman's (2001) "three strategies of community organization": locality development, social planning, and social action. Community organization strategies operate from the assumption that problems in society can be addressed by helping the community become better or differently organized, and each strategy perceives the problems and how or whom to organize somewhat differently. The concept of community as a social unit that we as outsiders interact with underlies this way of framing community practice.

In contrast, the essence of a community building orientation to practice, as defined here, lies in conceptualizing and relating to community as an inclusive, complex, and dynamic system of which we are a part. Such an orientation envisions community as a system that is multidimensional, involving people and organizations at many levels engaged in relationships with one another that are manifested in both actions and consciousness. Community building practice seeks to engage with these multiple dimensions of community, recognizing the range of perspectives and relationships that exist and integrating diverse strategies and methods of practice. The goal is to build the capacity of the entire system and all of its participants to operate as community.

The conceptualization of community building offered in this chapter both complements and differs from the broader view of community building put forward by scholars in fields such as urban and regional planning. Their macro-view tends to emphasize large, community-wide efforts at transformation, often in conjunction with well-funded community-based initiatives (Walsh 1997). As suggested in appendix 2, this macrolevel approach shares many characteristics and values with the approach I describe—for example, in emphasizing local problem solving and the role of multiple stakeholders and sectors in the community building process. Yet while this chapter focuses primarily on community building as an *orientation* to practice, the alternative view, well articulated by the Development Training Institute (Kingsley et al. 1998) and Angela Blackwell and her colleagues (Blackwell et al. 2002; also see appendix 2), includes elements, such as partner support for community economic growth and sustainability, consistent with a broader urban and regional planning perspective. Although it is beyond the scope of this chapter to discuss and illustrate that alternative approach, readers will recognize many shared values and dimensions in the pages that follow.

Following a critical review of the conceptualization of the community that underlies community organization strategies, I make the case, in this chapter, for a shift in perspective that substantially broadens our conception of community. I then offer a model for community building practice rooted in this new conceptualization, identifying its key elements and dimensions and highlighting the kinds of skills drawn on and developed in community building.

## The Community

In practice, we are generally taught to conceive of the community as being a neighborhood of people with whom we work; the people within a city or county dealing with a particular issue or problem to which our organization provides services; or people with a shared racial, ethnic, gender, or sexual orientation identity. In Ronald Warren's (1963) classic definition, *the community* in this sense is a fairly boundaried social or demographic unit involving a neighborhood or a people who share a common issue or interest with which practitioners interact to bring about change.

But this conceptualization of the community does not provide as complete a picture as we could use in our thinking and acting in practice; thus, it may at times limit the usefulness of our existing models for guiding community practice. Within this limited frame of reference of the community, we may neglect to take adequately into account, for example, the influence of our role as community practitioners, the organization we work with and its agenda, or the objectives of the sources that fund our work. Similarly, we may overlook how consciousness in the broader culture around a particular issue influences the experiences and priorities of those involved with that issue at the community level. By not explicitly acknowledging the multiple constituencies and interests that are engaged with and exist within the community as an integral part of the community, we run the risk of oversimplifying issues, seeing and attempting to address problems only at the community level, and being self- and society-serving, as opposed to community-serving, with our interventions (Rivera and Erlich 1995, McKnight 1987). Although the imperative "start where the people are" is familiar to most health educators and other social change practitioners, more often than not we start where we are funded to start, which has powerful ramifications for how we interact with the community; the strategies we employ; and what priorities or needs of the community will be elicited, supported, and sustained (see chapter 7).

## Community as a Multidimensional System

The way of conceptualizing community that I am proposing involves making a shift in perspective about what community is, a shift that expands the frame of what is included in community and reexamines how what we include is interrelated. This shift in perspective changes our focus from the community as a social-demographic entity or unit with which we interact to community as a multidimensional-dynamic whole or system of which we are a part.

I refer to community as *multidimensional* to describe the way in which the various dimensions that characterize community—such as people and organizations, consciousness, actions, and context—are integrally related with one another, forming the whole that is community. To develop an understanding of community, then, we need to articulate, visualize, and examine the unique qualities exhibited by each of these dimensions and how they come together to make up the complex and dynamic system of community.

Warren (1963, ix) identifies two dimensions of community involving the interrelations of units (whether individuals, groups, or organizations). The horizontal dimension involves "the relation of local units to one another"; this is what we think of as *the community*. The vertical dimension involves "the relation of local units to extracommunity systems" in the larger society and culture. This dimension might include, for example, the relationship between a local nonprofit organization and a state agency with which it has a contract. Clearly, Warren does not perceive relationships with more remote organizations to involve community, instead calling them "extracommunity systems."

In contrast, I am suggesting that by virtue of involvement in relationships with one another, every organization and every person at every level within both the horizontal and vertical dimensions is potentially a part of community. The people and organizations included in this new conceptualization of community represent multiple stakeholders with diverse interests, those referred to as the community in all their diversity as well as those formerly considered to be outside the community and who have been missing from the perceptual mix. As I have already indicated, and consistent with the vision of community building articulated by Black-well and her colleagues (2002, Walsh 1997; see also appendix 2), the latter include the organizations for which we work, the funders of our work and of services for the community, and us as practitioners. Those residing in the neighborhood or clos-est to the issue in terms of experience may be seen as being locally or intimately involved. Those farther removed who influence the issue or locality because they control resources could be seen as more remote. But all are integral to community.

Such an orientation has special relevance for the increasing numbers of us who, by virtue of our race, gender, or sexual orientation, consciously identify as part of the community in which we are working. But even those not so identified can benefit from this broader reconceptualization of community because it enlarges what we take into account when orienting ourselves in practice and thereby reveals additional avenues for practice activity.

For community to exist, there must be relationships between the people and organizations in these horizontal and vertical dimensions. These relationships involve actions and consciousness, which can be conceived of as dimensions of commu-nity as well. Warren (1963) has an interesting theory about community action. He hypothesizes that there is no preexisting community that takes action; rather, for each episode of action, an ad hoc body emerges or is formed. Looked at in this way, community can be described as dynamic and emergent in that it is continually being created and re-created, its parameters and relationships taking shape and chang-ing shape through the actions and interactions of people and organizations.

Those of us engaged in community occupy a variety of positions in relation to the issue or locality around which community is defined. Thus, we often have different interests, experiences, levels of power, and perspectives. These differences are reflected in our consciousness, which is manifested in the identities and val-ues we hold; the language we use to name and label; and the themes of the stories we tell regarding our selves and our roles, each other, and how we are related. Here and now, we decide what voices will be heard, what truths will be legitimized, and thus what story of community will be told. Interestingly, with the notable excep-tion of Paulo Freire's (1973) work, this dimension of community is generally not addressed in theories of community practice. This is particularly ironic in a soci-ety such as the United States in which we are bombarded each day with thousands of images, stories, and slogans designed to influence our thoughts and actions.

The inclusion of consciousness in our conceptualization of community is fun-damental to this shift from *the community* to *community* and therefore deserves fur-ther elaboration. In the view of the community as a functional unit, consciousness has no central role, which may lead us in practice to overlook the impact of the consciousness around the issue in the broader culture and in the community effort at every level. For example, beliefs about whether people who are poor deserve assistance have a direct impact on what kind of social and health policies and services are implemented, what barriers to access to these services are erected, and how people feel who are recipients and providers of those services. Because organizations and institutions are not machines but are made up of people, they "are conscious entities, possessing many of the properties of living systems" (Wheatley 1994, 13). If we view community as a multidimensional system, consciousness becomes one of the important dimensions to consider in community practice. Consciousness is the mesh that joins us in community, the full spectrum of perceptions, cultural constructs, and frameworks through which interaction with one another and our environment is filtered and shared. In our actions, this consciousness and these relationships are played out and emerge as the substance of what community is.

Finally, all of this takes place in the context of the larger society and cultures, our place in history's unfolding, and the physical environment of geographic regions and the planet. This dimension is the atmosphere in which community lives and breathes; it is one of the principle resources and shapers of community.

Conceptualizing community in this way enables us to see ourselves and each other as part of a dynamic system that is continually being created and re-created and that affects and is affected by our consciousness and actions. Everything within the dimensions is related, influenced by and influencing all of the dimensions and coming together to make a complex and inextricable whole. This is one of the qualities that makes community a system.

Another quality of community as a multidimensional system is the permeability of its boundaries. Taken together, what is within the dimensions at any given moment could be said to constitute the field of community. Yet what the community is or who and what are perceived to be inside or outside the community involves an ongoing process of negotiation. And different systems display different degrees of openness and closeness (Tappen 1995). Are people of mixed racial heritage considered to be part of a specific racial community? Are bisexual people included in the gay and lesbian communities? Are practitioners outsiders in the communities in which they work? Does an organization see the people it works with or serves as part of its community? These are difficult questions and are handled differently in different communities and at different times. How they are answered has profound and far-reaching ramifications for the character of community. How they are answered also has to do with the perspective from which they are answered. What community is can look very different depending on where one is sitting.

## Elements within the Dimensions of Community

The preceding description provides a good beginning for reconceptualizing community. Yet as most of us have experienced, the word community is often used even where little true community can be found. An organization, for example, may create token community involvement to satisfy a funding mandate or may use pre-cious community resources of time and energy without actually intending to share power or seriously consider recommendations. Similarly, a few community mem-bers seeking power may represent themselves as community leaders and, for their own political gain, wreak havoc with local organizations. In such instances, the community can be a less than community-like place. It is no wonder that we as com-munity practitioners are often met with suspicion and resistance in our attempts to engage with the oppressed or to encourage our organizations to work in partnership.

Community concerns not just engagement in relationship but the quality of the relationship. Calling something community does not necessarily make it so. There can be greater or lesser degrees of community. As Philip Selznick (1992) aptly points out, even though community is often found in common residence, com-mon residence is not necessarily an essential or defining feature of "community-ness." This is increasingly clear in an era in which many of us do not even know the names of our closest neighbors (see chapter 6). Selznick further suggests that "a group is a community to the extent that it encompasses a broad range of activ-ities and interests, and to the extent that participation implicates whole persons rather than segmental interests or activities. Thus understood, community can be treated as a variable aspect of group experience" (358). He goes on to argue that "a framework of shared beliefs, interests, and commitments unites a set of varied groups and activities. Some are central, others peripheral, but all are connected by bonds that establish a common faith or fate, a personal identity, a sense of belong-ing, and a supportive structure of activities and relationships. The more pathways are provided for participation in diverse ways and touching multiple interests . . . the richer is the experience of community" (358–59).

Community as variable provides an intriguing alternative conception in that it simultaneously acknowledges the dynamic nature of community and com-munity as a quality of experience, of which there can be more or less. Selznick refers to the indicators of community-ness as the elements of community: historicity, iden-tity, mutuality, plurality, autonomy, participation, and integration. The presence of these elements and their mix are what make for community. Although differ-ent communities will have different mixes, "a fully realized community will have a rich and balanced mixture of all of these seven elements" (364).

Along the same lines, John Gardner (1991) has written about the ingredients of community. These include shared vision, a sense of purpose and values, whole-ness incorporating diversity, caring, trust, teamwork, respect and recognition, com-munication, participation, affirmation, links beyond the community, development of new members, conflict resolution, investment in community, and community resources. There is a remarkable similarity in the qualities of community that Selznick and Gardner identify, indicating that as elusive as community might seem, per-haps we do know what composes it.

## Community Building Practice

The shift to a new way of conceptualizing community has important implications for community practice. First, it places *community*, not *the community* or *the community organizer*, at the center of practice. Rather than being the social unit with which practitioners interact as various strategies are employed, community becomes the milieu in which we as community practitioners interact with people and organizations and of which we are an integral part. With community at the center, a broad and inclusive continuum of community participants and stakeholders is encompassed in a way that extends power and recognition of contribution to each participant who builds and shapes community. Regardless of the context or level we occupy—whether as a person facing an issue, a resident in a neighborhood, a volunteer, a professional providing services, an administrator, a student, or a high-level official—we can be practicing community.

Second, thinking of community as multidimensional—involving people and organizations at many levels, consciousness, actions, and context—allows us to model greater complexity. By perceiving community as a complex whole, we develop our ability to perceive and work with the actual complexity that exists. This enables us to take more information and relationships into account when orienting ourselves in practice and suggests many possible levels and areas with which to engage and in which to work. Further, by highlighting the interrelatedness of the dimensions, we see how our efforts might have an impact on multiple dimensions simultaneously.

Third, if we perceive community not as an existing unit that needs to be organized differently but as a dynamic and emergent whole embodying varying degrees of community-ness that is continually being built or created, then the building of community will be one of the central concerns and activities of community practice. Community is created or built, or not, with each of our actions; with our consciousness concerning ourselves, others, and the issues; and with our relationships, whatever the task. As Michael Fabricant and Robert Fisher (2002) suggest, it attends heavily to process as "the basis upon which relationships are built" (6) Within this vision of community building, "process and content are inseparable" (Senge 1995, 52). Congruence between what we do and how we do it, a joining of ends and means, is essential if we aim to foster communication, participation, diversity, identity, a shared vision, and the other elements and ingredients of community. Opportunities for building and practicing community are continually available, whether in communicative-expressive events or functional activities such as meetings, document writing, telephone calls, theater productions, picnics and parties, marches and rallies, program operations, legislation, policy implementation, or budgeting.

Fourth, community practice then becomes less of an intervention or coming between and more of an interchange in which each of us is changed by coming together. Learning to engage with one another with respect and trust, developing partnerships, and attending to our consciousness and actions call upon us as whole persons, necessitating that we be open to learning and change within ourselves and not just try to create change outside ourselves in the community or in institutions. This change can involve conflict, emotion, identity crises, and ethical dilemmas; and it may require that we confront racism, classism, sexism, handicappism, professionalism, and homophobia in ourselves, others, and institutions as we struggle for wholeness incorporating diversity.

The essence of a community building orientation to practice is in how we conceptualize and relate to community. It is not a practice orientation that employs a particular strategy for intervening in the community. Rather, it is a theoretical orientation that begins from a theory of community as a multidimensional, dynamic, and emergent whole of which we are a part. This whole includes people, organizations, consciousness, actions, and context; and it can exhibit greater or lesser degrees of community-ness. The theoretical orientation proposed here seeks to build community by fostering the elements and ingredients of community and engaging with the multiple dimensions of community both as an approach to doing things and as a desired outcome.

## *Community Building: A Case Example*

To illustrate how a community building orientation might guide practice, I use the example of an AIDS organization in a midsized county that produced an AIDS walk. The purpose or need that inspired the idea for the event was to raise funds, but the success of the event within a community building orientation was linked to its effectiveness in building community through the blending and balance of the elements and dimensions of community. Thus, the purposes of the event from a community building perspective were to increase awareness of HIV, have an event in which people could participate, involve business and the media, develop credibility with funding sources and the larger society, increase the number of people actively involved in and having a stake in the issues and the organization, expand the capacity of the organization to be a resource and provide services for people with HIV and their loved ones, express and affirm values, recruit and involve volunteers, tell stories, celebrate working together, and remember.

Staying aware of all these facets while planning and developing an event is a skill involved in community building. It is helpful to have words and images that express and represent the multifaceted nature of the process and event to guide and shape the experience and all those involved as they work together. In this case, "Heart and Sole AIDSWALK" was used as the theme of the event, a phrase that referred to the activity of walking, articulated values and consciousness, served as a hook for both media and business sponsorship, mentioned AIDS as the issue, and grounded the ceremonial and identity aspects with rich imagery.

In every aspect, the elements of community were attended to and nurtured. The AIDS organization developed historicity by making the event annual and honored it by telling the story of those who had passed and how the people involved and the organization had changed over the years. Identity was fostered by printing the theme phrase on T-shirts and buttons, by encouraging team participation in the walk, and involving people in activities with meaningful roles. Mutuality was expressed through the involvement of volunteers (including people with HIV, who would benefit from the money raised) and the opportunities available to learn new skills and take leadership roles. Plurality was displayed and witnessed through the participation of diverse teams, walkers, speakers, and volunteers and through materials that spoke directly to diverse audiences (including people of color, non-English-speakers, women, lesbians, gays, and heterosexuals). Autonomy was manifested in the choice of whether and how to participate and in the opportunities available to the task area teams to be creative in how they went about their tasks. Participation was open, involved multiple opportunities for participation at varying levels of commitment, and was acknowledged and welcomed. Integration was created by bringing together diverse participants, groups, and businesses to do something meaningful that involved everyone actively.

Each of the dimensions was engaged with and drawn from in this community building process. People and organizations worked together in new ways to plan the event and develop skills and relationships. A lead team of staff and volunteers was assembled to develop the event in every aspect, including publicity and media, walk logistics, registration, communications, obtaining of sponsors, and coordination of walk-day volunteers. And many more volunteers were involved in each of the task area groups. The lead team developed ways of communicating and coordinating its efforts as a group that group members carried with them into the leadership of their task area groups. Finally, intensive volunteer trainings were conducted. Each person involved learned new skills and had a chance to build on existing ones by taking leadership and responsibility in a task area and facilitating the participation of others. Many of the people involved in this project have gone on to leadership roles in event and program planning and implementation in the organization and the larger community, and they are widely recognized as skilled leaders. Thank-you letters were sent to all of the people and organizations that participated, even as walkers and pledgers, to acknowledge the important role that everyone played in making the event successful on so many levels.

Another outgrowth of the event was that individuals, local groups and organizations, businesses, and the media developed a greater awareness of one another, of HIV in their community, and of their interrelatedness. The AIDS organization demonstrated its competence in planning and implementing a large-scale event.

The organization also showed that it had the support and involvement of the community it served, which enhanced its opportunities to be selected for funding, to be trusted to influence policy, and to be respected by others and used as a model for building community.

Action was taken by hundreds of people who volunteered, gathered pledges, walked, and sponsored walkers or the event. By taking action to support their values, these people and organizations became more involved and invested in the issue, were more likely to talk with others about their experiences and to educate others about HIV, and discovered others who shared their concerns. Many became ongoing volunteers and supporters of the organization. Not only were funds raised, but something was accomplished that extended the boundaries of community and was an expression of caring and a celebration of the power of taking action.

In the realm of consciousness, awareness around HIV was raised, values were established and reaffirmed, and communication was increased. The event, all of the preparations for it, and all of what followed from it influenced how the issues around HIV and AIDS were seen and framed. And the Heart and Sole theme and all that it connoted carried on throughout the year as people referred to the event and wore their T-shirts and buttons, becoming part of the language and imagery of the community. In the commons, the HIV community and organization developed a greater presence in the larger community and were able to garner broader participation in the event the following year.

Even though it rained on the day of the event, and three other walks were held that same day, people came and walked in the rain; and this walk was the one that received the media coverage. People continually remarked on how good it felt to be part of the walk and how smoothly everything went. What people talked about was how magical it was. The attention given in every detail to humanness infused the event with an aliveness that was the expression of caring in action, of the power of heart and sole.

This approach and event were successful precisely because all of the elements and dimensions were valued and engaged. The event was also successful in raising money for the services provided by the organization, more than $60,000 in the first year, making this one of the largest fundraising events ever in that city. Each activity or image served multiple purposes and was used consciously in that way. In large part, the point of what was being done, and certainly how it was being done, was the building of community.

## Health Educators and Community Building Practice

If a health educator operating from a community building practice orientation participated in a team producing an event such as the AIDSWALK, his or her focus might be on using the opportunity to educate, challenge, and enable everyone involved to be health educators on issues surrounding HIV and AIDS. He or she might provide opportunities for people to commit to the next step, whatever that might be for them, in educating and organizing around the epidemic.

The health educator would operate from an awareness that all of the people involved—whether as walkers collecting pledges or volunteers placing walk brochures at businesses—would be talking with many people about the walk. As a result, the health educator might explore a number of avenues to engage everyone as educators and organizers around the epidemic. On the individual level, this might include having some of the volunteer training sessions address how to talk with people about HIV and AIDS; inserting education information and a challenge in the walk brochure; and creating an information packet for volunteers to give to businesses, thus providing information on HIV for employers and employees. On the organizational or institutional level, the AIDSWALK event might be used as a catalyst for engaging businesses and workplaces in a critical rethinking of policies and practices that directly or indirectly affect employees and their families vis-à-vis HIV and AIDS. Opportunities for workplace-based HIV/AIDS education and outreach programs could be explored. Along with general HIV/AIDS information available at tables at the end-of-walk celebration, there might be sign-ups for groups or training for people who want more information to educate themselves or an opportunity to be trained as HIV educators and organizers. On the broader state and societal levels, opportunities would be made available for engaging interested participants in working against ballot initiatives that discriminate against people with HIV and AIDS or for healthier public policy in regard to AIDS and people with AIDS.

All of these ideas and avenues make creative, multiple use of opportunities to engage and involve people in meaningful and useful ways and help different parts of the system talk to each other. Health educators involved in community building practice find themselves working in any and all of the dimensions of practice and with people and organizations at many different levels. Whether planning a campaign, an event, or a program proposal; training peer educators and outreach workers; encouraging the participation of local community members in community advisory boards; conducting community assessments with people with HIV or AIDS; training professionals about how to incorporate health education and community organizing around the epidemic into their practices; using media advocacy to change the ways in which AIDS and people with AIDS are depicted in the mass media; or hosting celebrations for a job well done, we become community building practitioners through our perspective on community and the skills we employ, more than through the role we play.

## Skills and Principles for Community Building Practice

Because how we do what we do is essential to the building of community, it is critical that we develop translatable skills and principles for fostering community, participation, and creativity in planning and conducting activities and events. These skills and principles for building community must be relevant for use in a broad range of situations, with a broad range of people, and at many levels. They should also lend themselves to being taught to others through modeling and opportunity for practice. A preliminary list of skills for building community includes management of interconnectedness, communication, process awareness, process commentary, creative planning, and personhood.

- Management of interconnectedness involves systems thinking, direction, coordination, facilitation, appreciation, and affirmation.
- Communication through speech, writing, music, art, film, or movement, coupled with the willingness and ability to listen, see, and understand and to ask questions, makes human experience accessible and thus human community possible.
- Process awareness involves awareness of the dynamic quality of community and the ability to attend to the here and now on multiple levels and in multiple dimensions simultaneously.
- Process commentary involves the ability to articulate process and to bring the discussion of what's going on into the here and now.
- Creative planning involves the reconciliation and unification of multiple visions, where possible, toward the design of programs and the use of resources.
- Personhood involves clarity, strength, commitment, vision, integrity, flexibility, the willingness to take leadership, trust and respect, responsibility, follow-through, the ability to exchange positive energy, and the willingness to change.

We can develop and use these skills in every aspect of community practice, whether as health educators, social workers, volunteers, consumers, or administrators; whether working with peers, clients, constituents, managers, coalitions, state or county workers, legislators, or students.

Along with skills for building community, there are "operating principles for building community" that can be used to guide our practice (Brown et al. 1996, 525–29):

Focus on real work.
Keep it simple.
Act.

Build from good; expect better; make great.

Seek what unifies.

Do it when people are ready.

Design spaces where community can happen.

Find and cultivate informal leaders.

Learn how to host good gatherings.

Acknowledge people's contributions.

Involve the whole person.

Celebrate.

Practicing these skills and principles is a lifelong process, both professionally and personally. Ultimately, it is about the kind of community we want to be part of. These are things we already do, whether consciously or not, whether well or not. Practicing them consciously while seeking to build community is community building practice.

## References

Blackwell, A. G., S. Kwoh, and M. Pastor. 2002. *Searching for the Uncommon Common Ground: New Dimensions on Race in America*. New York: Norton.

Brown, J., B. Smith, and D. Isaacs. 1996. "Operating Principles for Building Community." In *The Fifth Discipline Fieldbook: Strategies and Tools for Building a Learning Organization*, edited by P. M. Senge, A. Kleiner, C. Roberts, R. B. Ross, and B. J. Smith, 525–29. New York: Currency Doubleday.

Fabricant, M., and R. Fisher. 2002. "Agency-Based Community Building in Low Income Neighborhoods: A Praxis Framework." *Journal of Community Practice* 10, no. 2: 1–22.

Freire, P. 1973. *Education for Critical Consciousness*. New York: Seabury.

Gardner, J. W. 1991. *Building Community*. Washington, D.C.: Independent Sector Leadership Studies Program.

Kingsley, G. T., J. B. McNeely, and J. O. Gibson. 1998. *Community Building: Coming of Age*. Washington, D.C.: Development Training Institute and the Urban Institute.

McKnight, J. L. 1987. "Regenerating Community." *Social Policy* 3 (winter): 54–58.

Rivera, F. G., and J. L. Erlich. 1995. "Introduction: Prospects and Challenges." In *Community Organizing in a Diverse Society*, edited by F. G. Rivera and J. L. Erlich. Boston: Allyn and Bacon.

Rothman, J. 2001. "Approaches to Community Intervention." In *Strategies of Community Intervention*, edited by J. Rothman, J. L. Erlich, and J. E. Tropman, 27–64. 6th ed. Itasca, Ill.: Peacock.

Selznick, P. 1992. *The Moral Commonwealth: Social Theory and the Promise of Community*. Berkeley: University of California Press.

Senge, P. M. 1995. "Creating Quality Communities." In *Community Building: Renewing Spirit and Learning in Business*, edited by K. Gozdz. San Francisco: New Leaders.

Snyder, G. 1990. *The Practice of the Wild*. San Francisco: North Point.

Tappen, R. N. 1995. *Nursing Leadership and Management: Concepts and Practice*. Philadelphia: Davis.

Walsh, J. 1997. *Stories of Renewal: Community Building and the Future of Urban America*. New York: Rockefeller Foundation.

Warren, R. L. 1963. *The Community in America*. Chicago: Rand-McNally.

Wheatley, M. H. 1994. *Leadership and the New Science*. San Francisco: Berret-Koehler.

# The Professional's
# Role in Community
*Part II*                                      # Practice

## Values, Core Assumptions,
## and Ethical Dilemmas

A PROFESSIONAL has been defined as "one who knows very, very well very, very little." Although professionals in fields such as community health education, health planning, and social work often pride themselves on being generalists rather than narrow technocrats, the humility implied in that definition is important, particularly in relation to our work with communities. For the more we appreciate the fact that we know "very well, very little" about communities, their needs, and their resources (at least in relation to how much communities tend to know), the more likely we are to engage in practice that is empowering and respectful of the communities with which we are engaged.

In part 2, we explore a number of roles and responsibilities of the professional as organizer as well as some of the value dilemmas and tough ethical questions with which he or she may be confronted. First, however, we take a step back with Ronald Labonte's careful look in chapter 5 at some of the assumptions underlying our notions of community and our related perceptions of community development work. Drawing on both his extensive work as a health promotion consultant internationally and his in-depth study of the Toronto Health Department, Labonte begins by asking professionals to free themselves from their often uncritical and romanticized notions of community. In a similar vein, he reminds us that community involvement and decentralized decision making, although wonderful concepts in theory, may translate into tokenism, both sapping a community's limited energy and inadvertently supporting government cutbacks. These issues deserve our serious and critical reflection.

Labonte then applies this attitude of critical rethinking to the whole domain of community development (which, he reminds us, has roughly the same meaning in Canada as community organizing does in the United States). Central to this discussion is the distinction he draws between *community-based* efforts and true *community development* work. In the former, Labonte suggests, health professionals or their agencies define and name the problem, develop strategies for dealing with it, and involve community members to varying degrees in the problem-solving process. In contrast, community development or organizing supports community groups as they identify problems or issues and plan strategies for confronting them. Building on these and related distinctions, Labonte suggests that community development approaches are far more conducive to the building of authentic partnerships. The latter require, among other things, that "all partners have established their own power and legitimacy" and that community workers support community group partners, whether or not the latter buy into the concerns and mandates of the professional or the agency.

Chapter 6 examines the increasingly challenging roles and functions of professionals as organizers in today's global economy. Marc Pilisuk, JoAnn McAllister, Jack Rothman, and Lauren Larin describe the critical bridging role that health educators and other social change professionals can play by engaging in active listening and dialogue with community members and enhancing community capacity. But the authors quickly turn their attention to challenges, including the delicate balancing act that professionals as organizers need to play as they weigh process versus task achievement and deal with identity politics, conflicting agendas, and differing criteria for success in organizing efforts.

The roles and functions described in this chapter would be difficult enough under the best of circumstances. But as Pilisuk and his colleagues suggest, they are made all the more difficult by the contemporary political, economic, and social context in which grassroots organizing takes place. The chapter therefore focuses most of its attention on contextual issues such as the fraying of the social fabric, the global causes of many local problems, the fragmentation among progressive groups and organizations, and the growing concentration and power of both the mass media and the interlocking and transnational corporate-government networks that dominate our political economy. Without minimizing the magnitude of these impediments to effective grassroots organizing, the authors point to strategies and approaches that are proving useful in confronting them. The growing use of media advocacy among community groups (see chapter 23), the effective linking of such groups with large public interest organizations, the coming together of autonomous smaller community organizing efforts to form social movements, and the development of an infrastructure for progressive social change organizations are among the new approaches advocated and discussed.

In chapter 7, Meredith Minkler and Cheri Pies revisit many of the issues and challenges raised in chapters 5 and 6, focusing special attention on the ethical dimensions of these issues. Six areas are explored: the problem of conflicting loyalties;

the difficulties involved in eliciting genuine rather than token community participation; cross-cultural misunderstanding and problems of real and perceived racism in organizing; the dilemmas posed by funding sources; the sometimes problematic, unanticipated consequences of our organizing efforts; and questions of whose common good is being addressed by the organizing effort.

Drawing on both theoretical literature and relevant case studies, the authors highlight the ethical challenges raised in each of these areas and pose hard questions for the professional as organizer regarding his or her assumptions, appropriate roles, and potential courses of action. Although several tools are provided, such as the DARE criteria for measuring empowerment and the publicity test of ethics for helping communities decide whether to accept money from a controversial source, the purpose of the chapter is to raise questions rather than answer them. A key message of the chapter—and indeed of this whole section of the book—is that careful questioning of our assumptions and values and careful exploration of the ethical dimensions of our work must be preliminary and ongoing aspects of our professional practice.

# Community, Community Development, and the Forming of Authentic Partnerships

**Chapter 5**

## Some Critical Reflections

It is hard to be critical of community when one spends most of the day working in the stuffy cubicles of a government building or in the isolated cubbyhole offices of universities. Community represents something more positive and affirming than the bureaucratic rigidities or academic competitiveness of one's daily working experience. It is difficult to question community's importance when the only positive comments about frontline workers' efforts come from small groups gathered in church basements or cluttered storefront agency meeting rooms. Yet questioning and critiquing the notion of community are precisely what I propose to do in this chapter. My concern is that an uncritical adoption of community rhetoric can, paradoxically, work against empowerment ideals that lie at the heart of many health practitioners' intent.

Let me clarify the meaning of a few key terms before proceeding. Several concepts bearing a community label are now common in the health sector, notably community organization, community mobilization, and community development. Different people use different terms to mean the same thing. In Canada, for example, community development is often used to describe what in the United States is called community organizing. For purposes of my argument, *community organizing* refers to efforts to create a new group or organization, often with the assistance of an outsider, such as a health promoter (Rothman 2001). *Community mobilization* describes attempts to draw together a number of such groups or organizations into concerted actions around a specific topic, issue, or event (Health and Welfare Canada 1992). Community development incorporates both but describes a particular health practice in which both practitioner and agency are committed to broad changes in the structure of power relations in society through the support they give to community groups (Labonte 1996).

This chapter examines the continued conceptual confusion that surrounds the term *community* and offers five cautions about its uncritical invocation in health and social practice. Drawing in part on insights gained through my recent study of the Toronto Department of Public Health (Labonte 1996), I argue that, even though the concept of community development continues some of this confusion, the practice of community development has considerable potential for fostering self-reliance and the creation of authentic partnerships with communities. The chapter concludes by presenting nine characteristics of authentic partnerships that health educators and other social change professionals are encouraged to strive for in our practice.

## The Contested Meaning of Community

Numerous historical developments have contributed to the conceptual prominence of community in health work. Although a detailed discussion is beyond the scope of this chapter, these factors include rising health care costs, the declining effectiveness and efficiency of medical treatment, and a growing appreciation of the role of individual and community factors in disease causation and prevention (Lalonde 1974, Hancock 1986).

As noted in previous chapters, the centrality of community and the importance of community organizing for health were reflected in such influential documents as the Ottawa Charter for Health Promotion (WHO 1986), which regarded "the empowerment of communities, their ownership and control of their own endeavours and destinies" as the heart of the "new" health promotion (3). Many commentators view community as the venue for, if not the very definition of, the new health promotion practice (Green and Raeburn 1988), a view commonly expressed by practitioners themselves (Feather and Labonte 1995). But there is little agreement on what community means. As Cheryl L. Walter suggests in chapter 4, a general weakness of professional-institutional discourses on community has been the largely atheoretical and uncritical way in which the term has entered common usage.

Initially in the health field, community was simply a reflexive adjective. In Canada, for example, hospitals became community health centers, nurses became community health workers, state health departments became community health departments, and health promotion and health education programs became community-based efforts. In the syntax of everyday language, community ceased to be a subject (a group of people acting with their own intent) and became an object (community as a target for health programs) or an adjective accompanying the real subjects. These continued to be health institutions, which had become, by linguistic sleight of hand, community-modified. The problem was not that community-enamored practitioners and their agencies did not know their grammar well. The problem was the way in which community became objectified as fact and posited as a solution to all health problems rather than treated as a definitional conundrum whose development is inherently problematic.

When community is defined at all, it is usually explained in the static vocabulary of data, creating categories based on identity (the poor community, the women's community, a particular ethnocultural community), geography (the neighborhood, the small town, a particular housing project), or issue (the environmental community, the heart health community, the social justice community). Often, community is simply assumed to be those persons using the services of an institution and living within administratively drawn catchment boundaries (the hospital community, the school community, the university community).

Community includes all of these elements—identity, geography, issue, even institutional relations—but it is also more. The word *community* derives from the Latin *communitas*, meaning "common or shared," and the *-ty* suffix, meaning "to have the quality of." Sharing is not some demographic datum; it is the dynamic act of people being together. Community is, in effect, organization. There is no "poor community" outside of poor persons coming together to share their experience and act upon transforming it. There is no "women's community" outside of two or more women sharing their reality, empowering themselves to act more effectively upon it. The Toronto Department of Public Health (1994b) came to define *community* as "a group of individuals with a common interest, and an identity of themselves as a group. We all belong to multiple communities at any given time. The essence of being a community is that there is something that is 'shared.' We cannot really say that a community exists until a group with a shared identity exists" (2).

Even recognition of the active, organizational nature of community, however, does not fully clarify the term. Community may be one of those "essentially contested concepts" so vast in territory (it routinely is used to describe any and every human group that falls between the individual and society) and so rich in evocation that it defies any rigid definition (Lyon 1989). But practitioners certainly need to be more critical in their use of the concept, and there are five considerations about its invocation that are helpful to ponder.

## Romanticization

Community, as implied in a World Health Organization (WHO) discussion paper (1984) and the Ottawa Charter (Epp 1986), can do no wrong. The building of stronger communities, for example, is often regarded as an elemental strategy for strengthening community health. Though it is important to accept community self-determination in principle, it is also vital to recognize that what communities do for their own health may be inimical to a broader public health. Nazi Germany was a classic example of a strong community. So, too, are many right-wing fringe groups, such as the Ku Klux Klan and other white-supremacist militia organizations. One could even argue that lobbyists against stricter pollution controls are a community, as are people who work together to block supportive housing for persons with mental disabilities or disabled elders. Neighborhoods, towns, cities, and states are filled with myriad communities, and they conflict with one another as often as they seek consensus and understanding. Under conditions of conflict, which community should be supported, and why? Without linking the question to a political theory of social organization and change and an analysis of social power relations, we cannot answer it; and thus, the notion of community becomes somewhat fatuous. Worse, it becomes romanticized in a way that can obscure real and important power inequities among different communities that may subtly imperil the health and well-being of less powerful groups—for example, the community of urban land developers versus the community of the homeless.

## Bureaucratization

Whose interests are most served by increasing community involvement in health? What exactly are health workers asking communities to become involved in? Apart from concerns about tokenism (participation without authority), community involvement in health programs may not always strengthen the community. Health professionals may bureaucratize thriving community initiatives if they are insensitive to the fact that a community organizing or community development approach to issues is intrinsically unmanageable by conventional planning standards, which rigidly specify goals, objectives, and outcomes before action can begin (Labonte 1993). Even when health agencies engender new initiatives, they may unintentionally sap the political vitality of community group leaders. One health educator was able to extract permission from her senior managers to involve local activists on a housing and health committee, but after a year little progress had been made (Labonte 1993). She had been involving community activists in her bureaucratic process of committee meetings, reports, and senior management approvals rather than helping the activists directly lobby decision makers and collaborate with them in a partnership for social change. This effectively, if unintentionally, silenced the political voice of some of the strongest community leaders.

## Antiprofessionalism

Just as health authorities can risk elitism in their desire to demonstrate health promotion leadership, community groups and some of their health worker supporters can undermine effective collaborations through a festering antiprofessionalism.

Professional is not the antithesis of community. Indeed, the Latin root of the word *professional* means to "profess" or "vow," a reference to the medieval practice of surrendering personal gain to the larger community of a religious order or workers' guild. It is true that health professionals, like others in the "poverty industry," can increase the victimization of people living in socially disadvantaged conditions through their attitudes and exercise of power over their clients. But to imply, as some have, that most past public health practice has been wrong or that, as John McKnight (1987) has argued, "resources empower; services do not" denigrates the community of health workers. It reinforces a we-they polarity and ignores the formative role that respectfully delivered, useful, and usable services have often played in developing new community organizations and overcoming the isolation of society's most marginalized or oppressed people (Hoffman 1989, Labonte 1993).

Many health professionals are also community activists; and all persons, employed or otherwise, are members of many different communities. If professionals respect the leadership prerogative of community groups, or if, as Walter suggests in chapter 4, they see themselves as part of the community, there is no reason for them to be self-deprecatory or to disparage the value of their own professional efforts. Indeed, community groups supported by health workers in Toronto specifically cite the professional status, legitimacy, and influence such workers bring to the relationship, which community groups use to enhance their own social change efforts (Labonte 1996). The process of policy change, for example, can be likened to a nutcracker (Labonte 1993). One arm is the data-rich reports, policy documents, charters, and frameworks produced by health professionals primarily for internal consumption and bureaucratic legitimacy. The other arm, exerting the greatest force, is community group pressure on politicians, cracking the issue against the more conservative arm of professional validation. Both arms are necessary, if different in their strategic placement and use, for creating healthy social change.

## Decentralization

The decentralization of decision making over public programs, another oft-cited tenet of community organization or community development, allows for the growth of programs unique to community groups and their perceived needs. But the concept must be tempered with the recognition that most economic and social policy is national and transnational in nature. Local decision making can only take place within narrow parameters at best and is unlikely to include substantial control over economic resources (see chapter 6). As a policy analyst with the Worldwatch Institute notes, small may be beautiful, but it may also be insignificant (Durning 1989). This is not to argue with the intractable nature of the health-damaging aspects of our present social structure. Just as apathy can become a barrier to the organizing efforts of less powerful groups, cynicism (the apathy of the better-off with bigger vocabularies) can undermine the efforts of health workers to support such organizing efforts. Nonetheless, practitioners must append a strong advocacy component for macrolevel policy changes at senior government levels to their drive for decentralized decision making. Otherwise, they may subtly privatize by rendering strictly local the choices available to people and mystifying the actual exercise of political power by national and transnational economic elites.

The rhetoric of decentralized local control may also inadvertently support growing social inequities by failing to defend social programs against fiscal restraint or regressive tax reform by more senior government levels (Labonte 1995). Indeed, part of the appeal of community, especially to neoliberals and neoconservatives, is that it can readily justify dramatic social service cutbacks in the name of increasing community control. It is instructive that, in Canada at least, decentralized community decision making in health care is becoming a fact only as public funding for health care is shrinking, hospitals are closing, and thousands of health care workers are losing their jobs.

## Self-Help

The promotion of self-help and mutual aid groups parallels the call for decentralized decision making. Professional coordination of self-help networks is sometimes advanced as a means of humanizing the welfare system and coping with program cutbacks driven by neoliberal economic policies. The first rationale is sound; the second accepts the reprivatization of social policy, better known as charity. Without question, self-help groups can be empowering and health-enhancing. But there is typically no recognition in government policies on health promotion and community development that self-help primarily taps the volunteer energies of women, society's traditional care providers. Will government support and professional coordination of self-help simply increase voluntarism at the economic expense of women? Moreover, the type of self-help usually being promoted is what is sometimes called "defensive"—groups of people with a common problem or disease provide peer support.

There is also a history of "offensive" self-help—those groups concerned with meso- and macrolevel social change strategies. These groups are less likely to receive government or other outside support because they are regarded as being too political, self-interested, or advocacy-oriented. Yet unless the right of groups to lobby for changes in government policy is recognized and supported in health promotion funding policy (although this again raises the dilemma of which groups are advocating for which issues), the self-help ethos restricts to a personal level problems that have both personal and political dimensions.

## Community Development:
## Assumptions, Cautions, and Potential

Many of the cautions just raised cut to the quick of community development as a specific health practice. (I remind American readers again that my use of this term includes much of what they may associate with community organization.) There is no theory of community development, anymore than there is a singular theory of or approach to health promotion. Rather, the term describes a range of practices within the many other sectors in which it has existed historically, such as international development, literacy, economic development, housing, and social work and social services.

Community development involves assumptions about the nature of society, social change, and the relationship among community developers, state agencies, and community groups. These assumptions are sometimes made explicit in community development and community organization literature and models (for example, Rothman 2001, Dixon and Sindall 1994). But they are rarely explicitly present in government or other health agency policy statements on community development and often remain unexplored among practitioners themselves (Labonte 1996). One succinct and representative statement of these assumptions comes from the Toronto Department of Public Health (1994b), which defines community development as "the process of supporting community groups in identifying their health issues, planning and acting upon their strategies for social action/social change, and gaining increased self-reliance and decision-making power as a result of their activities" (20). There are five important components of this definition.

*Community development describes a relationship between outside institutions and community groups.* The "doer" of community development in the health field typically is a health department or nonprofit health agency or organization. This may strike some readers as patronizing. Do not communities develop themselves? Yes, but when they do, they engage in what Walter (chapter 4) terms community building; rarely (if ever) do they describe it as community development. The latter term historically refers to the actions of institutions in relation to citizens, whether conceived of as interest groups or as persons living within some geographic space. When practitioners recognize themselves as the subjects of community development, they are forced to ask, "What do we intend by these relations?" Ideally, the answer should be to nurture relations with and among institutions and community groups that are more equitable in their power sharing. As health workers with the Toronto Department of Public Health (1994a) note, "The goal of community development . . . is really trying to establish a more equitable power relationship between institutions and community groups" (20). This requires practitioners to acknowledge the starting differences in power (status, authority, resources, legitimacy) that exist among themselves, their agency, and community groups. If practitioners presume without questioning that they are equal to community groups, they risk making invisible the types of power that they do hold over groups, thereby increasing the risk of abusing that power or failing to recognize the potential for making it available to groups for their own use (see chapter 7).

*Community development is always a matter of choosing some groups over others.* Accepting a professional interest in community development compels practitioners to ask, "Which groups are we interested in, and why?" Allison Watt and Sue Rodmell (1988) argue that health promotion implies an advocacy framework that supports those whose living conditions provide them with less material forms of power, such as income, authority over resources, or political legitimacy. One of the difficulties encountered in practice is that the choices made by health workers and their agencies are rarely made explicit or include only those groups that might agree to mobilize around particular health issues, such as heart health or antitobacco advocacy. This renders choice a matter of personal preference or institutional convenience.

There is an ethical concern in the first instance: public agencies should be publicly accountable. Favoritism in choice should be informed by an explicit analysis of the social determinants of health and theories of social change and power relations, not simply by ideologies kept from organizational or public view and debate. There are both ethical and political concerns in the second instance. One study of a Canadian health department found that social assistance recipients with the greatest health, organizational, and empowerment needs represented only 17 percent of practitioners' caseloads (Browne et al. 1995). Most health workers' time was spent with reasonably well-functioning and well-resourced middle-class individuals and groups, a finding common to many other local health departments (Labonte 1996). To the extent that community development is a public resource that can help to effect a redistribution in material resources, a high ratio of middle-class clients or groups represents an upward redistribution of resources that contradicts the social justice rhetoric of documents such as the Ottawa Charter.

*Community development involves making private troubles public issues.* Community development work is not support group work. We can distinguish a support group from a community group on the basis of whether its members primarily look inward to their immediate psychosocial needs or outward to the socioenvironmental context that creates those needs in the first place. To paraphrase C. Wright Mills (1956), community groups transform the private troubles of support groups into public issues for policy remediation. Support group work, or defensive self-help, is central to what many public health nurses, educators, social workers, and some community organizers do. It is fundamentally important work and necessary to community development; for without the support of a group, many historically marginalized people will lack the confidence to look outward to the harder-to-change sociopolitical conditions that created their marginality in the first place.

But whereas support group work concerns the creation of healthy (equitable) power relations within groups, community development concerns the creation of healthy (equitable) power relations among community groups and institutions, or offensive self-help. The reason for making this distinction is twofold. It prevents community development from becoming a term so large in practice that it no longer serves any useful conceptual purpose, a critique often, and aptly, made of health promotion. It also requires health professionals and their agencies to grapple with power relations at a higher level of social organization and not restrict themselves to the necessary but insufficient work of support group development.

*Community development is not simply bringing institutional programs into community settings.* We can distinguish between community-based and community development approaches to our work. The distinction lies in who sets the agenda and who names the issue or problem (see table 5.1). In the community-based approach, the agency finds existing individuals or groups and links its programs with them. It is an important approach to public health; but it is not community development, which attempts to support community groups in resolving concerns as group members define them. Of course, as already noted, not all groups or group concerns will or should be supported. Community development requires making choices that,

*Table 5.1*
Community-Based and Community Development Programming

| *Community-Based Programming* | *Community Development Programming* |
|---|---|
| The process in which health professionals and/or health agencies define the health problem, develop strategies to remedy the problem, involve local community members and groups to assist in solving the problem, and work to transfer major responsibility for an ongoing program to local community members and groups | The process of organizing and/or supporting community groups in their identification of important concerns and issues and their ability to plan and implement strategies to mitigate their concerns and resolve their issues |
| *Example:*   Nobody's Perfect or heart health programs | *Example:*   Healthy Communities projects |
| *Characteristics*<br>• The problem name is given.<br>• There are defined program time lines.<br>• Changes in specific behaviors or knowledge levels are the desired outcome.<br>• Decision-making power rests principally with the institution. | *Characteristics*<br>• The problem name starts with that of the community group, and then is negotiated strategically—that is, to a problem naming that advances the shared interests of the group and the institution.<br>• Work is longer term, requiring many hours.<br>• A general increase in the group's capacities is the desired outcome.<br>• Power relations are constantly negotiated. |

in turn, require explicit analyses of social power relations and agency-staff commitments to shifting these relations toward greater equity. But much community organizing and community mobilizing work in health concerns itself primarily with specific diseases, lifestyle behaviors, and those public policies that influence health risks (Labonte 1993, Labonte and Robertson 1996). These issues may not always be of concern to poorer groups or localities. When institutional support and financial resources for community work are streamed through these set agendas, the political empowerment work of groups or localities can actually be undermined.

Community development, however, can emerge from a community-based program, just as community-based programs sometimes arise in the context of a larger community development effort (Labonte and Robertson 1996, Hoffman and Dupont 1992). In the first instance, the practice issue becomes one in which health workers and their agencies accept as legitimate and find ways to support action on more structurally defined health problems (such as unemployment, violence, racism) that participants in community-based programs (such as heart health) might raise as concerns. In the second instance, the practice issue becomes one in which health workers and their agencies negotiate the content and timing of community-based programs with local citizens so that they fit into the context of other political mobilizations within localities.

*Community development promotes self-reliance, not self-sufficiency.* By defining community development as a process of creating more equitable relationships among groups and institutions, we can bury the myth of community self-sufficiency. According to that myth, the community group is able to mobilize or provide its own resources and the skills to enable it to function autonomously from others. This is often assumed to be the goal of community development or a measure of maximum community participation (Bjaras et al. 1991). But the health sector's rhetorical acceptance of terms such as *partnerships* and *intersectoralism* should lead practitioners and their agencies to foster equitable and effective interdependencies rather than promote the autonomy of localities. Self-reliance, as a contrasting concept, means that "the community group is able to negotiate the terms of its interdependence with external professionals, organizations and institutions" (Toronto Department of Public Health 1994b, 19). The goal of community development is not self-sufficiency; it is the ability of the group to negotiate its own terms of relationship with those institutions (agencies) that support it.

## Community Development and the Creation of Effective and Authentic Partnerships

An equitably negotiated arrangement among different groups is often referred to by the shorthand notion of partnership. Whether practitioners and their agencies rally behind the ideas of community organization, community mobilization, or community development, they are essentially entering a partnership with a variety of different groups or organizations.

## EFFECTIVE PARTNERSHIPS AND CONFLICT

Community development may strive for inclusivity in community building—for agreement among as broad a collection of community groups as possible. The reality, however, is that powerless groups usually seek to shift skewed social relations by limiting the power that other groups have over them. Powerless individuals often create their identity as a community group only in opposition to or conflict with groups that are more powerful than themselves. This dynamic has been at the base of the confrontational approach to community organizing favored by Saul Alinsky and his adherents (Alinsky 1971, Kling and Posner 1990) and has been used successfully to create communities from the seemingly intractable conditions of isolation and apathy (Ward 1987, Labonte 1993). More generally, research on social identity theory finds that group identities often require conflictual forms of "who's in–who's out" boundary setting (Abrams and Hogg 1990), and a large body of sociological theory argues that intergroup conflict is the norm rather than the exception and provides the necessary fuel for social change.

Even Barbara Gray (1989), whose work on collaboration theory is seminal to an understanding of partnerships, acknowledges that collaboration usually requires a period in which less powerful groups establish their legitimacy through conflictual relations with more powerful groups. But conflict may also be necessary during collaboration. One reason that environmental groups now participate in collaborative policy bodies with industry and government is that they have demonstrated that they are able, through direct conflictual actions, to prevent unilateral decisions by the other parties. Those environmental groups that participate in collaboration generally no longer engage in direct action. But if all environmental groups ceased conflict relations with industry or government, what would prevent a return to unilateral decision making by either of the two more powerful stakeholders?

## STRIVING FOR COLLABORATION

That intergroup conflict is healthy and perhaps essential to social change should not lead health workers to shun the necessity of uniting diverse, conflicting groups at some higher level of community. Community as an ideal—the moral resonance of the word—is what gives it power and appeal (Lyon 1989), even if this ideal must be approached with an analytical caution about how it can be used for anticommunity, right-wing political agendas. Nonetheless, as John Gardner (1991) remarks, pluralism without commitment to the common good is pluralism gone berserk. Pragmatically, the community born in conflict or struggle rarely survives eventual peace "unless those involved create the institutional arrangements and non-crisis bonding experiences that carry them through the year-in-year-out tests of community functioning" (14).

Gray (1989) provides a comprehensive partnership model for promoting those functions, which she describes as collaboration. Successful intergroup collaboration, defined as "a mutual search for information and solutions," has five features that characterize the process-as-outcome. First, recognition of stakeholder interdependence is enhanced. Second, differences are dealt with constructively. Third, joint ownership of decisions is developed. Fourth, stakeholders assume collective responsibility for managing the problem domain through formal and informal agreements. Fifth, the process is accepted as continually emergent.

There are several steps in effective collaboration, the first and most important being problem setting. This requires a "common definition of the problem," a "commitment to collaborate," and "identification of the stakeholders" (20). This stage subsumes a prenegotiation stage, the goal of which is to arrive at a common definition of problem and intent broad enough to get stakeholders to the table. The stage differentiates collaboration from the usual form of government or other health agency consultation, in which the issue and desired outcome are already defined.

Effective collaboration requires the efforts of persons whom Gray labels "midwives"—the community developers of organizations-as-communities. These midwives (functionally distant from all of the stakeholders) work with the stakeholders before they come to the table, seeking to find the "superordinate goal" that Muzafir Sherif (1966) years ago argued was the basis for initiating any reduction in intergroup conflict. This goal must be "compelling for the groups involved, but . . . unattainable by [any] one group, singly; hence it is not identical with 'common goal.' . . . [It must also] supersede all other goals each group may have" (88).

Whatever the superordinate goal is that initiates intergroup collaboration and conflict resolution, the conditions for authentic collaboration allow a sharper delineation of the differences among consultation, involvement, and participation (collaboration). Briefly, consultation involves seeking information from citizens but without ongoing dialogue. Involvement does involve dialogue, but such dialogue is typically controlled by the government or outside agency. Citizen involvement tends to be advisory only, centering on a problem or issue that the government or outside agency has predetermined or named. There is no agreement about power sharing. In contrast, true participation involves negotiated relationships with citizens, who are treated as constituencies and take part in naming the problem or selecting the issue. All affected groups participate, and resources are made available to enable the full participation of less powerful groups (Arnstein 1969, Doyle and Orr 1990, Labonte 1993).

What makes for the effective and authentic partnerships that community development creates? Building on the forgoing and drawing on Jean Panet-Raymond's

(1992) insights gleaned from attempts to forge relations between community health and social service centers and neighborhood volunteer centers in Quebec, we might say that partnerships exist only in the following cases:

1. All partners have established their own power and legitimacy. This often requires a period of conflict and some enduring strain between powerful and powerless groups. The provision of resources to these groups is one facet of community development work, as long as such resources remain in the autonomous control of the groups.

2. All partners have well-defined mission statements. They have a clear sense of their purpose and organizational goals.

3. All partners respect one another's organizational autonomy by finding a visionary goal that is larger than any one of their independent goals. This requires extensive midwifery to set the shared agenda. The achievement of this shared agenda is another facet of community development work.

4. Community group partners are well rooted in the locality. They have a constituency to which they are accountable.

5. Institutional partners have a commitment to partnership approaches in work with community groups.

6. Clear objectives and expectations of the partners are developed. The partners create a commitment among themselves to manage the problem domain jointly.

7. Written agreements clarify objectives, responsibilities, means, and norms. Regular evaluation allows for adjustments to these agreements.

8. Community workers have clear mandates to support community group partners without attempting to get them to buy into the institutional partner's mandate and goal. This distinguishes community development from community-based approaches to work.

9. All partners strive for and nurture the human qualities of open-mindedness, patience, respect, and sensitivity to the experiences of persons in all partnering organizations.

## Conclusion

Community is a potent idea, but its reality is a more modest process: people organize themselves, or are organized, into identity-forging, issue-solving groups. The multiplicity of people's group (community) experiences requires health practitioners and their agencies to specify clearly whom they mean when they invoke the term. Romantic notions of community are more likely to support neoliberal political agendas, the dismantling of social welfare programs, and the upward re-distribution of wealth and power than to empower localities in any significant way. As health practitioners attempt to organize people or support community groups, they must be wary of colonizing these groups with institutional, often disease-based ways of defining health issues. Moreover, they must locate their choice of issues and groups to support within some analytical framework of society and social change. This framework needs to take account of the many forms of power that partly constitute the relationship among institutions, health professionals, and community groups; for the essence of community development (community organizing) is the transformation of these power relations so that there is more equity within and among institutions and groups.

At base, community development opposes those inequalities between people that are created by people and their economic and political practices. For as French philosopher Raymond Aron once commented, "When inequalities become too great, the idea of community becomes impossible."

## Acknowledgments

Portions of this chapter are based on "Community Empowerment: The Need for Political Analysis," *Canadian Journal of Public Health* 80 (2) (1989): 87–88; and "Community Development and Partnerships," *Canadian Journal of Public Health* 84 (4) (1993): 237–240. Adapted and reprinted by permission of the Canadian Public Health Association.

## References

Abrams, D., and M. Hogg, eds. 1990. *Social Identity Theory: Constructive and Critical Advances*. New York: Springer-Verlag.

Alinsky, S. 1971. *Rules for Radicals*. New York: Random House.

Arnstein, S. 1969. "A Ladder of Citizen Participation." *American Institute of Planners* 35, no. 4: 216–24.

Bjaras, G., B.J.A. Haglund, and S. Rifkin. 1991. "A New Approach to Community Participation Assessment." *Health Promotion International* 6, no. 3: 199–206.

Browne, G., C. Roberts, J. Byrne, C. Byrne, J. Underwood, E. Jamiesen, M. Schuster, D. Cornish, S. Watt, and A. Gafni. 1995. "Public Health Nursing Clientele Shared with Social Assistance: Proportions, Characteristics, and Policy Implications." *Canadian Journal of Public Health* 86, no. 3: 155–61.

Dixon, J., and C. Sindall. 1994. "Applying the Logics of Change to the Evaluation of Community Development in Health Promotion." *Health Promotion International* 9, no. 4: 297–39.

Doyle, M., and J. Orr. 1990. *Opportunities for Community Empowerment and Community-Based Planning*. Toronto: Social Planning Council.

Durning, A. 1989. "Mobilizing at the Grassroots." In *State of the World*, edited by L. Brown, C. Flavin, and S. Postel, 156–73. New York: Norton.

Epp, J. 1986. *Achieving Health for All: A Framework for Health Promotion*. Ottawa: Health and Welfare Canada.

Feather, J., and R. Labonte. 1995. *Sharing Knowledge from Health Promotion Practice: Final Report*. Saskatoon: University of Saskatchewan, Prairie Region Health Promotion Research Centre.

Gardner, J. 1991. *Building Communities*. Washington, D.C.: Independent Sector Leadership Studies Program.

Gray, B. 1989. *Collaborating: Finding Common Ground for Multiparty Problems*. San Francisco: Jossey-Bass.

Green, L., and J. Raeburn. 1988. "Health Promotion: What Is It? What Will It Become?" *Health Promotion* 3, no. 2: 151–59.

Hancock, T. 1986. "Lalonde and Beyond: Looking Back at 'A New Perspective on the Health of Canadians.'" *Health Promotion* 1, no. 1: 93–100.

Health and Welfare Canada. 1992. *Community Mobilization*. Ottawa: Health and Welfare Canada.

Hoffman, K., and J. M. Dupont. 1992. *Community Health Centres and Community Development*. Ottawa: Health Services and Promotion Branch.

Hoffman, L. 1989. *The Politics of Knowledge: Activist Movements in Medicine and Planning*. Albany: State University of New York Press.

Kling, J. M., and P. S. Posner. 1990. *Dilemmas of Activism: Class, Community, and the Politics of Local Mobilization*. Philadelphia: Temple University Press.

Labonte, R. 1993. *Health Promotion and Empowerment: Practice Frameworks*. Toronto: Centre for Health Promotion/Participation.

———. 1995. "Population Health and Health Promotion: What Do They Have to Say to Each Other?" *Canadian Journal of Public Health* 86, no. 3: 165–68.

———. 1996. "Community Development in the Public Health Sector: The Possibilities of an Empowering Relationship between State and Civil Society." Ph.D. diss., York University.

Labonte, R., and A. Robertson. 1996. "Health Promotion Research and Practice: The Case for the Constructivist Paradigm." *Health Education Quarterly* 23, no. 4: 431–47.

Lalonde, M. 1974. *A New Perspective on the Health of Canadians*. Ottawa: Health and Welfare Canada.

Lyon, L. 1989. *The Community in Urban Society*. Toronto: Lexington.

McKnight, J. 1987. Comments at Prevention Congress III, Waterloo, Ontario.

Mills, C. W. 1956. *The Power Elites*. New York: Oxford University Press.

Panet-Raymond, J. 1992. "Partnership: Myth or Reality?" *Community Development Journal* 27, no. 2: 156–65.

Rothman, J., 2001. "Approaches to Community Intervention." In *Strategies of Community Intervention*, edited by J. Rothman, J. L. Erlich, and J. Tropman, 27–64. 6th ed. Itasca, Ill.: Peacock.

Sherif, M. 1966. *Group Conflict and Cooperation*. London: Routledge and Kegan Paul.

Toronto Department of Public Health. 1994a. *Making Choices*. Toronto: Department of Public Health.

———. 1994b. *Making Communities*. Toronto: Department of Public Health.

Ward, J. 1987. "Community Development with Marginal People: The Role of Conflict." *Community Development Journal* 22, no. 1: 18–21.

Watt, A., and S. Rodmell. 1988. "Community Involvement in Health Promotion: Progress or Panacea?" *Health Promotion* 2, no. 4: 359–68.

World Health Organization (WHO). 1984. *Health Promotion: A Discussion Document on the Concepts and Principles*. Copenhagen: WHO Europe.

———. 1986. *Ottawa Charter for Health Promotion*. Copenhagen: WHO Europe.

MARC PILISUK
JOANN McALLISTER
JACK ROTHMAN
LAUREN LARIN

| Chapter 6 | New Contexts of Organizing |
|---|---|

## Functions, Challenges, and Solutions

THE PROBLEMS addressed by grassroots organizing are increasingly affected by a global context. This raises new questions about the appropriate role and functions of health educators, social workers, and other social change professionals who are involved in these processes at the community level. Some functions of organizers in the areas of health and well-being remain unchanged even in a grossly changed modern environment. We will review these and then examine new functions we believe to be essential. For if the causes of local problems are found in global activities, then local projects will have to be linked to a larger movement for social change.

### Core Functions of Practice

Traditional functions of community building and social action organizing remain unchanged. As described in chapter 4, community building is based on the gradual nurturance of relationships within localities that bring about a sense of belonging. Whether organized around a cooperative housing unit or a shared experience as survivors of breast cancer, these relationships bring people together to share their supportive attentions and resources. Outcomes include a sense of personal and group empowerment. In contrast, social action approaches are oriented more toward organizing a disadvantaged or aggrieved people to take action on their own behalf (Fisher and Kling 1991; also see chapters 3 and 11). Expected outcomes include changing the policies and programs of organizations and governments; achieving a role in community decision making; and shifting power, status, or resources of individuals or communities.

The enduring truths about the importance of listening, raising questions that help to give voice to the voiceless, the adherence to nonviolent direct action—all remain a legacy of community organizing. To these elements the professional organizer has often added process consultation, alternative methods for resolving disputes, local coalition building, and the ability to evaluate the efficacy of conflictual versus consensual strategies. The goal of developing leadership rather than trying to lead has paid off among mentally disabled elders in single-room-occupancy hotels, alienated high-risk youth, and illiterate peasants. In community practice, the professional roles for health educators, social workers, and other professionals have also included helping create an organizational framework for decision making, locating information, and generally contributing to community building and empowerment.

## BEGINNING CONVERSATIONS, SHARING MESSAGES, AND TARGETING INFORMATION

One core function whose importance remains paramount involves beginning conversations and sharing messages. People who have a common problem often have little awareness that the problem is shared by their neighbors or that getting together to discuss their distress is possible. The organizer's first task is to begin such conversations—first with individuals, then with groups. Beginning these conversations requires active listening. In organizer Michael Miller's (1985) words, "By asking questions, the organizer draws out of the people their hopes, aspirations, fears, problems, vision [and] dreams" (1). In the process, the organizer may also learn about jealousies or rivalries within the group, members' past experiences with organizing, and their likes and dislikes. Such knowledge helps the organizer to bridge differences and affirm common aspirations. For Paulo Freire (1968, 1973), active listening also entails problem posing, or asking questions that cause a small group of people to reflect critically on their reality, their shared problems, the links between those problems, and their root causes. (See chapters 2 and 12 for a fuller discussion of this approach.)

As discussed in chapter 2, even when the topic for organizing has been externally determined (as, for example, when a health educator wants to help mobilize a community around tobacco advertising or violence prevention), starting conversations and engaging in active listening are critical first steps. When gangs are the primary basis for self-esteem among youth in a poor neighborhood, or when smoking is a popular means of coping in a work site characterized by boring, repetitive jobs and frequent layoffs, violence prevention or smoking cessation may take on a more complex reality. The organizer's role in such instances is to discover how the local community perceives an issue and then create a message that will pique the interest of members. The message must be broad enough to attract sufficient numbers of people, and it must be delivered clearly and strongly in ways to which the community can relate (Mondros and Wilson 1994). According to Nicholas Freudenberg (1984a, 1984b), the message must not only present information that the organizer feels is critical (for example, the potential hazards of a toxic waste dump that is being proposed in a low-income community) but should also reflect the concerns of community members that the health educator has uncovered through the needs assessment process. Active listening, in short, is important for reaching more people with "the message" and for bringing their messages back to the health department, nonprofit agency, or other external group. Through active listening, the health educator may discover potential bridges among these issues that further enable him or her to tailor messages to specific subgroups in the community (Freudenberg 1984b).

## BUILDING COMMUNITY CAPACITY

Although community members may identify a shared problem and express a desire to bring about change, they often do not know how or where to begin. As Miller (1985) notes, the fundamental task of organizers at this stage may be to help people think through what might be done, including, importantly, the gifts and resources they bring to the situation. Indeed, a major task of the organizer at this stage is to work with people in ways that enhance the capacities of the community to address its needs without continued reliance upon the organizer (Pilisuk et al., 1996).

This can be difficult because people who have internalized repressive messages may believe that their status is the inevitable consequence of the circumstances of their birth, class, gender, race, age, sexual orientation, or disability or that it was God's will. Some see change as wholly dependent upon powerful leaders. People may need to be introduced to or reminded of the power of people's movements. The well-versed organizer can point to the gains of the civil rights movement and similar movements that followed—for example, movements in which ordinary citizens participating in numerous local actions brought problems into the public spotlight, demanded change, and proposed solutions. Knowing about the history, continuity, and success of movements for change is a powerful enabler for people who do not believe in their own power (Moyer et al. 2001).

The organizer's special talent lies in a willingness to understand, and an unwillingness to collude with, such internalized oppression. The organizer needs to realize that helpful outsiders have come before and left the community without bringing about desired change or increasing community competence or problem-solving ability (Cottrell 1983). He or she will have to earn the people's trust and establish relationships with them in their surroundings. The organizer must also suspend the power, privilege, prestige, and protection offered by his or her own background and be willing to be less safe.

The health educator, social worker, or other social change professional may have practical skills in setting up an effective meeting, enlisting community participation in assessing needs and resources, and facilitating the process of developing goals and priorities. He or she may also be skilled at locating sources of information and other forms of power not known to the local community and helping get people admitted to a hearing or appointed to a local city or regional committee (Chavis et al. 1993, Johnson 1994). But ultimately it is more important to transfer such skills so that the community left behind is better able to organize itself in the future. There are many ways of doing this.

Most basic is to nurture the factors that help people remain involved. People come together with a shared local problem or goal. The glue that keeps them working together is the support and recognition they receive from the effort. If they share food, have been provided with child care, or meet a new friend, those elements are important. If they feel that they have an ally in their special need or even that they are linked to a broader social movement that values people over either government or corporate groups, such feelings make a difference (Pilisuk et al. 1996).

The health educator or other social change professional may teach community members how to conduct "barefoot epidemiology"—researching the etiology of health problems they have identified. He or she may help them understand the power structure as it relates to a particular issue, how to access information, and how to get invited onto task forces and other civic bodies. The outside organizer may do both formal and informal leadership training. Simple things such as roleplaying a planned meeting with local health department officials to enable group members to practice how they might best put forward their objectives can make a real difference, not only in the success of a given action but also in building community competence and the self-confidence of community members.

Nevertheless, health educators, social workers, and other professionals must be careful in their approach to leadership training and related activities. As discussed in chapter 7, teaching leadership skills has its own risks, as when indigenous leaders become distanced from others or use the skills they have acquired to manipulate other community members. An antidote to this deleterious outcome may be the organizer's emphasis on the importance of the different roles that individuals play in organizations and movements for change. According to activist and social change strategist Bill Moyer, activists and organizations play four different roles: citizen, rebel, reformer, and change agent. Each role is essential to effecting change and important at various stages of any social action. Understanding that different interests, skills, and tactics are necessary in seeking redress of social inequities increases the appreciation for collaborative efforts and may reduce reliance on a single leader (Moyer et al. 2001). Resources are best used to reinforce actions that build a sense of community, develop an organizing plan, find information, locate sources of power not known to the community, and maintain accountability to the community.

## Dilemmas Faced in Carrying Out
## Core Organizer Functions

These roles and functions of professionals engaged in community building and organizing have stood the test of time. Yet carrying them out is fraught with challenges, as this section will show.

### TASK VERSUS PROCESS CONSIDERATIONS
### IN MOVING INTO ACTION

A frequent dilemma for the professional as organizer involves curbing the temptation to do too much in the name of task accomplishment and losing sight of the equally important goal of enhancing the community's own problem-solving ability. This dilemma is particularly likely to surface because grassroots organizing exists in a world in which control of information is a form of power and concealment, a form of control. More than ever before, grassroots efforts that lack indigenous sophistication in obtaining information may require the technical assistance of outside professionals who can help the community uncover information about who controls social institutions, how decisions are made, and how dialogue is averted. The challenge for the organizer is to provide such information in ways that do not impose direction and thereby reduce the power of the community group for choice (Johnson 1994).

Effective and ethically sound organizing also often means relinquishing ownership of the problem and its definition. As discussed in other chapters, professional problem definition may result in the identification of a problem that is important to the outsider but not a major concern to residents (Miller 1985). Alternatively, professionals may identify a problem of real salience to the community yet define it in such a way that significant portions of the problem are omitted. Only after Act-Up, a grassroots organization of HIV-positive individuals and their friends, began organized direct action did health agencies begin to view AIDS as a serious national epidemic. Local action by patients with AIDS and with breast cancer called attention to the nonmedical, quality-of-life issues for persons facing these devastating diseases.

More frequently than they would like to admit, well-meaning health and social service professionals make assumptions about voicelessness and an inability to articulate individual and community problems and concerns. The Interagency Council on the Homeless (1992) offered important recommendations to a variety of federal departments and agencies concerning the integration of agency efforts, the expansion of housing options and alternative services, and the improvement of outreach and access for existing rehabilitative programs. What the report lacked, however, was an analysis of why people are homeless and a strategy for prevention. The latter was provided through a self-help movement of formerly hospitalized patients, who viewed the problem as one of power and empowerment. In the services that have evolved from their grassroots organizing, clients are treated to the previously often neglected practice of informed consent for any form of assistance. They come to understand how their prior diagnoses and institutional handling have diminished what resources they have. They gain strength by exercising actual control over decisions in the facilities they use; and many extend their grassroots efforts to political action on zoning restrictions, welfare reductions, or job training (Segal et al. 1991). The political nature of problems such as mental illness and homelessness leads to the inescapable conclusion that no solution can be found without the participation of those most affected in problem definition and in subsequent organizing and social movements (Yeich 1994).

## RECOGNIZING AND CONFRONTING
## COMMUNITY DIVISIONS AND IDENTITY POLITICS

Another dilemma faced by organizers is that communities are not of one mind. As discussed in chapters 5 and 7, for example, indigenous leaders may or may not be representative of their constituencies (Cnaan 1991, Friedmann et al. 1988). Race and gender prejudices often surface even among grassroots efforts intended to eliminate them. The organizer must address the sometimes divisive identity politics of the dispossessed (Delgado 1994). Men may try to speak for women or withdraw from action led by women. Long-term residents may resent immigrants, who are seen as competitors for jobs and services. Most American working people have never experienced a multiethnic framework of political solidarity, and the good organizer will have to rely upon broader ethical and ideological frameworks for guidance in how to work with them.

## ADDRESSING CONFLICTING AGENDAS
## AND CRITERIA FOR SUCCESS

Do social change professionals work for the organization that has hired them because of their credentials or for the community constituency? Do they define success by improvements in the situation of one particular target group in one community, despite the fact that such success may result in fewer local resources available to other groups with equally pressing needs? Do they support conflictual tactics, knowing that privilege rarely concedes without pressure; or do they advocate for consensual tactics that work against the exclusion of any parties? These and related questions are critical for health educators and other social change professionals and are discussed in more detail in subsequent chapters. Again, however, we suggest that, to make such decisions, leaders will have to rely upon broader frameworks that are both ethical and political.

The dilemmas are real, but the underlying principle is clear. Grassroots community organizing is not about creating clients for services (McKnight 1994) but about bringing people together and helping create conditions that facilitate empowerment and organization. For the outside organizer, this means, in part, thinking about where one's skills and orientation rest personally, politically, and professionally and being sensitive to whose purposes are served by an intervention and what its potential negative effects might entail. Conflict will occur when interventions challenge a society's status quo—for example, in matters of equity, social justice, or participation—and outside organizers need to be sensitive to their role in this process.

## New Dilemmas for Grassroots Organizing in the Global Society

The principles and practices just discussed represent a body of knowledge and experience predicated upon the premise that people who come together for the purpose of building a sense of community, identifying a shared purpose, or engaging in social action can produce vital changes in their well-being. Yet the global context of community organizing in the twenty-first century suggests that some of the roles and functions that organizers have traditionally played may need to be amended. The contemporary context introduces several dilemmas that require new functions for the organizer, several of which we highlight in this section.

### THE FRAYING SOCIAL FABRIC

Contemporary grassroots organizing takes place amid the fragmentation and decline of the supportive capacities of communities. Rapid change in industrial society has left the individual less securely embedded in a family, a workplace, a neighborhood, or a village (Putnam 2000). This condition both reflects and reinforces a disruption and decrease in the supportive capacity of communities.

Today's families in developed countries are smaller, less permanent, and more separated from extended kinship networks. Locally owned shops have been replaced by franchises of national or international chains, and the local doctor or lawyer has been replaced by corporate centers. People in need are more isolated from both each other and the resources they require (Bellah et al. 1985, Pilisuk and Parks 1986). Almost 17 percent of Americans change residences each year (Putnam 2000), contributing to a decreased psychological sense of community. As the supportive web of natural ties wears thin, the identity of individuals has been increasingly determined by their marketability within a global economy. People with little market value—children, frail elders, the poorly educated, the chronically ill, and the mentally disabled—have suffered the consequences, often falling between the cracks and becoming recategorized in the public dialogue as nonpersons. They may be sheltered or fed, imprisoned or deported, or herded out of public view.

Such conditions make it difficult for people to get together, talk over their problems, and organize for action (Pilisuk et al. 1996).

The fraying social fabric is compounded by war and a global economy, related phenomena that displace people. A U.S. Committee for Refugees (2002) survey estimated the number of refugees or internally displaced people at 25 million. Mostly women and children from the poorest parts of the world, they were displaced from fifty different countries affected by conflict. Such massive dislocations at the international level mean that significant numbers of diverse, persecuted people are seeking asylum in the United States.

Whether with isolated older residents or newly arrived immigrants from war-torn countries, organizing efforts are hampered when people have difficulty coming together because of geographic mobility, language barriers, or challenges related to living in locations of grave crisis. Thus, grassroots efforts to achieve specific ends must take into account the weakened fabric of social life.

### LOCAL PROBLEMS, GLOBAL CAUSES

Although unmet needs are experienced at the most local and personal levels, the resources needed to address them are increasingly far removed (Pilisuk 1986–87, Thurow 1996). With modern technology comes the intrusion of global forces into domestic settings. As products of technology dominate the ecology of each community, new needs are created.

Decisions affecting the level of contamination in the drinking water or even the general availability of safe drinking water are made in far-off corporate boardrooms and during visits by corporate lobbyists to colleagues holding political office. Efforts to gain a hearing in local newspapers or broadcast media have been increasingly frustrated by the remote ownership of consolidated media. On the other hand, the abusive conditions of children and young women in sweatshops in Indonesia or western Africa, once easily concealed from public view, now are routinely and rapidly transmitted via the Internet.

The global economy and modern technology have left a growing percentage of the world's population either unemployed or employed in alienating and underpaid forms of work. The global economy market has produced a greater polarization of income than at any time since records were assembled (Pilisuk 2001). Three billion people now live on less than $2 a day, while the world's 225 richest individuals have a combined wealth of $1 trillion—equal to the total annual income of the planet's 2.5 billion poorest people (Mueller 1999). In the United States, top executives in 2000 earned 531 times the wage of their average worker, and the gap continues to widen (Tobias 2003). Wars are fought in the developing world to determine whose interests will be served by local resources. Likewise, in the United States and some other postindustrial societies, corporate pressures to relax occupational and environmental standards are working to ensure ever-greater profits at the expense of workers, their families and communities, and the ecosystem (Brenner 1995). These trends, too, form a critical part of the context of contemporary grassroots organizing.

## INTERLOCKING GOVERNMENT-TRANSNATIONAL NETWORKS: THE CONCENTRATION OF UNACCOUNTABLE POWER

Taking action is impaired when those with authority for decisions about outcomes are either distant or unknown. These conditions—the impediments to contact among mobile populations and the remoteness of power—are endemic in post-industrial global society.

The globalization of capital has forged an even stronger and more intimate interdependence between governmental powers and conglomerate interests (Thurow 1996), often at the expense of local communities. The power of non-governmental bodies comprised of prominent members of corporations, think tanks, and government are proof that the corporate and financial worlds understand that the national policies of developed countries are crucial to the world's orderly transformation into a global market economy. Recent events, such as the U.S. General Accounting Office's inability to learn who was on the committee convened by Vice President Dick Cheney to shape a new national energy policy, underscore how deeply entrenched these interlocking corporate and government networks have become in our national and global economy. Further, with the progression of global trade agreements such as the North American Free Trade Agreement (NAFTA) and the authority of the World Trade Organization now overriding even governmental authority, corporate advantages have become embedded in a legal framework that is beyond the reach of most local communities.

Governments help to validate the belief that freedom for the individual and freedom for the corporation are identical and that what's good for General Motors is indeed good for the United States. But access to government and the media is severely limited for those without wealth (Bagdikian 2002). With the help of grassroots organizing, a group of Vietnam veterans may fast at the White House steps or a busload of disabled elders may descend on a state legislator. But larger financial interests employ permanent lobbyists and, more important, help choose the people who occupy public office.

The state does legitimate itself, of course, in part through programs such as Medicare, Social Security, worker's compensation, and consumer protection laws (O'Connor 1976). But such interests find form in grassroots actions long before they are represented by law. During times of severe fiscal retrenchment, moreover, groups that might otherwise be pushing for new protections and expanded programs instead find themselves lowering their sights to fight cutbacks in the already inadequate protections and safety net programs that are in danger of being stripped away.

## LACK OF COMMUNITY ACCESS TO INFORMATION
## ABOUT POWER AND CONTROL

The increasing distance between a community and the impersonal corporate ownership of that community's resources means that information about the causes of a local problem may be less available to local residents. Without such information, people easily blame scapegoats suggested to them by powerful interests in government, corporations, and the media. When a community hospital closes or a toxic waste facility is approved, most people who would be seriously affected know little about how to identify the responsible parties. The Internet, of course, is increasing people's access to previously unavailable information, which can spur and assist in organizing efforts (see chapter 18). But local communities, particularly if they are low income, tend to lack the research facilities and training needed to gather information that may be essential for informed action.

### TROUBLING EFFECTS OF THE MASS MEDIA

Who has power is heavily dependent on who participates in the dialogue (Pilisuk et al. 1996). Princeton scholar Cornel West (1993) argues that we need a massive revival of public conversation, through which people can find expression and work toward their collective best interests. Although a number of factors have contributed to the decline in such civic engagement, the effects of television have been particularly striking. Americans now watch television for approximately four hours daily; and as Putnam (2000) notes, "Television is . . . the only leisure activity that seems to inhibit participation outside the home. TV watching comes at the expense of nearly every social activity outside the home, especially social gatherings and informal conversations" (237). The decreased availability of people for group association is a fact of contemporary life that contributes to the weakening of the social fabric.

In addition to its role in decreased civic engagement, television, like the other mass media, is problematic in light of the hegemony it maintains over what is transmitted to the public (Bagdikian 2002). By the year 2000, just nine companies (among them Disney, AOL–Time Warner, and General Electric) dominated the national media in the United States, offering the great majority of television programs, films, radio, DVDs, CDs, books, and associated products. Indeed, the top six companies have annual earnings that are greater than the next twenty firms combined. As Ben Bagdikian (2002) argues in *Media Monopoly* (2002), this represents "a communications cartel of a magnitude and power the world has never seen" (xi).

With the media's heavy emphasis on "news," often presented in sensationalistic, rapid-fire fashion, people are becoming disempowered spectators of any but the most local of happenings (Pilisuk et al. 1996). Fragments of stories about a toxic spill, a famine in Africa, influence pedaling in government, and a local violent homicide: all are offered in the space of minutes, without serious inquiry into why these problems recur. Who loses? Who gains? What difference does it make to the viewer, or what difference might the viewer make to the situation? These un-addressed questions are vital to democratic participation (Hermann and Chomsky 1988). The highly touted information highway is already cluttered with mindless pitches to the marketplace, and the interactive highways still have far fewer on-ramps in poor communities.

When people believe that they cannot make a difference in a world characterized by injustice and inequality, they become easy prey to those who depict the disadvantaged and the displaced as undeserving and dangerous, responsible for the despair of people whose hard work has still not satisfied the marketed self-image of consumer (Katz 1995). Can grassroots groups overcome the disempowering effects of ever-more interconnected corporate and government interests? And can they gain access to the media to frame their own stories and effect changes in policy that can improve their health and quality of life?

### FRAGMENTATION AMONG PROGRESSIVE GROUPS AND THE NEED FOR IDENTIFICATION WITH A SOCIAL MOVEMENT

To answer these questions in the affirmative, grassroots groups and organizations, and the health educators and other professionals working with such organizations, need to come together through large networks and movements of their own. But we face a paradox. Many community groups and agencies working for causes that affect health and well-being are small. And while small size often means opportunity for involvement, it also means a great deal of inefficient effort in reinventing what other groups are already doing. Small groups are also frustrated when larger numbers are needed to make a difference. The contemporary environment of organizing is impeded by fragmentation and sometimes distrust among progressive groups. The politically progressive movement that some term "the left" doesn't encompass the full range of groups involved in health action but is a salient and sometimes definitive component. Getting a better handle on how to organize this amorphous group of concerned progressives can help us understand the issues involved in bringing coordinated effort to specific matters of promoting health and justice.

Jack Rothman (2002b), one of the authors of this chapter, recently conducted a survey of activists and leaders in more than forty grassroots organizations in the Los Angeles area (for example, the Industrial Areas Foundation founded by Saul Alinsky, the Association for Community Organization for Reform Now, Americans for Democratic Action, and the Mexican-American Legal Defense and Education Fund), asking them to identify what, in their experience, had contributed to lack of collaboration. Although the study was not limited to those engaged in community organizing to promote the public's health and welfare, many of the barriers and obstacles described are all too familiar to those engaged in community organizing and community building in health and related fields.

The obstacles identified included, for example, the lack of a common ideological framework and an associated organizational vehicle for supporting it and the tendency of many activists to reject collaborating with those who hold different positions from their own. A resulting niche mentality led to groups' preoccupation with single issues such as the environment, women, or particular health insurance initiatives, which in turn resulted in organizational isolationism.

Groups with compatible long-range goals often became antagonists because of differences surrounding immediate goals and tactics. For example, while agreeing to advance Latino interests, should you advocate or denounce bilingual education? And should a premium be placed on building grassroots constituencies or engaging in legal advocacy? Turf battles over money, resources, and media attention also were cited as obstacles to intergroup collaboration, with scarce funding from foundations and public agencies frequently forcing organizations to joust with one another over the same meager pool of available dollars. The structure of urban geography, which can create long travel distances, heavy traffic, and neighborhoods segregated by race and ethnicity or hemmed in by freeways, meant that many activists never even met one another. Finally, the immense number of task demands and time pressures on progressive leaders already suffering from scarce resources meant that scant time was available for coalescing with others. Stretched thin and often fatigued, leaders were not inclined to cross their defined mission boundaries.

## THE PARADOX OF INCREASED ACTIVISM

In light of such trends, we might anticipate a dramatic decline in participatory grassroots efforts. On the contrary, however, the number of both domestic and international grassroots groups has risen dramatically (Durning 1989, Lappé and DuBois 1994), and the proportion of Americans involved in voluntary associations remains well above that of most developed nations (Putnam 2000). This growth has occurred among all classes of people, and some among the poor have shown a remarkable ability to persist actively for decades (see chapter 3).

Grassroots groups are adjusting to the changed environment. Some have adopted sophisticated means to obtain, distribute, and use information. Some are building coalitions that cross the boundaries of geography and single issues and influence the policy process (Braithwaite et al. 2000, Kaye and Wolff 1995) or creating new forms of mutual aid once provided by intact communities (Pilisuk and Parks 1986, Putnam 2000). Finally, grassroots endeavors are helping to spread new symbols of value and legitimacy through social movements such as feminism, environmentalism, and cultural diversity (Buechler and Cylke 1996,

Hyde 1994). What began as local breast cancer support groups, for example, have evolved into coalitions demanding effective care and opposing environmental contaminators (Soffa 1994).

Broader ideologies, such as independent living, environmentalism, and feminism, have inspired local efforts for and by groups such as battered women. A shelter for battered women now provides community education about domestic violence, promotes state legislation, and organizes the surrounding community to challenge the belief that men have a right to dominate women (Garske 1996). Disability groups, too, demonstrate the power of grassroots efforts to reconstruct meanings that disempower them. Organizations like Disabled People's International and the World Institute on Disability have provided a focus for groups around the globe concerned with issues of access, public education to confront stereotypes, and changes in public policy that support the rights of people with disabilities (Dreidger 1989). The Americans with Disabilities Act could not have come to pass without working coalitions of grassroots groups (McQuire 1994). So despite formidable impediments, grassroots organizing is alive and well at the dawn of the twenty-first century.

## Expanding Roles and Functions to Address Global Impediments

Although most successful organizing efforts take place without the aid of social change professionals, the characteristics of postindustrial society, including the increase in information and skills needed to confront even local issues, have expanded the rationale for professional involvement. But what roles might health educators, social workers, and other social change professionals play as organizers; and what potential and dilemmas do these roles present in relation to the goal of fostering community empowerment? A few of these roles and their corresponding dilemmas and challenges are illustrative.

### CONNECTING COMMUNITY GROUPS WITH PUBLIC INTEREST ORGANIZATIONS

When grassroots groups seek broader policy changes, they need organizations that extend beyond the community confines. One important role for health educators or other social change professionals, therefore, may be to connect community groups with appropriate public interest organizations. Because local problems have distant causes, public interest groups such as the Center for Science in the Public Interest become important advocates that enhance grassroots activism at regional, national, and international levels. They often form broad-based coalitions and serve local community groups by making sophisticated information more widely assessible.

Nevertheless, although many public interest groups espouse the goal of participation, they frequently abandon it in practice and do little to empower their members. As David Bunn (1983) argues, difficulty with fundraising and pressures for immediate results and mainstream public credibility tend to push public interest groups away from grassroots strategies and toward a more corporate structure and strategy: "It is far easier to write a foundation grant proposal or to ask . . . law firms for major contributions than it is to organize a canvass or a community fundraising event. It is . . . faster to build a direct mail membership list than it is to organize and train community activists" (10–11).

Given these realities, the health educator or other social change professional may have an equally important role to play in working with public interest organizations to increase their responsiveness to community group members. With the latter, they can challenge the power of public interest groups to define the issues of dissent so that linking community groups with larger movements will result in real, rather than symbolic, participation.

## USING THE MASS MEDIA FOR
## POWER AND EMPOWERMENT

As noted, corporate hegemony over what the mass media transmit to the public is a major contributor to the voicelessness and lack of participation and power experienced by people and communities in postindustrial society (Bagdikian 2002). Yet even as media control is increasingly concentrated in a small number of corporations, new strategies are emerging that can help communities use the media to draw attention to their own issues, reframe the debate, and advance policies conducive to health. The most promising of these strategies is media advocacy, defined in chapter 23 as "the strategic use of mass media to advance a social or public policy initiative." A coalition of health, religious, and community organizations in Philadelphia that successfully prevented the test marketing of a new brand of cigarettes targeted to African Americans succeeded in part because of its effective use of local media. Through careful bridge building, goal setting, message framing, and selection of appropriate media outlets, the group not only prevented the test marketing of Uptown cigarettes in the city but also helped ensure that the new tobacco product was never even released (Wallack et al. 1993).

Health educators and other social change professionals have been among the key architects of media advocacy as a strategy for redressing power imbalances and promoting policies that improve the public's health (see Wallack et al. 1999). By becoming familiar with the concept and methods of media advocacy and sharing them with community groups, health education practitioners can play an important role in countering some of the disempowering effects of the mass media and helping communities use the media to further their own health and social goals.

## OVERCOMING DIVISIVENESS
## AND PROMOTING COALESCENCE

The study of activist fragmentation in Los Angeles identified a number of obstructions to collaboration among social change organizations (Rothman 2000a, 2000b). Despite these barriers and the difficulty of identifying cross-cutting issues, the groups expressed a common need for an infrastructure that could facilitate communication and capacity building across the network of progressive organizations. Such an infrastructure, which might be called a Center of Community Caring, would include components such as (1) a newsletter to keep organizations aware of each other's activities and upcoming events; (2) training programs for organizing skills such as fundraising, pressure tactics, using the media, and sustaining participation; (3) a directory of progressive groups to facilitate the identification of relevant organizations and networking with them; (4) a mutual-aid help line for sharing technical skills, loaning equipment, providing space, and reaching important contacts; (5) a central rapid-response hotline to disseminate information and quickly mobilize people across the progressive community for mass meetings, public hearings, and demonstrations; and (7) a common facility to provide meeting space for committees, conferences, and group events and to facilitate natural interaction (Rothman 2000a).

The experience shared in such group-building activities could slowly develop trust and association that would permit collaboration on more contentious issues that have been divisive in the past. Alongside the structure, groups meanwhile could continue at a full clip to pursue their own issues.

Such a facilitative infrastructure offers a modest but practical potential for countering fragmentation and strengthening collaborative progressive organizational capacity at the local level. Existing infrastructure from cross-cutting institutions such as community colleges and black churches could become a base from which to start. A center might have a beginning covenant such as "All people have a right to a livelihood, enough to eat, safe drinking water, a living wage, shelter, a safe and sanitary place to live and work, a clean and uncontaminated environment, education and health care, and participation in decisions affecting their lives." Health educators, social workers, and other social change professionals could usefully share their skills in the development of such a center.

### BECOMING PART OF A SOCIAL MOVEMENT

Communities, like individuals, need to know that they are not alone when their voices are raised. Some of the more effective coalitions have linked community efforts across the country and across continents to provide action on voter registration, the protection of women against violence, control of pollution, sweatshop labor, military intervention, and the monitoring of nuclear weapons laboratories. These alliances help keep alive a culture of caring and concern amid global trends toward competitive control. To stem the loss of community control over local resources, each separate project needs to be a source of education about where the control over resources really lies. Each local effort will have to offer a connection to other groups whose joint actions constitute a social movement to return a measure of global corporate accountability to the local community.

As we have noted, it is often difficult for individuals to see the connections among movements for change or even to identify with other activists. Media coverage of activism contributes to this estrangement. The media, particularly television, focuses almost entirely on protests and especially on the small percentage of protesters who are disruptive. Violence has a visual impact that is absent from public forums, meetings with government officials, lobbying for legislative change, or months of organizing constituencies and planning public events. Activists at any level can benefit from understanding the underlying process of social movements. In 1977, Moyer et al. (2001) developed the Movement Action Plan (MAP) to help activists see movements for change as long-term processes with distinct stages that are not defined by media attention. The eight-stage model shows how social action proceeds from problem recognition and analysis to a trigger event when the issue is put on the public agenda. Next are the tasks of bringing about broader support for change and, finally, getting policymakers' acquiescence to the people's demands. Developing a long-term perspective about social change and using analytical tools such as MAP can help local activists see their efforts in a broader context and resist the despair that comes from premature expectations of success.

## Concluding Implications for Practice

There are two ways to interpret the implications of global trends for grassroots efforts. The first applies to the means that the organizer must use to help community groups act in the face of a changed reality. These include building supportive ties into a project, obtaining information about power or ownership, and gaining access to media or governing bodies.

The second implication is to the ends that community organizing will have to address. At some appropriate point in each local action, the professional will need to help the community group articulate its analysis of the underlying reasons that resources to address their needs are scarce and how other groups like themselves are addressing this problem. The increasing control of local resources by national and global corporations is capping what any local group can accomplish. Affirmative action, fair wages and benefits, assured health care, aid for vulnerable populations, and conversion of military development to civilian uses are examples of issues that cannot be resolved at the community level, despite the fact that they are not likely to be resolved without local efforts.

The postindustrial milieu for grassroots organizing is one of exacerbated need in the face of new and often formidable impediments. The resurgence and dramatic growth of local organizing despite these obstacles are heartening and speak to the continued role of grassroots organizing as an essential part of the human story. Although most organizing takes place without the aid of professionals, outside organizers, including concerned health educators, social workers, and others, clearly have important contributions to make. The challenge and the dilemma for health educators, social workers, and others engaged in social change are how to lend their special gifts and resources in ways that strengthen rather than diminish community capacity in the process.

The traditional skills of the community organizer remain appropriate to current challenges but not sufficient to address the new global context. Just as community organizing gained efficacy by bringing people together, the new and more complex task lies in bringing coalitions of disparate organizations into a social movement that builds its power even as it attends to the most compelling needs of people in local communities.

## References

Bellah, R. N., R. Madsen, W. Sullivan, A. Swidler, and S. M. Tipton. 1985. *Habits of the Heart: Individualism and Commitment in American Life*. Berkeley: University of California Press.

Braithwaite, R. L., S. E. Taylor, and J. N Austin. 2000. *Building Health Coalitions in the Black Community*. Thousand Oaks, Calif.: Sage.

Brenner, M. H. 1995. "Political Economy and Health." In *Society and Health*, edited by B. Amick, S. Levine, A. Tarlov, and D. Walsh, 211–46. New York: Oxford University Press.

Buechler, S. M., and F. K. Cylke. 1996. *Social Movements: Perspectives and Issues*. Mountain View, Calif.: Mayfield.

Bunn, D. A. 1983. "Structural Development of a Grassroots Political Organization in Rural Communities of California." Master's thesis, University of California, Davis.

Chavis, D. M., P. Florin, and M.J.R. Felix. 1993. "Nurturing Grassroots Initiatives for Community Development: The Role of Enabling Systems." In *Community Organization and Social Administration: Advances, Trends, and Emerging Principles*, edited by T. Mizrahi and J. Morrison, 41–67. New York: Haworth.

Cnaan, R. A. 1991. "Neighborhood Representing Organizations: How Democratic Are They?" *Social Service Review* 65, no. 4: 614–34.

Cottrell, L. S., Jr. 1983. "The Competent Community." In *New Perspectives on the American Community*, edited by R. Warren and L. Lyon, 398–432. Homewood, Ill.: Dorsey.

Delgado, G. 1994. *Beyond the Politics of Place: New Directions in Community Organizing*. Oakland, Calif.: Applied Research Center.

Dreidger, D. 1989. *The Last Civil Rights Movement: Disabled People's International*. New York: St. Martin's Press.

Durning, A. B. 1989. *Poverty and the Environment: Reversing the Downward Spiral*. Washington, D.C.: Worldwatch Institute.

Fisher, R., and J. Kling. 1991. "Popular Mobilization in the 1990s: Prospects for the New Social Movements." *New Politics* 3: 71–84.

Freire, P. 1968. *Pedagogy of the Oppressed*, translated by M. B. Ramos. New York: Seabury.
————. 1973. *Education for Critical Consciousness*. New York: Seabury.
Freudenberg, N. 1984a. "Citizen Action for Environmental Health: Report on a Survey of Community Organizations." *American Journal of Public Health* 74, no. 5: 444–48.
————. 1984b. *Not in Our Backyards: Community Action for Health and the Environment*. New York: Monthly Review Press.
Friedmann, R. R., P. Florin, A. Wandersman, and R. Meier. 1988. "Local Action on Behalf of Local Collectives in the U.S. and Israel: How Different Are Leaders from Members in Voluntary Associations?" *Journal of Voluntary Action Research* 17, nos. 3–4: 36–54.
Garske, D. 1996. "Transforming the Culture: Creating Safety, Equality, and Justice for Women and Girls." In *Preventing Violence in America*, edited by R. L. Hampton, P. Jenkins, and T. P. Gullotta, 263–86. Newbury Park, Calif.: Sage.
Hermann, E. S., and N. Chomsky. 1988. *Manufacturing Consent*. New York: Pantheon.
Hyde, C. 1994. "Committed to Social Change: Voices from the Feminist Movement." *Journal of Community Practice* 1, no. 2: 45–64.
Interagency Council on the Homeless. 1992. *Outcasts on Main Street: Report of the Federal Task Force on Homelessness and Severe Mental Illness*. Washington, D.C.: Interagency Council on the Homeless.
Johnson, A. K. 1994. "Linking Professionalism and Community Organization: A Scholar/Advocate Approach." *Journal of Community Practice* 1, no. 2: 65–87.
Katz, M. 1995. *Improving Poor People*. Princeton, N.J.: Princeton University Press.
Kaye, G., and T. Wolff, T., eds. 1995. *From the Ground Up: A Workbook on Coalition Building and Community Development*. Amherst, Mass.: AHEC/Community Partners.
Lappé, F. M., and P. M. DuBois. 1994. *The Quickening of America: Rebuilding Our Nation, Remaking Our Lives*. San Francisco: Jossey-Bass.
McKnight, J. 1994. "Two Tools for Well-Being: Health Systems and Communities." *American Journal of Preventive Medicine* 10, no. 3: 23–25.
McQuire, J. F. 1994. "Organizing from Diversity in the Name of Community: Lessons from the Disability Rights Movement." *Policy Studies Journal* 22, no. 1: 112–22.
Miller, M. 1985. "Turning Problems into Actionable Issues." San Francisco: Organize Training Center. Unpublished paper.
Mondros, J., and S. Wilson. 1994. *Organizing for Power and Empowerment*. New York: Columbia University Press.
Moyer, B., J. McAllister, M. L. Finley, and S. Soifer. 2001. *Doing Democracy: The MAP Model for Organizing Social Movements*. British Columbia, Canada: New Society Publishers.
Mueller, C. 1999. "Wealth Distribution Statistics." Retrieved on July 6, 2003. http://www.cooperativeindividualism.org/wealth_distribution1999.html.
O'Connor, J. 1976. "What Is Political Economy?" In *Economics: Mainstream Readings and Radical Critiques*, edited by D. Mermelstein. 3d ed. New York: Random House.
Pilisuk, M. 1986–87. "Family, Community, and Government: The Value and the Limits of Local Caregiving." *International Quarterly of Community Health Education* 7, no. 1: 61–67.
————. 2001. "Globalism and Structural Violence." In *Peace, Conflict, and Violence: Peace Psychology for the 21st Century*, edited by D. Christie, R. Wagner, and D. Winter. Englewood Cliffs, N.J.: Prentice Hall.
Pilisuk, M., J. McAllister, and J. Rothman. 1996. "Coming Together for Action: The Challenge of Contemporary Grassroots Organizing." *Journal of Social Issues* 52, no. 1: 15–37.
Pilisuk, M., and S. H. Parks. 1986. *The Healing Web: Social Networks and Human Survival*. Hanover, N.H.: University Press of New England.
Putnam, R. 2000. *Bowling Alone: The Collapse and Revival of American Community*. New York: Simon and Schuster.

Rothman, J. 2000a. "Countering Fragmentation on the Left." *Social Policy* 30, no. 4: 42–46.

———. 2000b. "Why the Left Is Fragmented (and a Modest Proposal to Counter It). *Humanist* 60, no. 5: 40–42.

Segal, S., C. Silverman, and T. Temkin. 1991. *Enabling, Empowering, and Self-Help Agency Practice*. Berkeley, Calif.: Center for Self-Help Research.

Soffa, V. M. 1994. *The Journey beyond Breast Cancer: From the Personal to the Political*. Rochester, Vt.: Healing Arts Press.

Tobias, A. 2003. "How Much Is Fair?" *Parade* (March): 10–11.

Thurow, L. 1996. *The Future of Capitalism*. New York: Morrow.

U.S. Committee for Refugees. 2002. *World Refugee Survey, 2002: An Annual Assessment of Conditions Affecting Refugees, Asylum Seekers, and Internally Displaced Persons*. Washington, D.C.: U.S. Committee for Refugees.

Wallack, L., L. Dorfman, D. Jernigan, and M. Themba. 1993. *Media Advocacy and Public Health: Power for Prevention*. Newbury Park, Calif.: Sage.

Wallack, L., K. Woodruff, L. Dorfman, and I. Diaz. 1999. *News for a Change: An Advocate's Guide to Working with the Media*. Thousand Oaks, Calif.: Sage.

West, C. 1993. *Race Matters*. Boston: Beacon.

Yeich, S. 1994. *The Politics of Ending Homelessness*. Lanham, Md.: University Press of America.

MEREDITH MINKLER
CHERI PIES

# Ethical Issues and Practical Dilemmas in Community Organization and Community Participation

Chapter 7

THE SINGLE MOST IMPORTANT factor distinguishing true community organizing from other approaches, such as social planning (Rothman 2001) and public health consultation, is the active involvement of people, beginning with what they define as the needs and goals to be addressed. For although some degree of community involvement often occurs in the latter processes, increasing community capacity and problem-solving ability is usually not a primary objective.

From an ethical perspective, increasing community competence is important in part because it makes the community less vulnerable to outside manipulation in future encounters. A heavy emphasis on fostering community determination may at first suggest that the health or social change professional as organizer does not need to engage in extensive ethical reflection since many of the processes in which he or she is already involved make increased freedom of choice for the community a central goal. Yet despite these lofty goals and guiding principles, the practice of community organization is, in reality, one of the most ethically problematic arenas in which health educators, social workers, and other practitioners function.

All too often we find ourselves searching for answers to our ethical challenges in hopes that, by doing so, we can move ahead with plans and programs. But resolving these dilemmas may be less important than continuing our commitment to the process of articulating them as well as the values and assumptions that inform our practice. In the interest of real community participation and empowerment, how do we facilitate dialogue rather than direct it? How do we tease apart our own agenda from the community's? And what happens when there are multiple, and often conflicting, community agendas? These are just a few of the questions we face, and whether and how we think about them have critical implications for our work.

116

But ethical dilemmas in public health practice may not always be presented as straightforward cases of right and wrong or competing priorities. At times, we face practical situations that require us to balance the needs, rights, and perspectives of different individuals and groups. Within these practical situations may be embedded ethical issues—those that pose questions about appropriateness of behavior, the use of power, the margin of error allowed for ignorance, and so forth.

This chapter explores six areas in which health educators and other practitioners frequently experience tough ethical challenges and practical dilemmas in relation to the community organizing aspects of their roles: (1) conflicting loyalties, (2) dealing with funding sources, (3) eliciting real rather than symbolic participation, (4) addressing cross-cultural miscommunication and real or perceived racism, (5) the unanticipated consequences of organizing, and (6) the question of whose common good is being addressed. Case examples for each area highlight some of the challenges, with particular attention drawn to the ethical questions raised for practitioners as organizers.

## Conflicting Loyalties

Community health educators, social workers, and other professionals frequently find themselves simultaneously responsible to a health agency employer, the communities being served by that agency, and the funding sources supporting their project or program. Particularly when the health education professional is charged with facilitating consumer participation in the agency and acting as an advocate for the community, conflicting goals and loyalties may be problematic. As Jerry Grossman (1971) pointed out more than three decades ago, the health educator's role in helping people "set their own goals" often really means helping them set these goals "within the context of preexisting goals" (55). When agency agendas fail to match the needs and desires of the community, the health educator faces difficult ethical dilemmas involving the degree to which she or he feels comfortable about complying with agency expectations and directives.

Two ethical precepts that lie at the heart of community organizing and community building—self-determination and liberty—are helpful for thinking about and addressing such dilemmas. Both reflect an inherent faith in people's ability to assess their strengths and needs accurately and their right to act upon these insights in setting goals and determining strategies for achieving them.

In the language of health education, these ethical precepts are reflected in Dorothy Nyswander's (1956) early admonition to start where the people are. Yet when an HIV/AIDS prevention program has the goal of promoting safer sex, in part by mobilizing a community around the epidemic, and when the community in question is more concerned about drug abuse or violence, should the health education practitioner temporarily shelve the agency's formal agenda and truly start where the people are? Within the bounds of certain limiting conditions (discussed later in the chapter), our response to this question is yes. By choosing to start where the people are, the health professional commits to the principles of self-determination and liberty and the rights of individuals and communities to affirm and act on their own values.

Yet there is also a practical rationale for starting where the people are. When this ethical principle has been followed, trust in the community has been demonstrated, and the immediate concerns of people have received primary attention, community members frequently see that the organizer's original health concerns are relevant to their lives (see chapter 2).

An early case study demonstrates this phenomenon (Minkler 1978). The setting was a family planning agency in New York City where eight low-income African American and Puerto Rican women, all with large families, were hired to do community organizing around family planning in their communities. After meeting with the women, the agency's health educator quickly discovered that each had taken the job out of sheer economic necessity and was in fact quite suspicious of family planning on both health and political grounds.

Consequently, the health educator scrapped the agency's formal agenda and instead engaged the women in a dialogue about their own perceptions of the paramount needs in their communities. Using the issues they identified, such as irregular garbage collection and drug dealers in the schoolyard, the health educator began a discussion of various effective organizing techniques that the women might use to get action from appropriate agencies on these and other issues. Within weeks, the women, still on the payroll as family planning workers, were reporting success in stirring community interest and, in some cases, getting actual changes in undesirable environmental conditions.

Convinced at this point that the agency really was concerned with their communities' overall welfare, not merely with bringing down the birthrate, the women began to ask questions about birth control methods, their side effects, and the political ramifications of working in what was then a highly charged and sensitive area. Following these discussions, six of the eight women became convinced that family planning was in the best interests of their communities and began doing effective outreach and organizing in their neighborhoods.

If the health educator had failed to start with the concerns of the people she worked with, her chances of having effectively met the agency's health objectives would have been slim indeed. Yet by dropping the agency's formal agenda to assist the women in identifying and organizing around their own felt needs, she clearly took a risk. Objectives might have been set or actions taken that were incompatible with those of the funding agency.

A health educator working in a field such as HIV/AIDS prevention and serving a community with very high seroprevalence rates among youths may justifiably feel that continuing to work in this area is critical, even if the community does not share his or her perception of urgency. Such a situation may pose legitimate grounds for not starting where the people are. In such instances, however, the health educator, even when borrowing methods and tools from community organizing, would not be doing pure community organizing since the community's felt needs were not determining the goals set or the actions pursued.

Health educators or other professionals charged with organizing around a problem that has been externally identified by the health department or another outside agency may find a road around the choice between agency and community agendas. By carefully listening and asking thoughtful, probing questions (Miller 1993), the organizer may learn how the local community perceives the identified issue, what the community's primary issues are, and whether bridges or links can be found between these seemingly disparate agendas (see chapter 6).

The Asian Pacific Environmental Network (APEN), for example, wanted to organize a local Laotian refugee community in Richmond, California, around the high levels of potential toxins to which it was being exposed. Toxic spills from nearby oil refineries and other industries, contamination of the local fish on which many community livelihoods depended, and toxic waste in the plots of ground in which they grew vegetables were among the areas around which APEN, together with the university-based Labor and Occupational Health Program, hoped to organize (Center for Occupational and Environmental Health 1996). When meeting with local refugees, asking questions, and really listening to the answers, however, APEN staff learned that community members had far more urgent questions, such as how to grow better vegetable crops. APEN's organizing agenda was consequently put aside while the organizers addressed the community's concerns. This show of genuine appreciation and acceptance of the community's agenda increased APEN's credibility among the refugees, some of whom subsequently began mapping toxic waste sites in their community and in other ways taking first steps in organizing around environmental hazards in their neighborhood (Center for Occupational and Environmental Health 1996, Laotian Organizing Project Staff 2001).

Although we have focused primarily on the problem of conflicting loyalties between the community and a health educator's or other professional's agency, tensions may also surface when there are multiple communities or community factions with different and often conflicting agendas. A community committed to HIV/AIDS prevention, for example, may be deeply torn over an effort to organize around a needle exchange program. A low-income Hispanic neighborhood near a toxic waste dump may likewise be divided between those residents wishing to organize against environmental racism and those who see the dump as a source of needed employment. The outside health professional's efforts to organize in such situations may generate more conflict and confrontation than consensus among community members. Thus, the question of whether to intervene, and if so on what level and with what guiding ethical precepts, assumes added importance.

## Dilemmas Posed by Funding Sources

The ethical dilemmas posed by conflicting community or community-versus-agency loyalties may be complicated still further by the realities of funding availability. The nature and source of funding for organizing projects can severely limit the extent to which organizers can truly start where the people are. In the United States, nonprofit organizations with tax-exempt 501(c)3 status, for example, must agree not to engage in partisan politics and, with a few exceptions, not to take part in lobbying efforts. Although another tax category (501[c]4) permits somewhat greater degrees of lobbying freedom, even these organizations "must maintain, at least in rhetoric, a fuzzy line between non-partisan and partisan activities" (Paget 1990, 123). For the health educator or other social change professional working with either a 501(c)3 or a 501(c)4 agency, these constraints may greatly hinder efforts in organizing with communities around their political and social change agendas.

Where government funding has been received for a health promotion project that attempts to accent community participation, additional funding-related dilemmas also may arise. For example, the CDC's PATCH approach to community health promotion accented community involvement and participation, beginning with community needs assessment. According to Marshall Kreuter (1992), this approach works well when the planning process "leads to a priority problem for which resources are available." But "where the indicated problem is not a priority of the government, the community may have to choose between shifting focus to a health issue for which there are available resources or do without. This has been a long-standing problem with PATCH, and indeed all community based health promotion programs which require extensive technical assistance" (139).

Although PATCH and similar models are examples of a social planning approach rather than true community organizing (see chapter 2), the dilemmas they raise are nevertheless familiar to health educators and other social change professionals who engage in community organizing. Moreover, even when community members define their priority area for organizing and successfully seek government or foundation money to support their work, the community's priorities may shift over time, or members' interest may wane before project completion. Does the health educator or outside professional urge the community group to continue working on what is now a low priority in order to fulfill a funding mandate? Does she or he propose returning the remaining money to the funders? Or does the organizer ask the funding source to accept the community's change in direction and continue to provide overall project support, despite the group's failure to complete the efforts originally emphasized?

Still another funding dilemma involves the declining availability of both government and foundation funding and the resulting need to turn to other sources of support. In such a climate, community organizations and programs may find themselves considering or accepting financial support from sources they may not previously have countenanced—sources that sometimes have invisible strings attached. New York City's Coalition for the Homeless, for example, accepted a $100,000 grant from Phillip Morris, only to be pressured later to help defeat a bill mandating antismoking ads; Phillip Morris wanted the coalition to demand that the city council address more important issues, such as homelessness (Quindlen 1992)!

Even when no such strings materialize, the lack of funding from less problematic sources also may disturb organizers, who are caught between the desire to undertake a needed community project or event and the need to turn to less than ideal sources for support. The initial planners of the California AIDS Ride report that they were turned down by numerous potential corporate sponsors before turning to the alcoholic beverage company, Tanqueray, which became the major—and highly visible—sponsor of such rides in several cities around the United States, contributing an annual average of $900,000 in sponsorship cash between 1994 and 2001, when it ceased funding (Wilke 2001). But such funding often is critical for good causes. A Latina legislator in California understood this fact but nevertheless expressed frustration when she faced opposition from several major Latino organizations to her bill that would restrict the sale of Coca Cola and other sodas in public elementary and middle schools. From a public health perspective, the alarming increase in obesity and juvenile diabetes in this population should have made organizations such as the East Los Angeles Community Union (TELACU) strong supporters of the bill. But when we learn that these organizations each receive donations from soda companies (for example, a recent $50,000 gift from the Coca-Cola Foundation to TELACU for its scholarship fund), the motive for their opposition becomes clear ("New Hurdle for Soda Ban" 2003).

When a funding source poses a direct real or perceived conflict of interest for an organization, such problems may intensify. For example, early in its existence, Mothers against Drunk Driving (MADD) accepted a sizable donation from Anheuser-Busch, the nation's largest beer manufacturer. Subsequently, MADD's increasingly close affiliation with the alcohol industry was widely viewed as having compromised its ability to take a strong stand on the industry's role in the nation's alcohol problem (Marshall and Oleson 1994). In defense of MADD, William Dejong and Anna Russell (1995) have stressed the organization's leadership role in pushing for a national minimum drinking age and other policy changes opposed by the alcohol industry. Yet as these analysts also point out, MADD did not significantly strengthen its position on alcohol advertising until 1994, when it had cut its ties to an industry that, it belatedly concluded, "was truly not interested in solving problems due to the misuse of alcohol," despite its propaganda to the contrary (234).

For health professionals aware of the harmful effects of tobacco and heavy drinking, accepting such donations may be difficult indeed. Yet the community-based organizations or groups with which they work may either feel no conflict or agree with Saul Alinsky (1972) that, in organizing, the end (such as getting support for a battered women's shelter or an organizing project) justifies the means. To avoid situations like these, some health educators have begun working with alternative sponsorship projects, which link health and social programs and organizing efforts with alternative corporate or other sources of financial assistance, in the process dealing a public relations blow to alcohol and tobacco companies. Still other health educators have helped community coalitions and programs decide whether to accept funding from a controversial source by applying what has been called the publicity test of ethics. This simple test involves having a group ask itself whether its reputation or integrity would be damaged if the source of funding for a particular project became known.

Such strategies are important; but in a time of major fiscal retrenchment in health and social services and declining support for a host of worthy organizing endeavors, they do not begin to solve the problem of severe funding constraints. When the need is great, where should the line be drawn? And when community participation and empowerment are valued, who draws the line? In meetings with community members about a financial offer of assistance from a source that may pose ethical implications, health educators are often confronted with the reaction "We need the money—go for it!"

Are we truly promoting community participation and empowerment if we disregard the community's desire to accept needed resources from a source we may consider problematic? Or will the community's long-run agenda be undermined if taking the money may at some point constrain decision making, priority setting, or program direction? If what we are after is promotion of the common good, how do we accomplish this in a climate of declining public funding and the concurrent pull of likely support from potentially problematic sources? These are just a few of the kinds of questions health educators and other social change professionals need to ask themselves in relation to the funding of programs and organizing efforts with which they are associated.

## Community Participation: Real or Symbolic?

Community participation historically has been recognized as a central value in community health education practice. In the 1960s and 1970s, it gained increasing currency in the field of health planning as well, where calls for maximum feasible participation coincided with the birth of the neighborhood health center move-ment (Green 2003). More recently, as noted in chapter 2, community or public participation and the concept of empowerment have emerged as defining features of the health promotion movement (Robertson and Minkler 1994).

Despite increased rhetoric about participation in the health field, however, acting on the principle that calls for high-level community involvement has proved difficult indeed. As Gail Siler-Wells (1989) points out, "Behind the euphemisms of participation and empowerment [lie] the realities of power, con-trol and ownership" (142). And even as we attempt to blur hierarchical distinc-tions by talking, for example, about health care providers and consumers and calling for partnerships between health professionals and communities, these power imbalances remain (Minkler 1994).

In an early attempt to clarify these issues of control and ownership, health planner Sherry Arnstein (1969) developed what she called a ladder of participation. The bottom rungs of the ladder were two forms of nonparticipation: therapy and manipulation. In the middle were several degrees of tokenism—placation, con-sultation, and informing—points at which community members were heard and might have a voice, although their input was not necessarily heeded. Finally, the top rungs of the ladder were three degrees of citizen power: partnership, delegated power, and true citizen power.

Ann Robertson and Meredith Minkler (1994) argue that much current health promotion practice uses the rhetoric of high-level community participa-tion but in fact operates at the lower rungs of Arnstein's ladder as professionals "attempt to get people in the community to take ownership of a professionally defined health agenda" (305). In Ronald Labonte's (1990) words, such an approach "raises the specter of using community resources primarily as free or cheaper forms of service delivery in which community participation is tokenistic at best and co-opted at worst" (7).

In other instances, the community's input may be sought and then dis-counted, further reinforcing unequal power relationships between health profes-sionals and communities. The experience of some community advisory boards provides a good case in point. When taken seriously by professionals, community advisory boards or committees can make a real difference in how health educa-tors and other practitioners approach their community-based programs. When allowed to serve as true partners in decision making, such boards can provide valu-able information on community needs and strengths, the likely effectiveness of alternative organizing strategies, and the cultural nuances and sensitivities that need to be respected and addressed.

As Lawrence Green and C. James Frankish (1997) point out, however, far too often community boards are established in response to a funding mandate or sim-ilar inducement rather than out of a sincere concern for eliciting and acting on community advice. In such instances, community boards often perceive that they are expected to serve as rubber-stamp mechanisms for decisions that health professionals have already made.

Finally, even programs committed to community participation through advisory boards and the like may occasionally find themselves ignoring input that conflicts with predetermined projects and plans—sometimes at considerable cost. An unfortunate example occurred in what is in many respects a national model for effective health promotion on multiple levels: the California Tobacco Control Program (CTCP). We use this example to underscore that even the best programs can slip into paternalism, with negative results.

CTCP was created when a successful 1992 ballot initiative added a twenty-five-cent tax on cigarettes, allocating a quarter of the money generated to anti-tobacco health education and advocacy. The program has been extremely successful and is credited for the fact that the state's decline in cigarette smoking has recently been three times the national average (Skolnick 1994).

Part of CTCP's activity has involved supporting groups such as the African-American Tobacco Control Education Network (AATCEN), which has addressed the heavy targeting of cigarette advertising to people of color and helped to mount a culturally sensitive counter-advertising campaign. When professionals at CTCP first designed a proposed billboard aimed at the African American community, they asked AATCEN's advisory group for feedback. The billboard depicted a young African American man smoking a cigarette under the caption "Eric Jones just put a contract out on his family for $2.65. Secondhand smoke kills." Advisory group members perceived the proposed ad as racist and strongly urged that it not be used. Rather than heeding the group's concerns, however, CTCP ran the ad and received the same kind of negative reaction from community members (Ellis 1996).

The story behind the billboard is a sad and poignant reminder that it is not enough to talk the talk of community competence and community participation. We must indeed be willing to walk the walk—in this case, let an advisory board composed of African American community members teach the rest of us how to avoid stigmatizing their community in the name of health promotion.

It is easy to see how paying only lip service to the concept of community participation can make communities and community groups suspicious about the agenda of a community organizer. Without a strong commitment to real community participation, we risk undermining our future efforts and dissipating the often fragile trust that communities invest in us. The credibility of the community organizer can be easily undermined when community group members sense that their participation is only symbolic, thus leading them to question the commitment of the organizer and others to the community's real issues. Recognition of the importance of self-determination for communities, coupled with commitment to the concept of true partnership, must serve as guiding principles for ensuring meaning-ful community participation (see chapters 5 and 14).

Community organizers Herbert Rubin and Irene Rubin (2000) offer a use-ful tool for applying these guiding principles in the form of the DARE criteria of empowerment:

Who determines the goals of the project?
Who acts to achieve them?
Who receives the benefits of the actions?
Who evaluates the actions?

The more often we can answer these questions with "the community," the more likely it is that our partnerships and community organizing efforts will contribute to real community empowerment and high-level participation.

## Confronting Racism and Perceived Racism in Community Organizing

Because health educators and other professionals engaged in organizing fre-quently do not share the race, ethnicity, or cultures of the community groups with which they are involved, opportunities for cultural misunderstandings and for real or perceived racism are unfortunately plentiful. Further, since communities themselves are increasingly diverse, cultural misunderstandings and racism within the community are common. As noted in chapter 1, racism has been likened to "the gorilla in the living room," wreaking havoc while "everyone is trying to sit politely and ignore it." (Themba 1999, 92). Because community organizing and community building require strong commitments to active listening and dia-logue (see chapter 6), dealing openly with cross-cultural misunderstandings and racism as they arise should be of paramount concern. Yet "even under the best of circumstances, troubling situations can occur, particularly in a country with the historical baggage around race, ethnicity and racism carried in the United States" (Minkler in press).

In the course of his involvement with an organizing project in a racially and ethnically diverse inner-city community, a white physician working with one of this chapter's authors found himself facilitating a discussion in which a white mem-ber of the group began making disparaging comments about another race. The physi-cian, who was highly respected in the community, became visibly angry and stated loudly that he would leave immediately if further racist remarks were made. The forcefulness of his reaction shocked the group, which remained quiet for several moments before resuming the discussion. Although no racial or eth-nic slurs were heard again in the weekly meetings, neither did the group ever directly deal with the racist incident that had provoked the outsider's angry response. Was the physician's reaction appropriate? On the one hand, the vehemence of his response showed a level of intolerance for racism that sent an important message to the community members with whom he worked. On the other hand, the level of anger he displayed may have precluded any follow-up dialogue about the incident and its underlying causes. This kind of dialogue is necessary if race and racism are to be openly acknowledged and addressed.

In other cases, the outside organizer's racial-ethnic biases or lack of cultural competence may damage trust and good will in an organizing situation. For example, a well-meaning outside organizer who attempted to show cultural sensitivity by ordering Asian food for a community meeting whose attendees were largely Korean, Chinese, Thai, Laotian, and Filipino faced an angry reaction from some when the meal turned out to consist solely of Chinese food. Although the matter may seem minor, some group members thought that her food choice reflected the larger society's disrespectful tendency to lump together all Asians (and Asian Pacific Islanders). In this instance, the organizer took the important step of acknowledging her mistake and asking the group to decide on the food for subsequent meetings. In response, some offered to contribute their own favorite dishes, while others identified good and inexpensive restaurants serving their native cuisine; the next meeting included a plethora of diverse ethnic treats. Since the four most important words in community organizing may well be "refreshments will be served," taking care to involve communities in this way, and respecting community food preferences, is not an extraneous detail. Our handling of such situations can demonstrate a necessary cultural humility, if we approach them with a humble attitude characterized by acknowledgment of our own biases and ignorance, an openness to others' cultural reality, and a sincere desire to listen and to learn (Tervalon and Garcia 1998; also see chapters 1 and 14).

## Unanticipated Consequences of Organizing

The guiding principles of fostering self-determination and meaningful participation can go a long way in helping to avoid many of the problems that plague the community organizing process. Yet even when we follow these principles, our organizing efforts may result in unanticipated outcomes or by-products that may have negative consequences. We include two examples as illustration, one concerning injury prevention campaigns, the other related to training community health workers to enhance their skills in areas such as leadership and community organizing.

Many recent prevention and health promotion campaigns have done an excellent job of involving youth, people of color, and other traditionally neglected groups in the design and implementation of programs and materials aimed at reaching these populations more effectively (Eng and Parker 2002, Satterfield et al. 2002). Simultaneously, however, some have inadvertently reproduced and transmitted problematic aspects of the dominant culture. Caroline Wang (1992) has identified particularly poignant examples in her study of the stigmatization of people with disabilities, which is often communicated through well-meaning injury prevention campaigns. She tells of a MADD-sponsored billboard featuring a teenager in a wheelchair and the caption "If you think fourth period English is endless, try sitting in a wheelchair for the rest of your life!" Another includes the caption "One for the road" and shows a man on crutches and a partially amputated leg . As Wang points out, the implicit message in such ads is "Don't let this happen to you!" Although well intentioned, these messages reinforce already powerful negative prejudices in our society against people with disabilities. At a time when the disabled are organizing to assert their rights and break down negative societal stereotypes, such campaigns can be particularly demoralizing. As Wang notes, one person with a disability viewed the injury prevention ads and said, "I feel like I should be preventing myself!"

As we work to avoid negative and unanticipated consequences, the principle of high-level community involvement (in this case, reaching out to an overlooked community: people with disabilities) can stand us in good stead. Such an approach is illustrated in the close coordination between two strong advocacy and organizing groups based in the San Francisco Bay Area—the World Institute on Disability (WID) and the Trauma Foundation. Although the latter's raison d'être is injury prevention, its executive director, Andrew McQuire, has served as chair of the board of WID; and he and other foundation staff members are strong advocates for the recognition and treatment of disabled people as full participants in American society.

In some instances, of course, the very nature of the processes involved in community organizing can have negative unanticipated consequences. The training of health promoters or community health workers in both developing and postindustrialized nations provides a good case in point. From a health education and a community organizing standpoint, such activities makes eminent sense: they typically identify and build on the strengths of natural helpers in a community and address issues of homophily (for example, people often learn best and prefer to receive services from people who are like themselves in terms of race, social class, and so on). Moreover, many excellent models for community health worker training place a heavy accent on empowerment, often employing methods such as Paulo Freire's (1968, 1973) education for critical consciousness.

Yet as Freire (1968) himself has cautioned, leadership training can alienate the community members who are involved, making them strangers in their own communities. Once they have been trained and, in a sense, indoctrinated into the culture of the public health department or health clinic agency, community health workers may find it difficult to relate to or interact with their peers as they once had. Has their training given them a new vocabulary and consequently a different way of addressing identified problems? Do they feel some unstated pressure to fit into the agency that hired them, where most people are professionally trained and the culture of the office environment is different from the culture of the community or the neighborhood? Or is a community leader who tries to bring a particular health message to the community distrusted because he or she is now on the other side? How should we proceed when we are committed to involving indigenous community workers in the process of education and organizing yet know that such efforts may alienate these individuals from their communities and limit their credibility in the community?

Still another unanticipated consequence of training community members as health workers, group leaders, and organizers is that they may use the skills they have acquired to manipulate other members of the community. Almost forty years ago, Herbert Kelman (1965) warned that, as a consequence of the training received, a community leader "may be able to manipulate the group into making the decision he desires, but also to create the feeling that this decision reflects the will of the group discovered through the workings of the democratic process" (35).

There may always be some risk that community health workers or other recipients of training will misuse the tools we have helped them acquire. But numerous examples of effective community health worker programs and leadership training activities on the local level suggest that this strategy is, on balance, critical for improving health and contributing to individual and community empowerment, both in North America and around the world (Eng and Parker 1994, Ovrebo et al. 1994, Satterfield et al. 2002). The task for health educators and other social change professionals is to determine how best to help participants acquire the tools they need for effective leadership and organizing and to communicate the responsibilities this new training imposes as well as some of the difficulties and challenges communities may need to anticipate.

## Thoughts about the Common Good

Acknowledging and confronting the dilemmas posed by conflicting loyalties, potential funding sources, the task of creating real rather than symbolic participation in community organizing, and the unanticipated consequences of community organizing efforts may bring us close to greater community participation and ultimately greater empowerment of community groups. When we start where the people are, we make every attempt to respond to the needs, concerns, and agendas of a particular community, thereby affirming a commitment to self-determination and liberty as well as promoting the rights of individuals to act on their own values. Several question remain, however. Do we aim toward an ultimate end in our efforts to promote and preserve the common good of the communities with which we work? If so, whose common good is addressed? And who determines what constitutes the common good? Finally, should we also be concerned with notions of common good that transcend local communities?

Alinsky (1972) long argued that a cardinal rule in effective community organizing is to appeal to self-interest: people will not organize unless they see what is in it for them. In a country such as the United States, however, which is characterized by an emphasis on rugged individualism, stressing only self-interest may feed into an already impoverished notion of the common good. As Lester Thurow (1996) points out, the dominant American ideologies—capitalism and democracy— "have no 'common good,' no common goals toward which everyone is collectively working. Both stress the individual and not the group. . . . Neither imposes an obligation to worry about the welfare of the other. . . . In both, individual freedom dominates community obligations" (159).

In part because of the individual focus of these dominant ideologies, the debate over public or common good in the United States has been severely constrained. In Larry Churchill's (1987, 21) words, our notions of justice are based on "a moral heritage in which answers to the question 'what is good?' and 'what is right?' are lodged definitively in a powerful image of the individual as the only meaningful level of moral analysis" (21). Churchill goes on to argue that "a more realistic sense of community is one in which there are shared perceptions of the value of individual lives and a social commitment to protect them all equitably" (101).

The lack of a realistic sense of community and a well-developed notion of the common good may be particularly troubling for health educators and other social change professionals, whose world views and career choices are founded on a strong sense of social justice (Mondros and Wilson 1994; see also chapter 1). Moreover, as we have already suggested, although an appeal to self-interest may be pragmatic in helping to mobilize a community to achieve its self-interested goals, there are dangers in this limited approach. Key is the fact that a local community group may fail to see or reflect on the connection between its goals and concerns and the broader need for social justice in a democratic society. Consequently, even though a focus on self-interest may be necessary from an organizing perspective, it is too narrow to be sufficient.

We do, however, advocate against an overly simplistic utilitarian notion of the common good that focuses solely on achieving the greatest good for the greatest number, which may not truly reflect the end that those engaged in community organizing are attempting to realize. Instead, we look toward a definition of common or collective good that both speaks to local organizing efforts and includes a broader vision of society. This broader vision has frequently been absent from the Alinsky brand of organizing (Miller 1987) in which many community organizers are rooted.

Feminist leader Charlotte Bunch (1983) offers one approach that community organizers may usefully adapt and apply to create a bridge between local or small-scale organizing efforts and a broader social vision. She argues that any particular reform or change effort should be perceived and evaluated not as an end in itself but as a means toward a larger goal. For her, the latter is a revolutionary feminist agenda that leads to "a new social order based on equitable distribution of resources . . . , equal justice and rights for all, and upon maximizing freedom for each person to determine her own life" (204). If we replace the word *reform* with *community organizing effort* and *women* with *community members*, her criteria include the following questions: "(1) Does [the community organizing effort] materially improve the lives of community members and if so, which members and how many? (2) Does [participating in the organizing process] give community members a sense of power, strength and imagination as a group and help build structures for further change? and (3) Does the struggle . . . educate community members politically, enhancing their ability to criticize and challenge the system in the future?" (206–8). Overarching questions like these can help organizers engage the communities with which they work in the kind of broader reflection needed if we are indeed to build bridges between acting locally and thinking globally.

The end of the twentieth century and beginning of the twenty-first has been a time of renewed moral reflection in the United States (Elshtain 1995, Etzioni 1993, Lakoff 2002). As part of this reflection, scholars and social analysts along the political spectrum have begun reviving and refining a social vision of communitarianism in which, in Amitai Etzioni's (1993) words, the "restoration of the community [is] a core mission." For new left commentator Michael Lerner (in Labonte 1996), the effort is no less than an attempt to "shift the dominant discourse of our society from an ethos of selfishness and cynicism to an ethos of caring and idealism." For the more centrist Etzioni (1993), it calls for a return to the kind of community "in which people do not merely ask 'How are you?' . . . but care about the answer."

Health educators, community organizers, and other social change professionals must engage in discussion, reflection, and debate both to understand the issues and to bring their perspectives to a dialogue that will be critical to the future of communities, community organizing, and community participation. Through such discussions, we show how community organizing can serve as a bridge to thinking more deeply about the collective good not only of this or that community but also of the broader society.

## Conclusion

Throughout this chapter, we have been asking hard questions that go to the core of our practice as community organizers. As health educators and other social change professionals, we often operate on the implicit assumption that our interventions are ethically justifiable since they are derived from community-identified needs.

Yet the principles of starting where the people are and working closely with communities to translate their goals into reality, while critical to ethically sound practice, do not exempt us from the need to engage in frequent, thoughtful, ethical reflection. All too often, such reflection has been an afterthought, the result of unanticipated dilemmas and ethical issues. By making it an early and continuing part of our organizing efforts, we can enhance our ability to ensure that the actions we take in working with communities meet the criteria of ethically sound practice.

Although we have tried to address a number of specific ethical dilemmas in this chapter, many others cannot be anticipated, given the ever-changing context in which we work. We must commit ourselves to articulating the dilemmas we face in our practice as community organizers, with special attention to recognizing the contradictions with which we cope and understanding where our responsibilities lie.

It is critical, moreover, for us to identify and articulate not only the ethical dilemmas we face but also the underlying values that drive our work. How do we communicate the importance of the values of community participation and empowerment when we find ourselves in ethically challenging situations? When conflicting loyalties present us with the task of meeting different needs and different (and sometimes conflicting) agendas, how do we make explicit the values that help us do the right thing? When our agencies or funders propose what is really only symbolic or lip-service community participation, how do we formulate effective, value-based arguments to reinforce the importance of not only bringing community members to the table but also hearing their concerns and ensuring that their input is broadly reflected in the final product? Finally, what role can we play in helping community groups reflect on their own values as a means of grappling with difficult dilemmas concerning issue selection or whether to accept funding from a potentially ethically problematic source? And what role can we play in helping communities to explore the connections between their perceptions of their own common good and a broader vision of society?

Although we cannot anticipate the possible consequences of all our actions, we can anticipate that some consequences of our community organizing efforts will be different from our expectations. We must remind ourselves to expect the unexpected and to recognize that in the process we are likely to find ourselves in ethically challenging situations that require discussion, dialogue, and difficult choices.

### References

Alinsky, S. D. 1972. *Rules for Radicals*. New York: Random House.

Arnstein, S. 1969. "A Ladder of Citizen Participation." *Journal of American Institute of Planners* 35 (July): 216–24.

Bunch, C. 1983. "The Reform Tool Kit." In *First Harvest*, edited by J. Friedman. New York: Grove.

Center for Occupational and Environmental Health. 1996. "LOHP to Work with Local Laotian Community." *COEH Newsletter* (January): 2.

Churchill, L. 1987. *Rationing Health Care in America: Perceptions and Principles of Justice.* South Bend, Ind.: University of Notre Dame Press.

Dejong, W., and A. Russell. 1995. "MADD's Position on Alcohol Advertising: A Response to Marshal and Oleson." *Journal of Public Health Policy* 16, no. 2: 231–38.

Ellis, G. 1996. Personal communication, March 26.

Elshtain, J. 1995. *Democracy on Trial.* New York: Basic Books.

Eng E., and E. Parker. 1994. "Measuring Community Competence in the Mississippi Delta: The Interface between Program Evaluation and Empowerment." *Health Education Quarterly* 21, no. 2: 199–220.

———. 2002. "Natural Helper Models to Enhance a Community's Health and Competence." In *Emerging Theories in Health Promotion Practice and Research: Strategies for Improving Public Health,* edited by R. J. DiClemente, R. A. Crosby, and M. C. Kegler, 126–56. San Francisco: Jossey-Bass.

Etzioni, A. 1993. *Public Policy in a New Key.* New Brunswick, N.J.: Transaction.

Freire, P. 1968. *Pedagogy of the Oppressed,* translated by M. B. Ramos. New York: Seabury.

———. 1973. *Education for Critical Consciousness.* New York: Seabury.

Green, L. W. 2003. "Tracing Federal Support for Participatory Research in Public Health." In *Community Based Participatory Research for Health,* edited by M. Minkler and N. Wallerstein, 410–18. San Francisco: Jossey-Bass.

Green, L. W., and C. J. Frankish. 1997. "Implementing Nutritional Science for Population Health: Decentralized and Centralized Planning for Health Promotion and Disease Prevention." In *Beyond Nutritional Recommendations: Implementing Science for Healthier Populations,* edited by C. Garza, J. D. Haas, J. Habicht, and D. L. Pelletier, 230–45. Ithaca, N.Y.: Cornell University and the National Academy of Science.

Grossman, J. 1971. "Health for What? Change, Conflict and the Search for Purpose." *Pacific Health Education Reports* 2: 51–66.

Kelman, H. C. 1965. "Manipulation of Human Behavior: An Ethical Dilemma for the Social Scientist." *Journal of Social Issues* 21: 31–46.

Kreuter, M. 1992. "PATCH: Its Origins, Basic Concepts, and Links to Contemporary Public Health Policy." *Journal of Health Education* 23, no. 3: 135–39.

Labonte, R. 1990. Empowerment: Notes on Professional and Community Dimensions." *Canadian Review of Social Policy* 26: 64–75.

———. 1996. "Community Development in the Public Health Sector: The Possibilities of an Empowering Relationship between State and Civil Society." Ph.D. diss., York University.

Lakoff, G. 2002. *Moral Politics: How Liberals and Conservatives Think.* Chicago: University of Chicago Press.

Laotian Organizing Project Staff. 2001. "The Laotian Organizing Project: Exploring New Campaign Issues in West Contra Costa County." *APEN Voices* 6, no. 1: 9–14.

Marshall, M., and A. Oleson. 1994. "In the Pink: MADD and Public Health Policy in the 1990s." *Journal of Public Health Policy* 15, no. 1: 54–68.

Miller, A. S. 1987. "Saul Alinsky: America's Radical Reactionary." *Radical America* 21, no. 1: 11–18.

Miller, M. 1993. "The Tenderloin Senior Organizing Project." In *A Journey to Justice.* Louisville, Ky.: Presbyterian Committee on the Self-Development of People.

Minkler, M. 1978. "Ethical Issues in Community Organization." *Health Education Monographs* 6, no. 2: 198–210.

———. 1994. "Ten Commitments for Community Health Education." *Health Education Research* 9, no. 4: 527–34.

———. In press. "Ethical Challenges for the Health Educator As 'Outsider' in Community Based Participatory Research." *Health Education and Behavior.*

Mondros, J. B., and S. M. Wilson. 1994. *Organizing for Power and Empowerment*. New York: Columbia University Press.

"New Hurdle for Soda Ban." *San Francisco Chronicle*, July 24, 2003, p. A24.

Nyswander, D. 1956. "Education for Health: Some Principles and Their Application." *California Health* 14 (November): 65–70.

Ovrebo, B., M. Ryan, K. Jackson, and K. Hutchinson. 1994. "The Homeless Prenatal Program: A Model for Empowering Homeless Pregnant Women." *Health Education Quarterly* 21, no. 2: 187–98.

Paget, K. 1990. "Citizen Organizing: Many Movements, No Majority." *American Prospect* 1, no. 2: 114–28.

Quindlen, A. 1992. "Good Causes, Bad Money." *New York Times*, November 15, sec. 4, p.19.

Robertson, A., and M. Minkler. 1994. "New Health Promotion Movement: A Critical Examination." *Health Education Quarterly* 21, no. 3: 295–312.

Rothman, J. 2001. "Approaches to Community Intervention." In *Strategies of Community Intervention*, 6th ed., edited by J. L. Erlich and J. E. Tropman, 27–64. Itasca, Ill.: Peacock.

Rubin, H., and I. Rubin. 2000. *Community Organizing and Development*. 3d ed. New York: Macmillan.

Satterfield, D., C. Burd, L. Valdez, G. Hosey, and J. Shield. 2002. "The 'In-Between People': Participation of Community Health Representatives in Diabetes Prevention and Care in American Indian and Alaska Native Communities." *Health Promotion Practice* 3, no. 2: 166–75.

Siler-Wells, G. L. 1989. "Challenges of the Gordian Knot: Community Health in Canada." In *International Symposium on Community Participation and Empowerment Strategies in Health Promotion*. Bielefeld, Germany: University of Bielefeld, Center for Interdisciplinary Studies.

Skolnick, A. 1994. "Antitobacco Advocates Fight 'Illegal' Diversion of Tobacco Control Money." *Journal of the American Medical Association* 271, no. 18: 1387–89.

Tervalon, M., and J. Murray-Garcia. (1998). "Cultural Humility vs. Cultural Competence: A Critical Distinction in Defining Physician Training Outcomes in Medical Education." *Journal of Health Care for the Poor and Underserved* 9, no. 2: 117–25.

Themba, M. N. 1999. *Making Policy, Making Change: How Communities Are Taking Law into Their Own Hands*. San Francisco: Jossey-Bass/Chardon.

Thurow, L. 1966. *The Future of Capitalism*. New York: Morrow.

Wang, C. 1992. "Culture, Meaning, and Disability: Injury Prevention Campaigns in the Production of Stigma." *Social Science and Medicine* 3, no. 5: 1093–1102.

Wilke, M. 2001. "Tanqueray Rides down a New Road." Retrieved on July 14, 2003. http://www.commercialcloset.org/cgi-bin/iowa/?page=column&record=47.

# Part III

# Community Assessment and Issue Selection

FIELDS SUCH AS health education, health planning, and social work typically focus considerable attention on needs assessment, or the use of a variety of methods to determine the problems and needs of the groups with which the professionals work. Increasingly, however, we recognize the importance of shifting our gaze from a narrowly conceived needs assessment to a broader community assessment. Reflecting this change in emphasis, the first two chapters in part 3 suggest approaches to community assessment that go well beyond needs assessment as it is typically conceived and indeed reject the narrow needs assessment approach rooted in a "deficit thinking" mentality, which can harm rather than enhance our efforts at community organizing and community building for health.

In chapter 8, Trevor Hancock and Meredith Minkler pose a series of questions that get to the heart of the whys and hows of community assessment for health. Drawing on Hancock's extensive experience as a key architect of the Healthy Cities Movement worldwide, they suggest that the focus of such efforts should move from community health assessment to healthy community assessment if we are to pay adequate attention to the numerous factors affecting the health of communities. Arguing that community assessments are needed not only for the information they provide for and about change but also for empowerment, the authors make the case for assessment that is truly of, by, and for the community. Expanding on John McKnight's statement that "institutions learn from studies, communities learn from stories," they emphasize the need for collecting both stories and more traditional study data as part of a comprehensive assessment process.

As a framework for exploration, Hancock and Minkler use Sylvia Marti-Costa and Irma Serrano-Garcia's (1983) categorization of assessment techniques according to the degree of contact with community members that they entail. Their chapter makes a strong case for the use of multiple methods, with an accent on those that empower individuals and communities, in part through their active involvement in and ownership of the assessment process, such as the development and use of community indicators (Bauer 2003).

A critical part of the shift from a needs assessment to a community assessment focus involves appreciating that communities are not simply collections of needs or problems but vital entities possessing many strengths and assets. Chapter 9 presents a classic contribution to the community assessment literature: John L. McKnight and John P. Kretzmann's approach to mapping community capacity. Pointing out that the needs-focused approach to low-income communities has led to deficiency-oriented policies and programs, the authors propose instead a capacity-oriented model. Their community mapping technique looks first at primary building blocks (assets such as people and their talents and associations) located in the neighborhood and largely under its control. Consistent with Cheryl L. Walter's (chapter 4) expanded notion of community, however, they also consider nonprofit organizations, local businesses, and the like that are located in the neighborhood and that, although largely controlled by outsiders, nevertheless may constitute important secondary building blocks.

The sample neighborhood needs map and contrasting neighborhood assets map included in chapter 9 offer students and practitioners a graphic illustration of how changing our orientation from deficiencies to strengths can transform our perceptions of communities as well as those communities' images of themselves. Although the chapter addresses itself to geographic communities, the approach it demonstrates can be adapted for use in a workplace or a common interest community as well.

Closely connected to community assessment is working with communities in ways that enable them, rather than outsiders, to determine the goals and issues around which they wish to mobilize. In chapter 10, Lee Staples, author of the classic organizing manual *Roots to Power* (1984), draws our attention to this pivotal area as he explores the topic of selecting and cutting the issue. Echoing a theme that runs throughout much of the book, Staples argues that issues should indeed come from the members and potential members of a community. At the same time, he sees the outside professional as playing a critical role in helping community groups become familiar with the criteria of good issues so that they can select foci for action that measure up against these important yardsticks for success. As he suggests, a good issue is one about which the community feels deeply. But it also is an issue that is winnable, unites the community, provides opportunities for leadership development and broad-based member participation, and is consistent with the long-range goals and strategies of the organization.

Staples details the process that organizers refer to as cutting the issue, or deciding who gets what from whom and how and why they intend to get it. Using numerous examples from health and related organizing efforts in the United States, he describes and illustrates the issue-cutting process and how it fits within the conduct of a broader strategic analysis. Although largely based on a selection from *Roots to Power*, Staples's chapter has been significantly updated and revised and includes a wealth of new case studies that connect the principles with real-world community organizing for health.

## References

Bauer, G. F. 2003. "Sample Community Health Indicators on the Neighborhood Level." In *Community Based Participatory Research for Health*, edited by M. Minkler and N. Wallerstein, 438–45. San Francisco: Jossey-Bass.

Marti-Costa, S., and F. Serrano-Garcia. 1983. "Needs Assessment and Community Development: An Ideological Perspective." *Prevention in Human Services* 2, no. 4: 75–88.

Staples, L. 1984. *Roots to Power: A Manual for Grassroots Organizing*. New York: Praeger.

TREVOR HANCOCK
MEREDITH MINKLER

| Chapter 8 | Community Health Assessment or Healthy Community Assessment |
| --- | --- |

*Whose Community?*
*Whose Health? Whose Assessment?*

Mᴀɴʏ ǫᴜᴇsᴛɪᴏɴs need to be asked concerning the performance of a community health assessment. In this chapter, we discuss a number of these questions and provide some examples of assessment processes that we believe illustrate promising approaches. As our title implies, we believe that, to be truly empowering and health promoting, assessment should be of the community, by the community, and for the community.

### Why Assess?

In a seminal article, Sylvia Marti-Costa and Irma Serrano-Garcia (1983) argued that, far from being neutral or objective, needs assessment is an ideological process that can serve political purposes ranging from system maintenance and control to the promotion of social change and consciousness raising. At one end of the ideological continuum are needs assessments designed to support and justify the status quo. Although they may include some efforts at fine tuning the way in which the system functions, they do not question or wish to change the ideological commitments on which that system is based (Marti-Costa and Serrano-Garcia 1983). The health educator who is trying to increase attendance at agency-sponsored community health fairs, for example, might well conduct an assessment to determine whether the event's hours and location were problematic for local residents. But if the agency had already committed to health fairs as its modus operandi for community health outreach, the health educator would not be expected—or wanted—to determine residents' perceptions of whether the fairs really addressed their primary health needs.

In contrast, an assessment open to higher-level change would actively involve community residents in helping the agency or organization critically rethink its mission and activities. The purposes of such an assessment, as Marti-Costa and Serrano-Garcia (1983) have suggested, would be to accomplish the following:

Measure, describe, and understand community lifestyles
Assess community resources to lessen external dependency
Return needs assessment data to facilitate residents' decision making
Provide skill training, leadership, and organizational skills
Facilitate collective activities and group mobilization
Enable consciousness raising

The purposes of a needs assessment and the values and assumptions underlying this process, in short, heavily influence the choice of assessment techniques, the interventions proposed, the use of data obtained, and the perceptions of who owns the data in the first place.

Although Marti-Costa and Serrano-Garcia's framework was designed to stimulate critical thinking about the goals and purposes of needs assessment as they relate to social services programs, their message is equally relevant to community health assessment as an initial step in community organizing and community building. For example, a narrowly defined needs assessment designed and conducted by outside experts as a means of justifying and providing raw data for organizing around a predetermined community health need may be effective in achieving its objectives. But by failing to involve community members meaningfully in determining the goals of the assessment process, by focusing solely on needs rather than identifying and building on community strengths, and by failing to make empowerment of people a central goal of the assessment process, such an approach would fail to meet several critical criteria of community organizing and community building practice.

## The Rationale behind Community Health Assessment

Health professionals concerned with community organizing and community building have two reasons for implementing effective and comprehensive community health assessments: information is needed for change, and it is also needed for empowerment.

### INFORMATION FOR CHANGE

Information for change has three purposes: to stimulate change or action, to monitor change or action, and to assess the impact of change (Hancock 1989). Information that stimulates change must carry social and political punch. In addition, indicators must, of necessity, be sensitive to short-term change, given the short-term basis of much social and political action. Information that falls into this category includes stories and data about inequalities in health and the social and physical determinants of health in the community, preferably focusing on inequalities where there is a reasonable chance of seeing some change in a comparatively short period of time. Although it may be important in the long run to document differences in mortality rates for lung cancer or heart disease, for example, this needs to be balanced by information about people's perceived state of health, their social and physical living conditions, and their behaviors, all of which may be more likely to reflect changes in the short term after some policy or community action.

The change rationale for community assessment also requires information about the processes of change or action. In a discussion of healthy cities assessment, Leonard Duhl and Trevor Hancock (1988) note that, because the focus is on the processes involved in a given city or community, assessment is heavily dependent on stories and observations rather than hard data. Activities and related phenomena that appear to be precursors to change itself must be identified. These might include widespread community knowledge about the project, the establishment of participatory mechanisms such as intersectoral committees, evidence of the development of new skills among the population, and indicators of political commitment to the project at the local level. The linking rationale, which can be proved only in the long run, is that these activities will lead to other actions that will ultimately lead to better health.

Information that will assess the impact of change on health can function as a baseline of the individual and community dimensions of health. Here health is defined broadly to include physical, mental, and social well-being in both subjective and objective terms. Regular repetitions of the baseline measures via surveys and other instruments must be conducted to assess change.

### INFORMATION FOR EMPOWERMENT

An entirely different but equally important reason for wanting information about health is that knowledge is power and is therefore a component of empowerment. As noted in earlier chapters, the process of empowerment is central to, and indeed forms the core of, the WHO's (1986) definition of health promotion. Individuals and communities can become truly empowered only if they have the knowledge required to assess their situation and to take action, backed by sufficient power, to make change happen. The most obvious way of defining and obtaining information is to ask the community itself for its definition of a good or healthy community. In so doing, the health education or health promotion professional is helped to identify the most important components about which information must be collected. But by asking the community to define health, assess progress, and measure change, the outside professional is also furthering the process of empowerment.

If the community is to use information, that information, whether hard data or stories, must be physically, socially, and culturally accessible to the community. Information should be presented via local media and be placed in local community settings such as libraries, community centers, faith organizations, and schools as well as on easily accessed Internet sites.

Reports need to be written simply and in the dominant language of the community; even in postindustrial nations such as Canada and the United States, the latest available national figures suggest that between one-fifth and one-quarter of the population is either functionally illiterate or operating at the lowest level of literacy (Kirsh et al. 1993). Thus, in addition to written information, it is important to disseminate information in audio and video formats through the media that the majority of the population routinely use.

Information from the healthy community assessment also can and should be used as the basis for study groups, work circles, and other adult and popular education strategies, including literacy training and English as a second language (ESL) courses. A good example of this approach appears in the work of Leadership to Improve Neighborhood Communication and Services, a neighborhood affiliate of the Healthy Boston project in the linguistically diverse Allston-Brighton area. A community-wide assessment meeting, conducted in half a dozen languages and attended by more than three hundred people, uncovered concerns about inadequate housing, HIV/AIDS, and other topics. An effort then was made to incorporate some of these issues into the neighborhood's ESL programs. By combining ESL with leadership training, advocacy training, and field internships for more than forty residents, the project helped create a cadre of individuals who could serve as cultural liaisons between their cultural community and health and social service agencies as well as the larger city and neighborhood.

Knowing how well one's community functions, how much it cares about its citizens' well-being and quality of life, and how choices that affect health are made—and by whom—enables people to participate more fully and actively in the life of the community. This is a fundamental basis of health promotion and, even more broadly, of citizenship. And it underscores the importance of disseminating the information gleaned from a healthy community assessment through literacy training and a host of other channels.

## Whose Community, Whose Health?

We have referred thus far to "the community." But as earlier chapters have suggested, the real question is "Which community are we referring to?" Health educators and other health promotion professionals working with geographic communities often focus on a particular neighborhood, and this is indeed the level with which people tend to identify. Yet since one of the intents of the healthy city-community process is to stimulate local government involvement in and commitment to improving the health of the community, the boundaries for assessment may also often be municipal ones. The first challenge, then, is to assess the healthy community process and situation at both the municipal level and the level of the community or neighborhood.

The second challenge is to conceptualize health broadly enough so that we are able to look well beyond traditional indicators such as morbidity and mortality to embrace WHO's (1948) view of health as "a state of complete physical, mental and social well being, and not merely the absence of disease and infirmity." Community members know from their own experience that health is much more than the absence of illness or dysfunction, and they often have creative and meaningful ways of conceptualizing health for themselves. The challenge for the health professional is to pay more attention to how the members of the community define health and to incorporate their definitions for assessing the health of the community.

## Needs or Capacities?

Professor and community builder John L. McKnight (Kretzmann and McKnight 1993; see also chapter 9) describes the importance of the associational life, or the informal and formal community-based organizations and networks that form the underpinnings of the community. This is similar to what Robert Putnam (2000) calls civicness, or social solidarity. McKnight is particularly concerned about having professionals change their focus from individual and community deficits that require services to assets and capacities that enable community building (see chapter 9).

The implications of such a 180-degree shift in how we view people and communities are profound. For they suggest that we should reevaluate the entire way in which we conceive of the role of professionals in the community—as enablers and facilitators rather than providers of services—and the purpose of those services. From the perspective of assessment of the community's health, McKnight's approach has two important implications. First, it underscores the importance of assessing capacity, not merely needs; and second, it reminds us that the process of that assessment should itself contribute to the capacity of people and communities and to community health.

## Community Health Assessment or
## Healthy Community Assessment?

To understand the difference between a community health assessment and a healthy community assessment, it is necessary to begin with a clear understanding of what is meant by the term *healthy community*. The most commonly accepted definition was promulgated by Hancock and Duhl (1986) for WHO: "A healthy [community] is one that is continually creating and improving those physical and social environments and expanding those community resources which enable people to mutually support each other in performing all the functions of life and in developing to their maximum potential" (24).

Although there are several important points in this definition, key is that it is a definition of a process rather than a status. Thus, even though high health status and low mortality and morbidity are important, a healthy community is not necessarily one that has the highest health status in a conventional sense but one that is striving with every fiber of its being to be more healthy. Ideally, this is reflected in a commitment at all levels from the political to the personal, across all sectors, and involving all stakeholders and indeed all members of the community around the common focus of improving the health, well-being, and quality of life of the community and its members. The closer a community is to this ideal, the closer it is to being a healthy community.

Reviewing a wide range of literature, Hancock and Duhl (1986) suggest the following eleven key elements of a healthy community:

1. A clean, safe, high-quality environment (including housing quality)
2. An ecosystem that is stable now and sustainable in the long term
3. A strong, mutually supportive, and nonexploitative community
4. A high degree of public participation in and control over the decisions affecting one's life, health, and well-being
5. The meeting of basic needs (food, water, shelter, income, safety, work) for all the city's people
6. Access to a wide variety of experiences and resources, with the possibility of multiple contacts, interaction, and communication
7. A diverse, vital, and innovative city economy
8. Encouragement of connection with the past, cultural and biological heritage, and other groups and individuals
9. A city form that is compatible with and enhances the preceding parameters and behaviors
10. An optimum level of appropriate public health and sick care services accessible to all
11. High health status (both high positive health status and low disease status)

Only one of these eleven refers directly to health status, which is the usual focus of a community health assessment. As Hancock and Duhl contend, a community health assessment is just one component of a healthy community assessment. Furthermore, high positive health status and low mortality and morbidity are not the same. For example, a person can be healthy while dying, or a person who is a quadriplegic can be healthy in the sense that his or her mental and social well-being is high and physical health is as good as it can be.

A good place to begin a healthy community assessment is to consider the classical epidemiological elements of place, time, and person. Here, however, *place* refers to the geography and environment of the community, *time* refers to its history and development, and *person* refers to the demographic profile of the community. There is much that can be learned about the community's health by understanding these aspects of the community. The geography will reveal some of the factors likely to affect health, such as climate, natural resources (especially water and food sources), natural hazards, air and water quality, and wind direction, all of which usually define where low-income populations will live (downwind, downstream, and down-hill—or uphill if the hills are dangerous!). The community's history provides important information about the major economic, political, and social forces that have shaped its evolution and explain many of the present circumstances that influence the health of the community. Finally, the community's present demography (factors such as age and gender distribution and racial-ethnic and socioeconomic characteristics) provides further information that enables us to anticipate some of the health-related issues facing it.

Specific issues can be examined regarding each of the eleven components of a healthy community and others that are considered important by the community.

- Do people in the community have access to such basic prerequisites for health as food, shelter, education, clean water, clean and safe environments, and sustainable resources?
- What is the degree of equity (or inequity) in the community?
- How strong is civic or associational life?
- How do urban design and architecture affect health in this community?
- What is being done to improve health?
- How rich is the cultural life of the community—its artistic, creative, and innovative elements?
- What is the environmental quality of the community, what is its impact on regional and local ecosystems, and what is being done to minimize that impact?
- Does everyone have access to basic primary care?

Several illustrations are useful in demonstrating what such an approach to assessment might look like. The quality-of-life indicators in Pittsburgh, Pennsylvania, for example, include the amount of overcrowded housing, the high school dropout rate, mass transit miles per capita, and the child abuse rate (University of Pittsburgh 1993). Similarly, the "sustainable Seattle" indicators include wild salmon runs through local streams, gallons of water consumed per capita, usage rates for libraries and community centers, and "provocative" indicators (items for which the quality and validity of the data may be in doubt but that make people think, such as the amount of beef eaten per capita compared to the amount of vegetables eaten). Finally, a community in Hawaii identified the presence of Manapua trucks (small fast-food trucks that visit local communities) as an indicator of declining community health for four reasons: they replace home cooking and family dining, the nutritional quality of the food they provide is poor, they make it easier for children to buy cigarettes, and they harm local businesses by undercutting them and taking money out of the community. As these examples suggest, communities can offer thoughtful indexes of local health status.

A healthy community assessment also needs to look at the processes underway in the community that are believed to be related to health and the extent to which health is taken into account or is a focus for action. On the level of the city or formally defined municipality, for example:

- Does the municipal council take health into account in its policy deliberations?
- Is there a mechanism for health impact assessment?
- Do the local planning department and other government bodies understand the affects of planning and design on health?
- Is the economic sector (for example, the chamber of commerce, business improvement associations) part of the process?
- Do businesses understand the importance of health for their activities?
- Do they understand the importance of equitable access to the basic determinants of health for the entire population?
- Are neighborhood and resident groups involved? In what way?
- Are environmental groups and organizations involved? School boards? Faith organizations? The police? Local politicians at all levels of government?

Finally, a healthy community assessment takes the time to determine not only formal leadership at the local level but also those informal leaders who can be identified through methods such as reputational and decisional analysis. The former technique involves having knowledgeable community members formally or informally nominate residents who play a powerful role in community affairs (Israel 1985). The latter technique has informants describe recent community decisions and the roles played by various key participants in actually bringing about those decisions. Among the questions that may to help identify informal leaders are the following (Israel 1985, Minkler and Hancock 2003, Sharpe et al. 2000; see also appendix 1):

- Whom do people in this neighborhood go to for help or advice?
- Whom do children go to?
- When the community has had a problem in the past, who has been involved in working to solve it?
- Who gets things done in the community?

By studying the processes of community action and change on multiple levels and uncovering multiple players in these processes, the healthy community assessment greatly broadens its potential for subsequently involving these diverse stakeholders in building a healthier community.

We have argued so far that several categories of information for and about health are needed for assessment at the local level. These include the following (Hancock 1989):

- People's perceptions of the strengths and resources of their communities as well as their individual and collective health and well-being
- Stories about the formal and informal processes of developing healthy cities and healthy communities
- Data and stories about the community's physical and social environment
- Data and stories about inequities in health and the prerequisites necessary to address these inequities
- Health status data, at the neighborhood or small-area level, incorporating mortality and morbidity data and both subjective and objective assessments of physical, mental, and social well-being

This is a much broader approach than is usually taken when professionals develop a community health status report, which is for the most part concerned with only the last of these categories. A healthy community assessment is much more than a community health assessment.

## How Do We Assess?

Knowing what to assess is only part of the approach to healthy community assessment; we also need to determine how the process can contribute to the health of the community. This question of the process of assessment is vital, requiring that we consider carefully both the type of information that is collected and the degree of contact with the community during the data collection process.

### THE TYPE OF INFORMATION COLLECTED

As McKnight is fond of pointing out, "Institutions learn from studies; communities learn from stories." Just as there is a critical difference between needs assessment and community assessment, important differences exist between the two main

types of information for health on the community level: studies and stories. Studies are usually data-rich and, with the important exception community-based participatory approaches to research (discussed later in the chapter; see also Green
and Mercer 2001, Minkler and Wallerstein 2003), tend to be carried out by academics and professionals working *on* rather than *with* communities. The data are
analyzed to yield information, but the knowledge that is acquired is seldom trans-
the community; and as a result, there is little increase in wisdom. Stories,
nt the accumulated and almost folkloric wisdom of a commu-
knowledge that can be adapted and applied by other com-
ontain information in the form of hard data. Thus, for the
little interest for academics and professionals. But if one accepts
ower and that stories are a means of transferring knowledge
n communities, the empowering potential of stories as a source
out health becomes apparent.
and studies have important roles to play in our efforts to assess
health and well-being at the local level. People can learn much about the health
of their communities by listening to and telling stories, whether around the
kitchen table, at community meetings, through the media, or through events that
celebrate successes or acknowledge loss. More structured means of exchanging stories
can occur, taking the form of newsletters; videos (Chavez et al., in press); collections
of stories (Ontario Healthy Communities Coalition 1994); or workshops at conferences or at regional, national, or international meetings.

Stories can form the basis of studies, with qualitative ethnographic research
often providing a more formal means of listening to and learning from stories.
The work of Penelope Canan (1993) and her colleagues in Molokai, Hawaii, is
illustrative. When the researchers asked villagers what they valued about their
communities, one of the things they identified was the slow pace of life. When
then asked how to measure pace of life, community members suggested count-
ing the number of alarm clocks in each village: if the number of alarm clocks went
up, the villagers were clearly losing their slow pace of life. As this story shows,
people know what is important to them, and they have the ability to identify innovative and meaningful measures that make sense in their own community.
Ethnographic studies and other means of gathering and really listening to people's
stories can provide critical information for an assessment of community health
and well-being.

Of course, quantitative approaches and studies have an important role to play
in assessing communities and community health. Such approaches can provide
documentation of health inequalities within and between communities, which are
often starkly dramatized through studies of infant mortality rates and the like. Quantitative methods often have the advantages of perceived scientific rigor, large denom-
inators, and forms of data analysis that make the findings readily accessible to

policymakers and others who need the numbers to make a case for new legislation or other proposed actions. For quantitative studies to live up to their potential as an empowering community assessment, however, they must transfer information and knowledge to members of the community and, ideally, involve community members in the research process as well. This approach, which in the health field is increasingly termed *community-based participatory research*, is defined by Lawrence Green and his colleagues (in Green and Mercer 2001) as "systematic inquiry, with the participation of those affected by the issue being studied, for the purposes of education and taking action, or effecting social change" (1927).

Two case examples illustrate how we can achieve more empowering and participatory approaches to research. The Grandparent Caregiver Study (Roe et al. 1995), based in Oakland, California, was primarily concerned with exploring, through both quantitative and qualitative measures, the health and social status of African American grandmothers who were raising young children as a consequence of the crack cocaine epidemic. Before any instruments were developed or data collected, however, local community-based organizations were sought out for their input and a community advisory committee established. Consisting primarily of older African American women, the committee was heavily involved in decision making about all aspects of the proposed study, including the topics and questions to be included. Once the initial data were collected, moreover, findings were presented first to the study participants themselves, both verbally and in an easy-to-read, nontechnical report. At a luncheon in their honor, where all but two of the seventy-one study participants were present, the women were consulted about where they wanted to see the information taken and which findings they felt most needed to be highlighted (and in one case, held back) to benefit the community in the best way (Roe et al. 1995).

A similar accent on listening to the community, building its concerns into the research, and then giving back findings to facilitate empowerment appears in the *State of the City* report developed by the Healthy City Office in Toronto, Ontario (Toronto Healthy City Office 1994). The study began by determining what people said was important to the health of the city. The Healthy City Office then collected both data and stories that illustrated the extent to which the city was or was not healthy in the seven areas identified (housing, education, the economy, and so on). In addition to producing a thick report containing many pictures, charts, quotations, and stories, as well as hard data, the office generated a citizen's guide in plain language, containing highlights of the report as well as pertinent questions. The intention was to make the citizen's guide a basis for study circles that would enable residents to ask and discuss questions about the health of their own neighborhood or community as well as the health of the city as a whole.

In short, a balance of studies and stories make up the information needed to assess communities and community health. How this information is collected, the purposes for which it is sought, and whether the findings are then returned to the community play critical roles in determining the empowering potential of the assessment process.

## THE DEGREE OF CONTACT WITH THE COMMUNITY

Numerous techniques and approaches can be employed to obtain the types of information needed, and a comprehensive list is beyond the scope of this chapter. A helpful framework for thinking about these alternative methods, however, is provided in Marti-Costa and Serrano-Garcia's (1983) suggestion that assessment techniques be grouped into categories defined by the extent to which they involve contact between the outside professional and members of the community. Since contact with and high-level involvement of community residents in the assessment process are vital parts of community organizing and community building for health, special attention should be given to methods that foster community involvement and consciousness raising as part of the assessment process. At the same time, as already noted, the utility of studies that produce hard data, including some that may involve no-contact or minimal-contact methods, should be considered.

NO-CONTACT METHODS. Demographic and social indicators, such as divorce and unemployment rates and morbidity and mortality statistics, are often the first types of data looked at by health professionals charged with conducting a community needs assessment. Presented in the form of rates and percentages, small-area analyses, or dynamic modeling, studies using such data often have the advantages of a large numerical base or a representative sample and an aura of scientific objectivity. No-contact methods such as multivariate analysis can document factors such as the influence of race and class on mortality rates in neighboring communities, thus providing information that may be vital in demonstrating health inequalities in a format that legislators and advocacy groups can use in fighting for health resources.

But use of such methods is based on the assumption that "the community needs and problems that appear in official statistics are representative of community problems" (Marti-Costa and Serrano-Garcia 1983, 81). That assumption, of course, is not always warranted. Statistics on mental health treatment, for example, may indicate a dramatic change in the types of mental illnesses in a given community when what, in fact, has changed are the service categories for which mental health agencies receive funding. Mental health professionals thus may simply be labeling what they see creatively in order to continue treating persons they believe to be in need.

In addition to statistical studies, no-contact methods often include document reviews, with pertinent documents including community newspapers or newsletters, written progress reports from health departments or other agencies, and community bulletin boards, whose contents may offer a taste of the kinds of issues and resources represented in a given community. Like outside collection of health and other demographic and social indicator data, such methods, when used without community involvement, lack the potential to facilitate local empowerment or mobilization.

Increasingly, however, the term *no-contact methods* is becoming something of a misnomer. With the advent of accessible computer technology, for example, opportunities are expanding for community members to be involved in the collection and use of data that were formerly within the exclusive purview of researchers and health professionals. Resources such as the Community Tool Box (http://ctb.ku.edu), which includes more than six thousand pages of how-to information to assist communities and professionals in issue identification and a host of other areas are among a wealth of new Internet-based systems that greatly enhance the ability of local communities to effectively study, mobilize around, and address shared concerns (see chapter 18). By helping community members become conversant with such tools and their applications in the assessment process, professionals can greatly expand the empowering potential of many so-called no-contact methods.

MINIMAL-CONTACT OBSERVATIONAL METHODS. A variety of observational methods may be useful for the health professional who wishes to gain some early impressionistic sense of the community with which he or she will be working. One such technique involves the initial use of a neighborhood "windshield tour" or walk-through. Using this approach, the health educator or other social change professional walks or drives slowly through a neighborhood, ideally on different days of the week and at different times of the day, on the lookout for a variety of potentially useful indicators of community health and well-being. As described in appendix 1, observing the condition of houses and automobiles, the nature and degree of activity level, social interaction among residents, and similar indicators can provide valuable impressionistic information (Eng and Blanchard 1990–91), as can sitting in a neighborhood coffee shop or observing at a community forum or a PTA meeting. Looking at the content of bulletin boards in community centers, libraries, faith-based organization buildings, and local stores or the public notices stapled to utility poles or fences also can provide valuable clues to local hot issues in the community (Minkler and Hancock 2003, Sharpe et al. 2000).

As in the case of no-contact methods, minimal-contact approaches increasingly are being used in ways that promote community involvement and hold the potential for facilitating empowerment. Health department–sponsored efforts such as the Healthy Neighborhood Project described in chapter 14 (see also El-Askari et al. 1998), for example, train neighborhood residents to use walk-throughs, asset mapping (see chapter 9), and other techniques, viewing their community through fresh eyes as they gather impressionistic data, which then can be shared and compared with that of other members of the assessment team. Once again, if our goal in community assessment is not solely to stimulate, monitor, and assess the impact of change but also to further empowerment, exploiting opportunities for increased community contact and involvement is critical.

INTERACTIVE CONTACT METHODS. This category of methods includes techniques such as key informant interviews, door-to-door surveys, and a variety of small-group methods for eliciting data and stories about a local community. Included in this last approach are three methods that particularly deserve mention. The first, discussed in detail in chapter 12, is Paulo Freire's (1973) education for critical consciousness. Using a problem-posing method, group members are asked questions that cause them to reflect critically on their lives and the life of their community. The generative themes that emerge from this process and that capture the hopes and concerns of the people frequently offer rich insights into group members' assessments of community and community health.

A second small-group method with particular utility in community assessment is Andre Delbecq and colleagues' (1975) nominal group process. A structured process designed to foster creativity, encourage conflicting opinions, and prevent domination by a few vocal individuals, the nominal group method is especially helpful in encouraging the participation of marginal group members.

The third approach, the focus group, holds perhaps the greatest current appeal among small-group methods used in community assessment. The focus group brings together, under the direction of a professional moderator, a small group of community members who, in a confidential and nonthreatening discussion, address a series of questions concerning their feelings about their community (Krueger and Casey 2000). Employed by health agencies, philanthropic foundations, community-based organizations, and local policymakers, focus groups have considerable potential for providing the stories and perceptions that can greatly enrich the overall community assessment. A number of other contact methods lend themselves to use with either small or larger groups, and two of them—photovoice (Wang 1999) and community asset mapping (Kretzmann and McKnight 1993)—are discussed later in the book (in chapters 19 and 9, respectively).

Another increasingly popular method, however, involves working collaboratively with communities to develop community health indicators (CHIs) that characterize a neighborhood or a community as a whole rather than simply the individuals or subgroups of which it is comprised (Cheadle et al. 1992, Hancock et al. 1999). As Donald L. Patrick and Thomas M. Wickizer (1995) suggest, such indicators take several forms and may be thought of as "a community analogue to health-risk appraisal for individuals" (72). The number, type and visibility of no-smoking signs in workplaces; the proportion of space in grocery stores devoted to low-fat foods (Patrick and Wickizer 1995); and the proportion of a community's children under age two with up-to-date immunizations all are examples of potent community health indicators.

A limited set of quantitative and qualitative measures which indicate the current health status of the community, CHIs can also suggest how the community's health status, broadly defined, is changing over time (Bauer 2003). Hancock and his colleagues (1999) suggest that good community indicators should reflect both health determinants (such as environmental quality and social cohesion) and process dimensions (such as education and civil rights). Finally, to be relevant to both policymakers and the general public, community indicators should have several key qualities (Hancock et al. 1999):

- Face validity: they make sense to people
- Theoretical and empirical validity: they measure an important health determinant or dimension
- Social value: they measure things people care about
- Valency: they are powerful and carry social and political punch

Many of these considerations were demonstrated in the community indicators project coordinated by Georg Bauer (2003) and involving a community-based organization in Oakland, California (the Community Health Academy); community residents; and representatives of the county health department and the University of California at Berkeley's School of Public Health. Meeting monthly as a small working group and guided by theoretical frameworks from community organizing and ecological perspectives on community health and sustainability, the group developed an initial list of ten categories of indicators, with more specific indicators under each. "Intention to stay in the neighborhood" thus was used as an indicator of "community attraction," while "street violence" appeared under "community health and safety." These indicators, in turn, were used as the basis of a community survey in which residents were asked to indicate both their level of concern about each given item and their level of interest in taking action. Findings such as the fact that almost three-quarters of residents assigned high importance to "street violence" and that more than half reported high interest in action on this item (Bauer 2003) helped point the way toward subsequent issue selection and community mobilization.

Throughout this chapter we have reinforced the importance of asking—and having community members ask themselves—the kinds of questions that provoke meaningful discussion about community, health, and healthy communities. Whether in the context of focus groups or key informant interviews or as part of large town hall meetings or community dialogues, such questions might include the following (Minkler and Hancock 2003, Sharpe et al. 2000; see also appendix 1):

- What do you like best about living in this community?
- What would you like to see changed?
- Is this a good place to raise children? Why or why not?
- Do people in the neighborhood socialize with one another often? Do you socialize with others here?
- If youth get into a fight in this community, are adult residents likely to intervene?
- How would you characterize the relationship between members of different racial or ethnic groups in the neighborhood?
- Who gets things done?

Questions like these often generate a wealth of initial data and stories about a community and also may help identify a core group of informal leaders who then may be brought together, engaged in a similar dialogue, and encouraged to be key participants in a community organizing or community building project (see appendix 1). The results of such data collection may be presented either in narrative form or in charts and graphs that summarize key findings (Minkler and Hancock 2003, Sharpe et al. 2000). As already suggested, however, the richest and most honest answers may emerge when local residents themselves conduct the interviews and then help analyze the results.

Although contact methods, by definition, involve community residents, their potential for truly facilitating empowerment depends on how these methods are employed. Focus groups and key informant interviews, for example, can be disempowering if they only seek information about community needs and problems and ignore or discount participants' knowledge of their community's resources and assets. In contrast, you can contribute to community capacity building when you ask questions that encourage residents to reflect on and contribute to a broader understanding of community strengths. Question such as "What are the things you like best about your community?" "What makes this a good or healthy community in which to live?" and "How have people here come together in the past to make a decision or solve a problem?" are among those that can help residents think positively about the strengths of their communities. Community asset mapping techniques, as described in chapter 9, similarly represent a powerful means for community members to work together in identifying the strengths and potential building blocks of their neighborhood, not merely its problems and deficiencies. By revealing an outsider's appreciation of the community and engaging informants in a process of thinking critically about the strengths and competencies of their community, such techniques and questions can make a real difference in the information obtained and in the community's willingness to be actively involved in the assessment process.

MULTIMETHOD ASSESSMENT. Clearly, no one method or approach to community assessment can capture the richness and complexity of communities and community health. A strong case should therefore be made for the use of multiple methods—what researchers refer to as *triangulation*. The CDC's PATCH model (Kreuter 1992) and the collaboratively developed *Assessment Protocol for Excellence in Public Health* (APEXPH) (1991) both include elaborate multimethod approaches to community assessment as a precursor to action plans for addressing priority health issues. Directed respectively to state and local health departments, both models emphasize the collection of hard data on a community's health status and needs, information on health department organizational capacity, and community participation in the identification of health issues and community resources and in the development of health promotion strategies (Nelson 2001).

The promise of methods such as PATCH and APEXPH has not always been fully realized. In an early PATCH application in Chicago, for example, a community opinion survey's finding that violence and drugs were of major concern to residents was put on the back burner by health professionals so that they might attend to the problem of heart disease, for which funding was available (Bogan et al. 1992). Similarly, Marshall Kreuter (1995) notes that, in a few PATCH sites, what was being called community participation "was often a collection of health officials and formal interest groups talking to one another, with little or no attention being paid to the perceived needs of those they were supposed to be serving" (7).

Partially in response to such concerns, the National Association of County and City Health Officials (NACCHO) worked collaboratively with the CDC to develop a new approach known as Mobilizing for Action through Planning and Partnerships (MAPP) (http://www.naccho.org/tools.chm). Using this strategic planning tool, public health leaders help communities prioritize public health issues as well as resources for addressing them. Case vignettes, as well as a variety of user-friendly assessment techniques and resources, are available at the web site for those wishing to apply this multimethod approach.

On a more modest scale, the assessment component of Ronald L. Braithwaite and colleagues' (1994) community organization and development (COD) approach for health promotion offers a useful multimethod strategy. Specifically designed to foster community empowerment in low-income communities of color, the COD model stresses participatory ethnography through which community members are involved with outside health educators in developing a systematic description of the health needs and resources of their neighborhoods. Personal interviews, surveys, videotaped documentation of the perceptions of local leaders, and focus groups designed to identify and prioritize health concerns are among the methods used. The development of a community resource inventory and the conducting of community forums are among the participatory activities included in this component of the assessment.

But the COD approach also includes the obtaining of geographic and demographic information from local community planning and development agencies, including block statistical maps identifying census tracks and a variety of health indicator data. The result is a rich portrait of a community and its health profile and priorities, which then serves as the basis for community action and change (Braithwaite et al. 1994). Regardless of the scale on which a community assessment is conducted, it is likely to be most effective if it combines multiple methods, respects both stories and studies, and places its heaviest emphasis on eliciting high-level community participation throughout the assessment process.

## Conclusion

This chapter has built on the ideological framework provided by Marti-Costa and Serrano-Garcia (1983), as well as on more recent insights developed through the Healthy Cities Movement, to propose an empowering approach to community assessment for health. Both stories and studies are vital if we are to stimulate, monitor, and assess the impact of change and at the same time facilitate the empowerment that comes with knowledge, specifically with the transfer of knowledge to communities. Likewise, no single assessment tool or technique is sufficient in and of itself to capture community or community health sensitively and accurately. That is better accomplished by multiple methods, especially those that empower individuals and communities while making explicit the realities of the community, its resources, and its health.

### References

*Assessment Protocol for Excellence in Public Health.* 1991. Washington D.C.: Centers for Disease Control and the National Association of County Health Officials.

Bauer, G. 2003. "Sample Community Health Indicators on the Neighborhood Level." In *Community Based Participatory Research for Health*, edited by M. Minkler and N. Wallerstein, 438–45. San Francisco: Jossey-Bass.

Bogan, G., III, A. Omar, S. Knobloch, L. Liburd, and T. O'Rourke. 1992. "Organizing an Urban African-American Community for Health Promotion: Lessons from Chicago." *Journal of Health Education* 23, no. 3: 157–59.

Braithwaite, R. L., Bianchi, and S. E. Taylor. 1994. "Ethnographic Approach to Community Organization and Health Empowerment." *Health Education Quarterly* 21, no. 3: 407–16.

Braithwaite, R. L., S. E. Taylor, and J. N. Austin. 2000. *Building Health Coalitions in the Black Community.* Thousand Oaks, Calif.: Sage.

Canan, P. 1993. Presentation at Emory University/CDC workshop on quality-of-life indicators, Atlanta, Georgia.

Chavez, V., B. A. Israel, A. Allen, R. Lichtenstein, M. DeCarlo, A. Schulz, et al. In press. "A Bridge between Communities: Video-Making Using Principles of Community-Based Participatory Research." *Journal of Health Promotion Practice.*

Cheadle, A., E. A. Wagner, T. D. Koepsell, A. Kristal, and D. Patrick. 1992. "Environmental Indicators: A Tool for Evaluating Community-Based Health Promotion Programs." *American Journal of Preventive Medicine* 8, no. 6: 345–50.

Delbecq, A., A. H. Van de Ven, and D. H. Gustafson. 1975. *Group Techniques for Program Planning: A Guide to Nominal Group and Delphi Processes*. Glenview, Ill.: Scott, Foresman.

Duhl, L., and T. Hancock. 1988. *A Guide to Assessing Healthy Cities*. Copenhagen: FADL.

El-Askari, G., J. Freestone, C. Irizarry, K. L. Kraut, S. T. Mashiyama, M. A. Morgan, and S. Walton. 1998. "The Healthy Neighborhoods Project: A Local Health Department's Role in Catalyzing Community Development." *Health Education and Behavior* 25, no. 2: 146–59.

Eng, E., and L. Blanchard. 1990–91. "Action-Oriented Community Diagnosis: A Health Education Tool." *International Journal of Community Health Education* 11, no. 2: 93–110.

Freire, P. 1973. *Education for critical consciousness*. New York: Seabury.

Green, L. W., and S. L. Mercer. 2001. "Can Public Health Researchers and Agencies Reconcile the Push from Funding Bodies and the Pull from Communities?" *American Journal of Public Health* 91, no. 12: 1926–29.

Hancock, T. 1989. "Information for Health at the Local Level: Community Stories and Healthy City Indicators." Unpublished paper.

Hancock, T., and L. Duhl. 1986. *Healthy Cities: Promoting Health in the Urban Context*. Copenhagen: World Health Organization Europe.

Hancock, T., R. Labonte, and R. Edwards. 1999. "Indicators That Count! Measuring Population Health at the Community Level." *Canadian Journal of Public Health* 90, supp. 1: 22–26.

Israel, B. A. 1985. "Social Networks and Social Support: Implications for Natural Helper and Community Level Interventions." *Health Education Quarterly* 12, no. 1: 65–80.

Kirsch, I. S., A. Jungeblut, L. Jenkins, and A. Kolstad. 1993. *Adult Literacy in America: A First Look at the Results of the National Adult Literacy Survey*. Washington, D.C.: U.S. Department of Education, National Center for Education Statistics.

Kretzmann, J. P., and J. L. McKnight. 1993. *Building Communities from the Inside Out: A Path toward Finding and Mobilizing a Community's Assets*. Evanston, Ill.: Center for Urban Affairs and Policy Research.

Kreuter, M. 1992. "PATCH: Its Origins, Basic Concepts, and Links to Contemporary Public Health Policy." *Journal of Health Education* 23, no. 3: 135–39.

———. 1995. "A Brief, Biased, and Limited History of Community-Based Strategies to Prevent and Control Chronic Disease." Paper presented at the National Chronic Disease Conference, Atlanta, December 7.

Krueger, R. A., and M. A. Casey. 2000. *Focus Groups: A Practical Guide for Applied Research*. 3d ed. Newbury Park, Calif.: Sage.

Marti-Costa, S., and I. Serrano-Garcia. 1983. "Needs Assessment and Community Development: An Ideological Perspective." *Prevention in Human Services* 2, no. 4: 75–88.

Minkler, M., and T. Hancock. 2003. "Community-Driven Asset Identification and Issue Selection." In *Community Based Participatory Research for Health*, edited by M. Minkler and N. Wallerstein, 135–54. San Francisco.: Jossey-Bass.

Minkler, M., and N. Wallerstein, eds. 2003. *Community Based Participatory Research for Health*. San Francisco: Jossey-Bass.

Nelson, J. O. 2001. "Community Health Assessment and Improvement." In *Community Health Education Methods: A Practitioner's Guide*, edited by R. J. Bensley and J. Brookins-Fisher, 1–18. Boston: Jones and Bartlett.

Ontario Healthy Communities Coalition. 1994. *Stories to Guide Action*. Toronto: Ontario Healthy Communities Coalition.

Patrick, D. L., and T. M. Wickizer. 1995. "Community and Health." In *Society and Health*, edited by B. C. Amick, S. Levine, A. R. Tarlov, and D. C. Walsh, 46–92. New York: Oxford University Press.

Putnam, R. 2000. *Bowling Alone: The Collapse and Revival of American Community*. New York: Simon and Schuster.

Roe, K. M., M. Minkler, and F. F. Saunders. 1995. "Combining Research, Advocacy, and Education: The Methods of the Grandparent Caregiver Study." *Health Education Quarterly* 22, no. 4: 458–75.

Sharpe, P.A., M. L. Greany, P. R. Lee, and S. W. Royce. 2000. "Assets-Oriented Community Assessment." *Public Health Reports* 113, nos. 2 and 3: 205–11.

Toronto Healthy City Office. 1994. *The State of the City.* Toronto: Beacon.

University of Pittsburgh. 1993. *Pittsburgh Benchmarks: Quality-of-Life Indices for the City of Pittsburgh and Allegheny County.* Pittsburgh: University Center for Social and Urban Research.

Wang, C. C. 1999. "Photovoice: A Participatory Action Research Strategy Applied to Women's Health." *Journal of Women's Health* 8, no. 2: 185–92.

World Health Organization (WHO). 1948. *Constitution of the World Health Organization.* New York, April 7.

———. 1986. *Ottawa Charter for Health Promotion.* Copenhagen: World Health Organization Europe.

JOHN L. McKNIGHT
JOHN P. KRETZMANN

| Chapter 9 | Mapping Community Capacity |
|---|---|

No ONE CAN DOUBT that our older cities these days are deeply troubled places. At the root of the problem are the massive economic shifts that have marked the past two decades. Hundreds of thousands of industrial jobs have either disappeared or moved away from the central city and its neighborhoods. And while many downtown areas have experienced a renaissance, the jobs created there are different from those that once sustained neighborhoods. Either these new jobs are highly professionalized and require elaborate education and credentials for entry, or they are routine, low-paying service jobs without much of a future. If effect, these shifts in the economy, and particularly the disappearance of decent employment possibilities in low-income neighborhoods, have removed the bottom rung from the fabled American ladder of opportunity. For many people in older city neighborhoods, new approaches to rebuilding their lives and communities, and new openings toward opportunity, are vital.

### Traditional Needs-Oriented Solutions

Given the desperate situation, it is no surprise that most Americans think of lower-income urban neighborhoods as problems—areas noted for deficiencies and needs. This view is accepted by most elected officials, who codify and program this perspective through deficiency-oriented policies and programs. Then human service systems—often supported by foundations and universities—translate the programs into local activities that teach people the nature of their problems and the value of services as the answer to their problems. As a result, many low-income urban neighborhoods are now environments of service where behaviors are affected because residents have come to believe that their well-being depends upon being a client. They see themselves as people with special needs to be met by outsiders. And gradually, they become mainly consumers of services with no incentive to be producers. Consumers of services focus vast amounts of creativity and intelligence on the survival-motivated challenge of outwitting the system or on finding ways—in the informal or even illegal economy—to bypass the system entirely.

There is nothing natural about this process. Indeed, it is the predictable course of events when deficiency- and needs-oriented programs come to dominate the lives of neighborhoods where low-income people reside.

## The Capacity-Focused Alternative

The alternative is to develop policies and activities based on the capacities, skills, and assets of low-income people and their neighborhoods. There are two reasons for this capacity-oriented emphasis. First, all the historic evidence indicates that significant community development takes place only when local community people are committed to investing themselves and their resources in the effort. This is why you can't develop communities from the top down or from the outside in. You can, however, provide valuable outside assistance to communities that are actively developing their own assets.

Second, there is little prospect that large-scale industrial or service corporations will locate in these low-income neighborhoods. Nor is it likely that significant new injections of federal money will be forthcoming soon. Therefore, it is increasingly futile to wait for significant help to arrive from outside the community. The hard truth is that development must start from within the community; and in most of our urban neighborhoods, there is no other choice.

Unfortunately, the dominance of the deficiency-oriented social service model has led many people in low-income neighborhoods to think in terms of local needs rather than assets. These needs are often identified, quantified, and mapped in needs surveys. The result is a map of the neighborhood's illiteracy, teenage pregnancy, criminal activity, drug use, and so on.

But in neighborhoods that include effective community development efforts, there is also a map of the community's assets, capacities, and abilities. For it is clear that even the poorest city neighborhood is a place where individuals and organizations represent resources upon which to rebuild. The key to neighborhood regeneration is not only to build upon those resources that the community already controls but to harness those that are not yet available for local development purposes.

The process of identifying capacities and assets, both individual and organizational, is the first step on the path toward community regeneration. Once this new map has replaced the one containing needs and deficiencies, the regenerating community can begin to assemble its assets and capacities into new combinations, new structures of opportunity, new sources of income and control, and new possibilities for production.

## Mapping the Building Blocks for Regeneration

It is useful to begin by recognizing that not all community assets are equally available for community-building purposes. Some are more accessible than others. The most easily accessible assets, or building blocks, are located in the neighborhood and controlled by those who live there. The next most accessible are those assets that are located in the neighborhood but controlled elsewhere. The least accessible are those located outside the neighborhood and controlled by outsiders. Therefore, we will map community assets based upon the accessibility of assets to local people.

### PRIMARY BUILDING BLOCKS:
### ASSETS AND CAPACITIES IN THE NEIGHBORHOOD,
### LARGELY UNDER NEIGHBORHOOD CONTROL

This cluster of capacities includes those that are most readily available for neighborhood regeneration. They fall into two general categories: the assets and capacities of individuals and those of organizations or associations. The first step in capturing any of these resources is to assess them, which often involves making an inventory.

INDIVIDUAL CAPACITIES.   Our greatest assets are our people. But people in low-income neighborhoods are seldom regarded as assets. Instead, they are usually seen as needy and deficient, suited best for life as clients and recipients of services. Therefore, they are often subjected to systematic and repeated inventories of their deficiencies with a device called a needs survey.

The starting point for any serious development effort takes the opposite approach. Instead, there must be an opportunity for individuals to use their own abilities to produce. Identifying the variety and richness of skills, talents, knowledge, and experience of people in low-income neighborhoods provides a base upon which to build new approaches and enterprises.

To begin identifying the skills and abilities of individuals, organizers can develop an inventory of capacities—a simple survey designed to identify the multitude of abilities within each individual. Neighborhood residents have used capacity inventories to identify the talents available to start new enterprises. For example, people have begun a new association of home health care providers and a catering business. Public housing residents in a number of cities have formed local corporations to take over the management of their developments. They immediately needed to identify the skills and abilities of neighbors in order to be effective. The capacity inventory provided the necessary information, allowing people to become producers rather than problems.

PERSONAL INCOME.  Another vital asset of individuals is their income. It is generally assumed that low-income neighborhoods are poor markets. Some studies suggest, however, that people have much more income per capita than observers often assume. Nonetheless, it is often used in ways that do not support local economic development. Therefore, effective local development groups can inventory the income, savings, and expenditure patterns of their neighborhoods. This information is basic to understanding the neighborhood economy and developing new approaches to capturing local wealth for local development.

THE GIFTS OF LABELED PEOPLE.  Even the most marginalized individuals have rich potential waiting to be identified. Human service systems have labeled these people *retarded, mentally ill, disabled, elderly,* and so on. They are likely to be dependent on service systems, excluded from community life, and considered burdens rather than assets to community life.

In recent years, a growing number of unique community efforts have incorporated these labeled people into local organizations, enterprises, and community associations (O'Connell 1988a, Walsh 1997). Their gifts and abilities have been identified and the people introduced to groups who value these contributions. The results have been amazing: the underdeveloped hospitality of neighborhood people has been rediscovered; and the gifts, contributions, and capacities of even the most disabled people have been revealed.

INDIVIDUAL LOCAL BUSINESSES.  The shops, stores, and businesses that survive in low-income neighborhoods—especially those smaller enterprises owned and operated by individual local residents—are often more than economic ventures. They are usually centers for community life as well. Any comprehensive approach to community regeneration will inventory these enterprises and incorporate the energies and resources of these entrepreneurs into neighborhood development processes. The experience and insight of these individuals might also be shared with local not-for-profit groups and students.

HOME-BASED ENTERPRISES.  It is fairly simple to inventory the shops, stores, and businesses in low-income neighborhoods. But as neighborhoods become lower income, informal and home-based enterprises often increase. Local development groups have begun to make an effort to understand the nature of these individual entrepreneurs and their enterprises. After gathering information about them, development groups can identify the factors that initiated such enterprises and the additional capital or technical assistance that could increase their profits and the number of people they support.

## ASSOCIATIONAL AND ORGANIZATIONAL CAPACITIES

Beyond individual capacities are a wide range of local resident–controlled associations and organizations. The following is an initial inventory.

CITIZENS' ASSOCIATIONS. In addition to businesses and enterprises, low-income communities have a variety of clubs and associations that do vital work in assuring productive neighborhoods. These groups might include service clubs, fraternal organizations, women's organizations, artistic groups, and athletic clubs (see appendix 1). They are the infrastructure of working neighborhoods. Those involved in the community building process can inventory the variety of these groups in their neighborhoods, the unique community activities they support, and their potential to assume a broader set of responsibilities (O'Connell 1988b). Then these groups can become part of the local asset development process or perhaps affiliate in other ways (for example, by creating a congress of neighborhood associations).

ASSOCIATIONS OF BUSINESSES. In many older neighborhoods, local business people are not organized. Where they are organized, they are not informed about effective joint partnerships in neighborhood economic development. Connecting local businesses with each other and expanding their vision of self-interest in community development are major efforts of effective community building activities.

FINANCIAL INSTITUTIONS. Relatively few older neighborhoods have a community-oriented financial institution, such as a bank, a savings institution, or a credit union. But where they do exist, they are invaluable assets.

One ambitious and successful example of a locally controlled financial institution is the South Shore Bank in Chicago. The bank has been a continuing experiment in how to capture local savings and convert them to local residential and commercial development. A related effort in Bangladesh, called the Gameen Bank, is a successful experiment in very small capitalization for small community enterprises. Similar experiments involving credit unions are taking place in the United States. All of these inventions are new tools to capture local wealth for local development. Their presence or potential is a central resource for the future of a developing community.

CULTURAL ORGANIZATIONS. People in low-income neighborhoods are increasingly giving public expression to their rich cultural inheritance. Celebrating the history of the neighborhood, and the peoples who have gathered there, is central to forming a community identity and countering the negative images that originate outside the community. Neighborhood history fairs; block and neighborhood celebrations featuring the foods, music, dancing, and games of diverse peoples; cross-cultural discussions and classes; oral history projects; theatrical productions based on oral histories—all hold great potential for building strong relationships among residents and for regaining definitional control of the community. In many neighborhoods, local artists are central to the creation of these expressions.

COMMUNICATIONS ORGANIZATIONS. Strong neighborhoods rely heavily on their capacity to exchange information and engage in discussions. Neighborhood newspapers, particularly those controlled by local residents, are invaluable public forums. So, too, are less comprehensive media such as newsletters, fliers, even bulletin boards. In addition, both local-access cable TV and local radio hold promise as vehicles relevant to community building.

RELIGIOUS ORGANIZATIONS. Finally, any list of organizational assets in communities would be woefully incomplete without the local expressions of religious life. Local parishes, congregations, and temples have involved themselves increasingly in the community building agenda, sometimes through community organizations or community development groups, sometimes simply by building on the strengths of their own members and networks. In fact, the ability of local religious institutions to call upon related external organizations for support and resources constitutes a very important asset.

SUMMARY. In summary, then, the primary building blocks include those community assets that are most readily available for rebuilding the neighborhood. These involve both individual and organizational strengths. Our initial list includes

| *Individual Assets* | *Organizational Assets* |
|---|---|
| Skills, talents, and experience of residents | Associations of businesses |
| Individual businesses | Citizens associations |
| Home-based enterprises | Cultural organizations |
| Personal income | Communications organizations |
| Gifts of labeled people | Religious organizations |

## SECONDARY BUILDING BLOCKS:
## ASSETS IN THE COMMUNITY,
## LARGELY CONTROLLED BY OUTSIDERS

Although the people who live in the neighborhood possess much individual and associational capacity, other kinds of capacity are directed and controlled from outside, even though they are physically part of the community,. To capture these assets for community building purposes, neighborhood actors not only conduct inventories but construct strategies designed to enhance the regenerative uses of these assets. The examples that follow fall into three categories: private and not-for-profit organizations, public institutions and services, and other physical resources.

### PRIVATE AND NONPROFIT ORGANIZATIONS

*Institutions of higher education.* Private and public junior colleges, colleges, and universities remain in, or adjacent to, many older urban neighborhoods; but they are often quite detached from the local community. Community building groups are creating new experiments with partnerships in community development between local institutions of higher education and those who are mobilizing community capacities.

*Hospitals.* Next to public schools, hospitals are the most prevalent major institution remaining in many older neighborhoods. They are a tremendous reserve of assets and resources to support initiatives in community enterprise. In a few cases, hospitals have created innovative local partnerships. Creative development groups are exploring the nature of the development assets controlled by their local hospitals.

*Social service agencies.* Although they are often dedicated to the delivery of individual service to clients (an activity that does not necessarily contribute to community building), local social service agencies do have the potential to introduce capacity-oriented strategies to their programs. Many, in fact, have begun to see economic development and job creation as appropriate activities, while others have entered into networks and partnerships with community organizations and neighborhood development groups for community building purposes.

### PUBLIC INSTITUTIONS AND SERVICES

Of the range of public institutions and services that exist in low-income communities, a few deserve to be highlighted for their community building potential.

*Public schools.* Big-city schools have often become so separate from local community initiatives that they are a liability rather than an asset. The Carnegie Commission on Public Education has said that the primary educational failing of the local public school is its separation from the work and life of the community. Therefore, localities need to teach their schools how to improve their educational function by connecting themselves to community development efforts. As an integral part of community life rather than an institution set apart, the local public school can begin to function as a set of economic and human resources aimed at regenerating the community (McKnight 1987).

*Police.* As with all other local institutions, the police need to participate in the neighborhood revitalization enterprise. Much of the hesitation surrounding new investment of all kinds relates to issues of security. Therefore, local police officials should be asked to join the asset development team, acting as advisers to and resources for development projects. In a number of instances, responsive police departments have joined forces with local community organizations and other groups to devise and carry out joint safety and anticrime strategies.

*Fire departments.* In both small towns and large cities, the local fire department boasts a tradition of consistent interaction with the community. Because of the sporadic nature of their important work, firefighters are often available for a variety of activities in the neighborhood. Retrieving and building upon that tradition are important strategies for community building.

*Libraries.* Many older neighborhoods contain branches of the public library, often underfunded and underused. But when seen as not only a repository for books and periodicals but also the center of a neighborhood's flow of information, the library becomes a potentially critical participant in community regeneration. For example, neighborhoods that choose to enter into a community planning process will need localized information on which to base their deliberations. The availability of library-based personal computers can enhance access to a variety of relevant data bases. The library can also provide space for community meetings and initiate community history and cultural projects.

*Parks.* In many low-income communities, the local parks have fallen into disrepair and are often considered uninviting and even dangerous. But when local citizens organize themselves to reclaim these areas, they can be restored not only physically but functionally. As symbols of community accomplishment, they can become sources of pride and centers for important informal relationship building. Often, groups of existing associations will take joint responsibility for renewing and maintaining a local park.

PHYSICAL RESOURCES

Besides the private and public institutions in the neighborhood, a variety of physical assets are available. In fact, many of the most visible problems of low-income neighborhoods, when looked at from an asset-centered perspective, become opportunities instead. A few examples follow.

*Vacant land, vacant commercial and industrial structures, vacant housing.* The vacant lots in older urban neighborhoods are often seen as blights, as are empty industrial and commercial sites and buildings. In some U.S. cities, however, local groups have found creative and productive methods to regenerate the usefulness of both the land and the buildings. They identify potential new uses, create tools to inventory and plan for local reuses, and organize the redevelopment process. Similarly, abandoned housing structures are often structurally sound enough to be candidates for locally controlled rehabilitation efforts.

*Energy and waste resources.* The costs of energy and waste collection are relentless resource drains in older neighborhoods. As their costs escalate, they demand a disproportionate and growing share of the limited income of poorer people. As a result, maintenance of housing is often foregone, and deterioration speeds up. But in some neighborhoods, this problem has become an opportunity. New local enterprises are developing to reduce energy use and costs and to recycle waste for profit. These initiatives need to be identified, nurtured, and replicated.

SUMMARY

These secondary building blocks are private, public, and physical assets, which can be brought under community control and used for community building purposes. Our initial list includes

| *Private and Nonprofit Organizations* | *Public Institutions and Services* |
| --- | --- |
| Higher education institutions | Public schools |
| Hospitals | Police |
| Social service agencies | Libraries |
| | Fire departments |
| | Parks |

*Physical Resources*

Vacant land, commercial and industrial structures, housing
Energy and waste resources

### POTENTIAL BUILDING BLOCKS:
### RESOURCES OUTSIDE THE NEIGHBORHOOD,
### CONTROLLED BY OUTSIDERS

In this final cluster are resource streams that originate outside the neighborhood but might be captured for community building purposes. There is a sense in which all local public expenditures are potential investments in development. In low-income neighborhoods, however, they are usually expenditures for the maintenance of an impoverished area and unemployed individuals. We need tools and models for converting public expenditures into local development investments. In addition to the public institutions just cited, two other public expenditures are critical.

WELFARE EXPENDITURES. In Cook County, Illinois, thousands of dollars are expended annually by government for low-income programs for every man, woman, and child whose income falls below the official poverty line. This substantial investment is distributed so that, on a per capita basis, poor people receive the disproportionate share of this money in the form of services rather than as actual income. This creates an impoverished family dependent on services. Creative community groups are developing new experiments in which some of these welfare dollars are reinvested in enterprise development and independence.

PUBLIC CAPITAL-IMPROVEMENT EXPENDITURES. Every neighborhood is the site of substantial infrastructure investments. In downtown areas, these dollars leverage private investment. In neighborhoods, the same funds are usually applied only to maintenance functions. Effective community development groups are creating experiments to convert local capital improvement funds into development dollars.

PUBLIC INFORMATION. Wherever we have seen community innovation in local neighborhoods, the people there have had to gain access to information not normally available. What is the vacancy ratio in the worst buildings? How many teachers have skills that could help our development corporation? When do the crimes occur that threaten our shopping center? How much property is off the tax rolls? What does the city plan to invest in capital improvements? Unfortunately, most useful development planning data are collected for the use of downtown systems. But as neighborhoods become responsible for their future, information must be decoded and decentralized for local use. Some neighborhoods have done pioneering work in developing methods to translate systems data into neighborhood information. This neighborhood information is an invaluable asset in the development process.

SUMMARY. These potential building blocks include major public assets, which ambitious neighborhoods might begin to divert to community building purposes. At the beginning, at least, they include the following:

Welfare expenditures
Public capital information expenditures
Public information

## Two Community Maps

This chapter begins to map the assets that exist in every neighborhood and town. It is a new map that can guide us toward community regeneration. But there is another map, an old map of neighborhood deficiencies and problems. As we noted at the outset, it is a needs-oriented neighborhood map created by needs surveys. This is a powerful map, teaching people in low-income neighborhoods how to think about themselves and the place where they live.

The needs-oriented map is initiated by groups with power and resources that ask neighborhood people to think of themselves in terms of deficiencies in order to access the resources controlled by these groups. Among the groups that ask neighborhood people to inventory their problems, needs, and deficiencies are government agencies, foundations, universities, United Ways, and the mass media. Indeed, the institutions that produce this map not only teach people in low-income neighborhoods that their needs, problems, and deficiencies are valuable. They also teach people outside these neighborhoods that deficiencies, problems, and needs are the most important things about low-income people and their neighborhoods. In this way, low-income people, helping institutions, and the general public come to follow a map that shows that the most important part of low-income neighborhoods is the empty, deficient, needy part. Figure 9.1 illustrates an example of a neighborhood needs map.

It is true that this map of needs is accurate. But it is also true that it is only half the truth. It is like a map of the United States that shows only the portion of the country east of the Mississippi River. The United States also lies west of the Mississippi River, and a map omitting the west is obviously inadequate in the most fundamental ways.

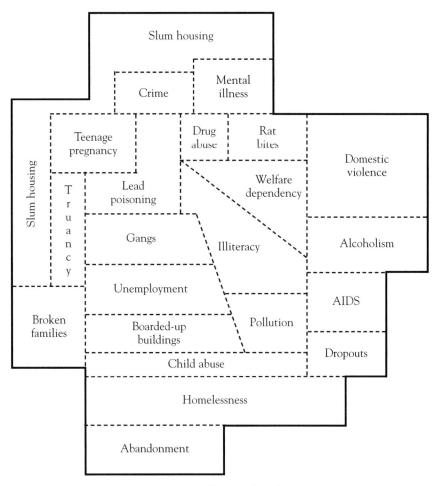

*Figure 9.1.* Neighborhood needs map.

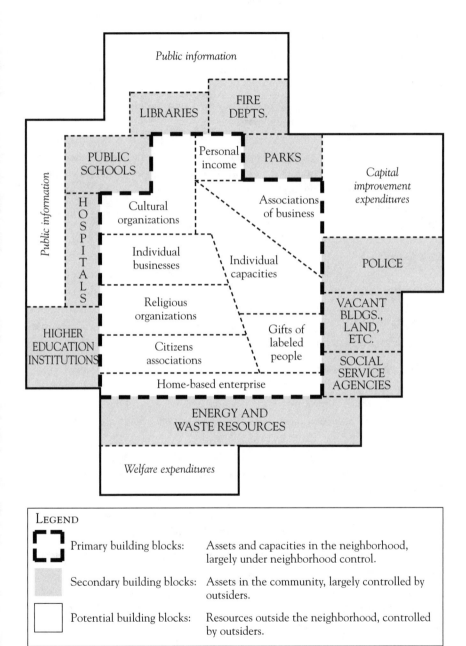

Figure 9.2. Neighborhood assets map.

Similarly, every neighborhood has a map of riches, assets, and capacities. It is important to recognize that this is a map of the same territory as the neighborhood needs map. It is different because it shows a different part of the neighborhood. But the most significant difference in this capacity map is that it is the map a neighborhood must rely on if it is to find the power to regenerate itself.

Communities have never been built upon their deficiencies. Building community has always depended on mobilizing the capacities and assets of a people and a place. That is why a map of neighborhood assets is necessary if local people are to find the way toward empowerment and renewal. Figure 9.2 illustrates an example of a neighborhood assets map.

Finally, it is important to remember that this assets map is very incomplete because it is new. It does not even begin to identify all of the assets of every community. Therefore, we know that as more and more neighborhood regeneration processes are created, residents will identify many more skills, capacities, riches, assets, potential, and gifts to place on the map.

## Using the Capacities Map

Most of the assets just listed already exist in many low-income neighborhoods. They are waiting to be inventoried and turned toward the goal of rebuilding communities. Different communities will approach this challenge with different strategies. Leaders in every community, however, will need to consider at least three questions central to the rebuilding task.

1. Which organizations can act most effectively as asset development organizations in our neighborhood?
2. What kinds of community-wide research, planning, and decision-making processes can most democratically and effectively advance this rebuilding process in our neighborhood?
3. Having inventoried and enlisted the participation of major assets inside the community, how might we build useful bridges to resources located outside the community?

## Asset Development Organizations

To begin with, who might lead the community building process? Where might the necessary asset development organizations be found?

Two kinds of existing community associations are particularly well suited to the task of knitting together a neighborhood's various assets and capacities. The first, already central to the lives of many older city neighborhoods, is the multi-issue community organization, built along Saul Alinsky's organization of organizations model. Community organizers already understand the importance of associational life to the well-being of the neighborhood and to the empowerment of the local residents. A number of these community organizations are beginning to incorporate a capacity-oriented approach to community building in their ongoing activities.

The second potential asset development organization is, of course, the community development corporation. Groups that are dedicated to community economic development have often worked hard to assemble the business assets available to the neighborhood. Many have championed strategies emphasizing local purchasing and hiring and have encouraged homegrown enterprise development. All of these approaches can only be strengthened as the local development corporation broadens and deepens its knowledge of community capacity.

Together or separately, these two types of community-based organizations are well suited to the challenge of asset development. But in many communities, neither the multi-issue organizing group nor the development corporation may exist. In these settings, neighborhood leaders face the challenge of creating a new asset development organization. This new organization may be built on the strengths and interests of existing citizens' associations and will challenge those associations to affiliate for these broader purposes.

## The Community Planning Process

Having identified or created the asset development organization, community leaders face the challenge of instituting a broad-based process of community planning and decision making. Capacity-oriented community planning will no doubt take many different forms. But all of them will share at least these characteristics in common:

1. The neighborhood planning process will aim to involve as many representatives of internally located and controlled assets as possible in the discussion and decisions. In fact, the map of neighborhood assets provides an initial list of potential participants in the planning effort.
2. The neighborhood planning process will incorporate some version of a community capacity inventory in its initial stages.
3. The neighborhood planning process will develop community building strategies that take full advantage of the interests and strengths of the participants and will aim toward building the power to define and control the future of the neighborhood.

## Building Bridges to Outside Resources

Finally, once the asset development organization has been identified and has begun to mobilize neighborhood stakeholders in a broad-based process of planning, participants will need to assemble the many additional resources needed to advance the community building process. This will involve constructing bridges to persons and organizations outside the neighborhood.

It is clear that no low-income neighborhood can go it alone. Indeed, every neighborhood is connected to the outside society and economy. It is a mark of many low-income neighborhoods that they are uniquely dependent on outside and human service systems. What they need, however, is to develop their assets and become interdependent with mainstream people, groups, and economic activity.

Organizations that lead developing communities often create unique bridges to the outside society. These links are not to government alone. Instead, they create bridges to banks, corporations, churches, other neighborhood advocacy groups, and so on (McKnight 1987). These bridged relationships in the nongovernmental sector are vital for opening new opportunities to local residents and enterprises.

The task of the asset development organization, then, involves both drawing the map and using it. It involves leading the community interests into capacity-oriented planning and creating the organizational power to enable that process to become the map of the neighborhood's future. The challenge facing the asset development organization, and all of the participants in the neighborhood planning process, is both daunting and filled with promise. But meeting this challenge to rebuild our neighborhoods from the inside out is crucial to the hopes and aspirations of city dwellers everywhere.

## Acknowledgments

Adapted from J. L. McKnight and J. P. Kretzmann, *Mapping Community Capacity* (Evanston, Ill.: Northwestern University, Center for Urban Affairs and Policy Research, 1988) by permission of the authors.

## References

Alinsky, S. D. 1972. *Rules for Radicals*. New York: Random House.

McKnight, J. 1987. *The Future of Neighborhoods and the People Who Reside There: A Capacity-Oriented Strategy for Neighborhood Development*. Evanston, Ill.: Northwestern University, Center for Urban Affairs and Policy Research, Neighborhood Innovations Network.

O'Connell, M. 1988a. *Getting Connected: How to Find Out about Groups and Organizations in Your Neighborhood*. Evanston, Ill.: Northwestern University, Center for Urban Affairs and Policy Research,. Neighborhood Innovations Network.

———. 1988b. *The Gift of Hospitality: Opening the Doors of Community to People with Disabilities*. Evanston, Ill.: Northwestern University, Center for Urban Affairs and Policy Research,. Neighborhood Innovations Network.

Walsh, J. 1997. *Stories of Renewal: Community Building and the Future of Urban America*. New York: Rockefeller Foundation.

| | Selecting and |
|---|---|
| *Chapter 10* | Cutting the Issue |

IN COMMUNITY ORGANIZING, issue campaigns are both ends and means. Organizations are formed as vehicles to address issues, and the issues that they are created to resolve help the organizations grow and flourish. The capacity of an organization to deal successfully with an issue is a function of its level of organizational development. Like the people within them, organizations grow through experience and practice; issue campaigns are the lifeblood of the process. Through them, new people are attracted, existing members remain active, and leadership abilities flower. The interrelationship between organizational development and issue campaigns cannot be overemphasized. The group builds in order to win and, by winning, builds an even stronger power base.

Good issue campaigns should have the twin goals of winning a victory and producing organizational mileage while doing so. Therefore, when choosing an issue, the organization must be concerned with not only whether it can be won but also how the campaign can be used to develop the group. The choices frequently will be difficult, and decisions should be made carefully.

The issues should come from the members and potential members rather than from outsiders. As discussed in chapter 6, issues are found by talking with people and testing various themes. This kind of testing can be done in a variety of settings where significant numbers of people are found, such as organizational meetings, actions, and events. Door knocking and house meetings are two of the best ways of revealing and testing new issues. Among health educators, social workers, and other professional change agents, focus groups or community forums have also achieved popularity as methods for finding and testing issues and community-perceived needs. (See chapter 8 for a fuller discussion of some of these methods.) Regardless of the method chosen, the role of the organizer is to listen actively (Miller 1993), ask questions, agitate, and in other ways engage in the issue-cutting process.

There are no shortcuts for testing new issues. Sometimes it may be tempting simply to discuss a potential issue among the top leadership, but this common mistake overlooks one key factor. The highest leaders may be so committed to the organization that their notion of self-interest has broadened to the point where they are no longer typical of members. Thus, they may be very poor judges of what issue campaigns will appeal most widely and deeply to the rest of the membership. Within the organization, issues should be tested and selected with as much bottom-up participation as possible. To do otherwise is to risk a campaign without a large base of committed people.

Of course, at times the organization will have little choice but to respond to a particular issue. For instance, the threatened closure of a large public hospital in a low-income community without other reliable sources of medical care almost chooses itself as a salient issue for community mobilization. The positive aspect of such a situation is that many people will be angry and ready to take action. The danger is that the group may be forced to bite off more than it can chew. Regardless, in such instances the organization really cannot afford to walk away if it hopes to retain its credibility.

Many organizations will also choose to be involved in more than one issue campaign at a time. This usually is desirable, providing the organization has a multi-issue focus that helps create a broad base of participation and a wide range of influence. But the group must be aware of the danger of spreading itself too thin in the process. There is no simple answer to the question of how many issues an organization should take on. Resources are a key factor, as are the level of organizational development and the demands of the other issue campaigns. Another significant factor is timing. It is certainly possible to run several campaigns simultaneously if some are relatively quick hits while others are more protracted. In the final analysis, each situation must be assessed individually within the context of the two primary goals of winning basic issues of immediate concern to the members and further developing the organization.

The normal rules for decision making will vary according to the particular organization's structure. Fundamentally, however, the process should be democratic and involve as many members as possible. In addition to being a worthy organizational end in itself, a democratic process will help ensure that a broad base of members begins to feel ownership of the issue campaign and the developing strategy. Large numbers of people will usually be necessary both to achieve a victory on the issue and to develop increased organizational mileage.

In addition, the decisions should be made on a strategic basis. A strategy is simply a well-thought-out plan to achieve a specific goal or set of goals. Strategic thinking is systematic, logical, and analytical; it is highly rational and focuses on a methodical line of action necessary to achieve the desired result. Formulating a successful strategy requires the ability to anticipate likely outcomes. Each possible option for organizational action will produce a reaction; strategic analysis predicts the most probable results of each alternative. Based on those predictions, participants can make the wisest-possible choices and decisions.

As organizations mature, their leaders and members will be able to take on increasingly more complex issue campaigns with strategies that unfold in a series of steps, each predicated on the outcome of the last. Like a chess master, the best strategists will be able to think through the implications of most variables and be able to lay out the stages of the campaign to an end point well in the future.

Since organizational resources are limited and every issue cannot be addressed, it is not sufficient simply to choose an issue and then develop a strategy. That approach locks the organization into a campaign before all factors can be evaluated. Rather, issues should be chosen on the basis of a strategic analysis that determines in advance whether they are winnable and capable of building the organization. When community groups and organizers are assessing the potential of a possible issue campaign for developing the organization, the following questions will help focus attention on the most vital considerations. Of course, the complete answers to many of them will not be known until after the organization actually engages in the campaign. Indeed, the questions should be reexamined in even greater detail as part of a systematic postcampaign evaluation process. Nevertheless, much can be determined and predicted ahead of time. The list that follows illustrates the kind of thinking called for in a strategic analysis:

- Is the issue consistent with the long-range goals of the organization?
- Will the issue be unifying or divisive?
- Will the campaign help the organization grow?
- Will the campaign provide a good educational experience for leaders and members, developing their consciousness, independence, and skills?
- Will the organization receive credit for a victory on the issue, improve its credibility, and increase its overall visibility?
- How will the campaign affect organizational resources?
- Will the campaign develop new allies or enemies?
- Will the campaign emphasize direct action and produce new tactics or issues?
- Will the campaign produce a significant victory?

## Consistency

Is the issue consistent with the long-range goals of the organization? How will this issue campaign fit in with the overall organizational agenda? Will it help move the organization along that path, or will it involve a detour or even a basic change in direction? For instance, a health access organization in a low-income neighborhood might be considering involvement in a campaign to fight cutbacks in bus service—an issue of concern to many members. Although not dealing specifically with health in the narrow sense, the transportation issue may have a direct impact on many of the organization's low-income constituents. One of the many factors the group should consider before making a decision on this issue will be the campaign's impact on future organizational directions. Will other health access issues be neglected while the transportation campaign is undertaken, or will this fight complement other organizational actions? Does this signal the start of a new multi-issue approach? Will this campaign build the power of the organization to represent the interests of low-income residents better than other issues might? Beyond these questions, what are the long-range goals, and how have they been determined?

## *Unity or Division*

Will the issue be unifying or divisive? Serious internal splits will weaken an organization, so it is important to consider how a potentially divisive issue relates to the organization's ultimate goals. Sometimes people on each side of an issue may argue that it is intimately entwined with the organization's long-term goals. One faction may contend that, by taking a position, the organization will virtually destroy itself, while others argue that if a stand is not taken, the organization will not be worth saving. These situations often have no easy solution, and feelings will run high; but a clear understanding of one fundamental principle is essential: any issue campaign that weakens the organizational base jeopardizes the attainment of all other goals.

An organization that bites the bullet on too many divisive issues may find itself with a pure ideological record but only a handful of self-righteous true believers. An organization needs to stand up for its principles and goals; but to be effective, it also needs lots of people standing up with it. One important safeguard is a democratic decision-making process. Both organizers and leaders need to avoid imposing their own ideological goals and visions on the rest of the organization. When controversial, divisive issues arise, organizers and leaders need to come to grips with their own feelings and try to separate them from their roles within the group. When this is not possible, the division should be acknowledged honestly; and those whose positions run counter to the group's consensus should withdraw as much as possible from the issue or in some cases even leave the group.

Any good campaign on a significant issue will attract new people who agree with the organization's position and action. But it will also, to a lesser degree, flush out some members who did not really understand or accept the basic aims of the organization to begin with. Such minor losses of membership are healthy and should be expected.

Often, a possibly divisive issue can turn out to be unifying if it is cut in a positive way. An inner-city community hard-hit by epidemics of drug use and HIV/AIDS may be heavily divided over whether to mobilize in favor of a needle exchange program when the issue is cut in terms of condoning or not condoning the use of illicit drugs. But when the health educator or other social change professional can provide evidence that needle exchange programs reduce the spread of HIV without encouraging drug use, the issue can be cut instead in positive terms of disease prevention.

Problems of divisiveness are often more complex for multi-issue organizations than for single-issue groups since the former usually have a more diverse, multi-constituency base. Again, the interests of different constituent groups need to be weighed against the group's long-term goals.

Organizations also need to be aware of possibly counterproductive external divisions. Sometimes, for example, opponents will be able to divide an organization from its potential allies. Tobacco companies thus frequently provide funding for Cinco de Mayo parades and other cultural events in heavily Latino areas. In so doing, these companies may drive a wedge between community groups and health educators working together to fight the increased targeting of people of color in cigarette advertising and others in the community who want the tobacco companies' financial backing for these prized cultural events (see chapter 7). Obviously, questions of unity and divisiveness must be considered carefully before any issue is selected. A mistake in this area can have a profound and lasting impact on the organization.

## Growth

Will the campaign help the organization grow? An organization's ultimate source of power is its membership. The best campaigns will appeal to a broad range of people and attract new members. Such campaigns will also provide ample opportunity for direct participation by large numbers of people through direct actions and other organizational activities. The recruitment and involvement of large numbers of people will provide much of the leverage necessary to win the issue campaign while simultaneously expanding and building the membership base.

In addition to increasing membership, a good campaign should involve and develop new leaders—a principle that is not emphasized adequately in many organizations. Organizational leadership should be spread among many people rather than be lodged in the hands of a few. This collective form of leadership depends on the infusion of new people, who bring added skills and energy to the group. A good issue campaign should be able to attract new leaders and involve them in important roles. In some cases, they will be people who have never before been active with the organization, whereas in other instances former second-line leaders will move into positions of increased responsibility and prominence. Most organizations will periodically suffer the loss of some leaders, and the infusion of new leadership blood through issue campaigns can compensate for such losses.

Some issues are particularly effective in expanding organizational membership and leadership because they appeal to more than one natural constituency. Environmental issues increasingly fall into this category. Although they continue to appeal primarily to young, white, middle-class constituencies, some environmental groups have begun in earnest to tackle the environmental racism reflected in the disproportionate location of toxic waste dumps in low-income communities of color. And across the United States, low-income communities of color have themselves organized locally against their status as "the unchallenged dumping ground for toxic waste" (see chapter 6). By forging links with these local efforts and moving concerns about environmental justice to the top of the agenda, larger environmental organizations can expand their constituencies while tackling one of the most critical environmental problems facing low-income communities.

Finally, organizations that hope to expand their geographic turf can do so most easily through systematic recruitment on a hot issue. Much of the suspicion and resistance common to such an expansion effort will melt away in the face of a hot issue and an appealing action plan to deal with it.

## Education

Will the campaign provide a good educational experience for leaders and members, developing their consciousness, independence, and skills? In organizing, the principles of adult education leader John Dewey (1946) should be borne in mind: people learn best through action and experience. An issue campaign can provide an educational experience that dozens of consciousness-raising sessions, workshops, or seminars could never accomplish. In a campaign, learning takes place within the context of actual life experience; there is a unique opportunity for the development of political awareness and analytic, strategic planning abilities. Skills can be learned in a wide range of areas, including, but not limited to, recruitment, the holding of effective meetings, direct-action tactics, negotiation, work with the media, and supportive grassroots fundraising. Developing these abilities and skills will lessen the organization's dependence on organizers and other outside professionals.

Learning should take place in a three-step process that involves as many people as possible: analyzing situations and making plans accordingly, carrying those plans into action, and evaluating the results. Organizations often tend to concentrate on developing top leadership while overlooking the rest of the membership, but that is a serious mistake. It is important to use campaign opportunities to educate the membership at large, especially second-line leaders who will be moving into top positions in the future.

Obviously, it is not always functional to have the entire membership involved in intricate strategic planning; but the leadership can poll people about various options, and briefings before all actions can explain the strategic line of thinking to everyone. The more people feel they are part of the process of making organizational decisions and plans, the greater will be their sense of ownership and investment in the campaign, creating a more committed and loyal membership.

The evaluation of issue campaigns provides an excellent opportunity to develop increased political awareness and more sophisticated analysis of how social systems work. For instance, a campaign against an increase in electric rates can lead to increased knowledge of how a private utility corporation functions, how electric rates are structured, and how the regulatory process works. The immediate campaign provides a specific context and experience within which these larger issues can be raised. This process, organizers hope, will lead to new campaigns on the larger issues themselves. The battles of Association of Community Organizations for Reform Now (ACORN) against utility-rate hikes, for example, have developed into statewide initiative campaigns to change the rate structure and replace appointed regulatory bodies with elected representatives. As people develop a better understanding of their organization's potential to bring about small but important changes in their lives, they will become more committed to building an organization that can win larger victories and achieve more significant systemic changes.

## Credit

Will the organization receive credit for a victory on the issue, improve its credibility, and increase its overall visibility? Although we may resent the person who always wants the acclaim when good things happen, an organization should be aggressive about taking credit when it is due. For one thing, an organization's ability to raise funds and secure additional resources may be linked to the credit it gets for its victories. For another, new members may be attracted by the organization's publicity and winning image. And the group may be able to establish greater respect and credibility as a result of receiving credit.

Organizations may receive both internal credit within the community and external credit outside it. External credit most typically is secured through the press and electronic media. Most groups are very conscious of the type of press and media coverage they receive and go to some pains to secure it. Unfortunately, it is not always forthcoming. When this happens, the group still may receive proper credit "on the street" in its own community.

Sometimes the organization must help the process along at the local level. For example, a community group may have successfully pressured city officials to improve trash collection in the neighborhood. The mayor, who ordered the sanitation commissioner to correct the problems only after being confronted by angry organization members (an event that the press failed to cover), may have gotten credit in a news story for "taking bold, aggressive action to improve neighborhood conditions." Leaders and members could attempt to tell the real story through phone calls, the group's newsletter, and word of mouth. There might also be an effort to enlighten the media by framing the story in a new way and use media advocacy to highlight the community group's message (Wallack et al. 1999; see chapter 23 for a full discussion of this strategy.) Regardless of the method or methods chosen, however, the organization would be able to get some measure of credit within its own community.

A distinction should be made between credit and credibility; the two go together frequently but not necessarily. A group that has credibility will be taken seriously. In the preceding example, the group lacked external credit but undoubtedly increased its credibility with the mayor. On rare occasions, things may work the other way. A group may get credit for a victory when in fact it played a minor role. For instance, a piece of health legislation for which an organization lobbied may have passed a legislative body simply as a bargaining chip in a power struggle played out between two politicians. The organization may claim and receive credit for the bill's passage; but if the group plays this game too often, as many are tempted to do, it may actually lose credibility among legislators who know the real story. There also is the added danger that leaders and members will believe their own press clippings, even when they are untrue. This can lead to overconfidence, confusion about the group's true source of power, and a drift away from direct-action tactics.

Many leaders and members may be inclined to say, "Who cares who gets the credit as long as we get a victory on our issue?" But to build organizational mileage, credit and visibility are important. Although this result is difficult to predict, the best campaigns should have the potential for giving the organization increased visibility, credit, and credibility.

## Resources

How will the campaign affect organizational resources? The availability of organizational resources will, of course, greatly affect the outcome of an issue campaign. But the reverse is true; campaigns, both successful and unsuccessful, will often have a lasting impact on an organization's resources. Clearly, internal and external visibility, credit, and credibility will have a direct bearing on fundraising efforts. The organization that can attach an impressive list of victories and an array of good press clippings to a funding proposal will stand a good chance of receiving external funding. Private foundations or large individual contributors often have favorite issues, such as health care or education. An organization should never prostitute itself by choosing issues simply to get funded, but a working knowledge of the fundraising potential of a campaign is certainly a legitimate factor for leaders and members to consider when making a decision.

Of course, the effect of issue campaigns on external funding can cut both ways. For example, an organization that funds part of its staff through local government moneys had better be aware of the implications of taking on the mayor in a nasty fight. This type of example is the major reason that organizations should think long and hard before accepting any government funds. Or a group funded by a conservative foundation should not be surprised when a militant campaign for health care for the homeless leads to a cutoff of funding. Organizations may choose to engage in those campaigns anyway, in spite of the risk. But the funding implications of campaigns should be considered and weighed carefully before any decisions are made. There may be sound organizational reasons for taking on a campaign that jeopardizes funding, but there is no excuse for not anticipating and preparing for the contingencies of such decisions beforehand.

Door-to-door canvassing for large numbers of small contributions falls somewhere between external and internal fundraising. Although many factors affect a canvasser's ability to raise money, organizational name recognition and issues that appeal to the donor's self-interest are usually key ingredients for success.

Finally, internal fundraising, both through membership dues and various grassroots events, will be affected by issue campaigns. Obviously, the greater the organization's visibility, credit, and credibility in its own community, the greater will be its ability to raise funds. Certain issue campaigns will generate more new members than others; and people will be more willing to buy a raffle ticket, attend a fundraising event, or make a donation if they care about the issues the organization is tackling. Internally divisive issues will naturally split the organization's grassroots funding base.

Beyond direct funding, other organizational resources will be affected by any issue campaign. These range from supplies, use of equipment, and technical expertise to, most important, the time of leaders, members, staff, and volunteers. Successful campaigns will frequently attract future donations of supplies and equipment along with an increase in the number of volunteers. As organizer and advocate Herbert Chao Gunther (see appendix 10) explains, "More than anything else, Americans want be on the winning side."

Just as leaders and members develop political and organizational skills through actual campaigns, so do staff members learn through direct experience. A good issue campaign should provide an opportunity to increase the knowledge and skills of new staff and challenge the abilities of the veterans. Generally, success breeds success in organizing, with the best staffs developing in the most effective organizations. Like any other organizational resource, staff must be cultivated, nurtured carefully, and used wisely.

Once there is an answer to the question "Do we have the resources necessary to win?" another question remains: "Is this the best use of our resources, and what will be the effect of this campaign on the rest of the organization?" Even though the resources to win on an issue may exist, the organizational payoff may not be worth the sacrifices. Choosing to work on a particular issue may mean not taking on several others or becoming involved in an all-consuming effort that forces the neglect of other issues and activities. Thus, when community groups and organizers are examining potential issues, it is not enough to analyze whether the issues are winnable; the overall impact on funding and other organizational resources should be considered as well.

## Allies and Enemies

Will the campaign develop new allies or enemies? An old labor union saying goes, "Make no permanent friends or enemies." These still are wise words for both unions and other social action organizations, particularly when dealing with politicians. Allies and opponents can, and frequently will, shift from issue to issue. Nevertheless, relationships may be established that have lasting effects, especially between organizations. Texas Industrial Areas Foundation (IAF) leader Ernesto Cortes, Jr., (1993) has described how in 1975 San Antonio's Communities Organized for Public Service (COPS) staged major and highly publicized actions against several prominent downtown business leaders who had refused to work with COPS on a budget for improving conditions in the city's neglected West Side. The actions were successful, and dialogue was begun between the business leaders and COPS. Two decades later, one of the major business leaders involved in the earlier confrontation and its follow-up was serving as chair of the board of a job training program designed and implemented in part by COPS. He had also played a key role earlier in bringing the other business leaders to the table with COPS and the local IAF organization to plan a community assessment in the areas of income and job training. In Cortes's words, "Establishing and maintaining relationships with both adversaries and allies is a critical component of the capacity to survive the contradictions of politics. . . . If you cannot have a real conversation with your opponent, he or she will never become your ally" (5).

Organizations that work together formally in coalitions or more loosely as allies on an issue campaign have an opportunity to cooperate on specific actions, activities, and tasks. A relatively new and unknown organization might derive both concrete assistance and a measure of needed legitimacy from working with another large, established organization. Both positive and negative experiences are bound to have some carryover effect; and where the former is true, the stage is set for future joint efforts. The development of such relationships can be a source of increased organizational mileage.

But sometimes an organization also helps define itself and what it stands for through the opposition it tackles (Wallack et al. 1999). United Indian Nations, the Circle of Strength/Healthy Nations Project, several local Native American health centers, and other local and national organizations concerned about the health of multicultural communities thus underscored their commitments in this area when they organized a campaign against Hornell Brewing Company. The company had expropriated the name and image of a revered Native American spiritual leader, Crazy Horse, to sell forty-ounce malt liquor to young people, targeting inner-city communities. Denouncing the use of the Crazy Horse name as insulting and degrading to Native Americans, and unable to convince the brewing company to cease using the label, the groups formed the Campaign against Cultural Exploitation. The latter organized a widely publicized boycott of both Crazy Horse malt liquor and the manufacturer's popular Arizona Ice Tea.

As this example illustrates, organizations establish much of their identity through the kinds of issues and targets they pick and the types of campaigns they wage. When community groups are making these decisions, it is important to look at the long-term organizational significance of the friends and enemies who are chosen.

## Tactics

Will the campaign emphasize direct action and produce new tactics or issues? The best victories will be those achieved through the direct action of large numbers of people. Campaigns featuring a high level of direct action enable the leaders and members to experience their own collective power. The organizational lesson is "We won because lots of us stuck together and fought like hell."

Direct-action organizations are always searching for imaginative new tactics. The elements of surprise and unpredictability are important for most good actions, and innovative tactics can make the difference between success and failure. The Gray Panthers in Denver, Colorado, amply demonstrated this principle after encountering resistance from city officials to the organization's request for a longer stoplight at a major intersection. Many elderly senior center participants, especially those with disabilities, had been unable to get from their bus stop to the senior center across the intersection before the light changed. The Panthers organized a demonstration in which some three hundred seniors, many of them with canes and wheelchairs, all attempted to cross with the light at the same time. The ensuing traffic tie-up effectively made its point, and the officials reversed themselves by giving into the Panthers' original demand. Although the tactics do not necessarily have to be brand-new, they should be unexpected by the opposition (Alinsky 1972). Potential issue campaigns may hold possibilities for standard tactics that an organization has not used before—sit-ins or vigils, for example—and opportunities to engage in these tactics will broaden the experience and repertoire of the group's leaders and members.

In other instances, it may be necessary to develop a new variation of an old tactic or something entirely new. ACORN's campaigns against abandoned housing illustrate that a wide range of innovative tactics is often available. When city officials in Little Rock, Arkansas, refused to board up vacant buildings, ACORN members did it themselves and presented the city with a bill for materials. The press covered the action; the city paid up and improved its performance. Faced with a similar situation in New Orleans, Louisiana, ACORN members provoked city officials to act by tearing down an unsalvageable eyesore. In more than a dozen cities, ACORN members have squatted in vacant houses, moving in, beginning repairs, and demanding title to the properties.

In addition to producing new tactics, a good campaign may also create opportunities for new but related campaigns. Sometimes a logical progression can be seen ahead of time. For instance, the primary value of a campaign to establish a landlord-tenant commission is that it sets up future campaigns and establishes a new arena in which to resolve grievances. In other cases, a campaign may set the stage for escalation. For example, neighborhood efforts to obtain street repairs can progress to campaigns for fairer allocation of community development block grant money. Victory on one issue lays the groundwork for future battles. The potential for either spinning off or escalating campaigns can be an important factor in an organization's evaluation of how much mileage any one issue might produce.

## Victory

Will the campaign produce a significant victory? There may be times when a group is forced to take on an issue and fight the good fight even though prospects for success are dim. But to grow and flourish, organizations need victories. In the vast majority of cases, issues should not be chosen unless there is a real possibility for victory, especially when the organization is new.

What constitutes a significant victory? Despite the importance of external credit and credibility, the organization's members are the final judge of whether a victory will make a substantial difference in their lives. At one level, the test is whether an issue is important and whether it can be won. At another level, the test is whether the organization can be strengthened in the process, thereby increasing its power and the members' capacity to gain a greater measure of control over their lives in the future.

Of course, there will be times when almost-certain victory evaporates into defeat. In other instances, a campaign will lose momentum, getting bogged down by forces beyond the organization's control. Such occasions often precipitate an organizational crisis when the energy and anger that are usually focused on the opponent turn inward. In-fighting, scapegoating, low morale, and other internal problems can result. At just such a juncture, a "fight in the bank" can provide the needed remedy. The idea is to delay taking action on an easily won issue until a propitious moment. Then when the organization finds itself caught in an impasse or defeated on an issue campaign, it draws on the fight in the bank to gain a quick, easy victory with all its attendant benefits (Alinsky 1972).

When community groups and organizers are considering questions of organizational mileage, it is important to make one further distinction between types of issues. Recruitment issues lend themselves to systematic outreach efforts that can attract large numbers of new participants and members. Examples include any issue that great numbers of people care about deeply—for instance, the closing of a neighborhood health center or the discovery of a plan for a new hazardous waste dump near a low-income residential area. These issues can help build the organization, providing a steady influx of new leaders and activists.

Maintenance issues, in contrast, do little to build the organization numerically but may provide mileage in other ways. These are issues that do not have a strong self-interest draw for lots of people but nevertheless concern the organization's leadership and core group of activists. Often maintenance issues present opportunities to develop better social policy. Frequently, such issues involve taking positions on a specific piece of legislation. Maintenance issues can provide mileage by producing victories, establishing new allies, increasing visibility and credibility, generating new resources, and developing increased political skills.

Organizational mileage is enhanced when maintenance campaigns are politicized and unite different neighborhoods. For example, vacant lots are a traditional neighborhood concern, and campaigns to clean them up are a common focus for sustaining local group activity. But the efforts will produce more organizational mileage if a number of neighborhood groups combine to advocate a city ordinance that charges landlords the cost of cleanups and places liens on their property for unpaid bills. Winning the ordinance creates new campaign opportunities, targeting individual landowners and demanding city enforcement. Serious problems can arise, however, when organizations stop recruiting and concentrate too heavily on maintenance issues that involve only a small core of activists.

## Cutting the Issue

Winning victories, empowering people, and bringing about change are what organizing is all about. But without good strategic thinking, none of this is possible.

Before organizers and community groups make an action plan, a preliminary phase of strategy development is critical. One of the central components of this strategic development is cutting the issue.

To develop the basic outlines of an issue, community groups and the organizers working with them should explore four questions. Who makes up the constituency that will participate? What are their goals? Who are the targets of their action? How will the community group members gain the necessary leverage or handle to move into action effectively? Thus, the process of cutting the issue lays out the basic dynamics of the conflict: who wants what from whom, and how and why they intend to get it (Katz 1980).

## CONSTITUENCY

People will participate in an issue campaign if they feel it is in their own self-interest to do so. That self-interest can be tested through the application of Saul Alinsky's (1972) criteria of whether the issue is immediate, specific, and winnable.

Obviously, issues will appeal differently to various constituencies. For instance, antitobacco organizing has been an issue of deep concern to many middle-class activists. Yet in a low-income neighborhood where issues of basic survival confront people daily, tobacco may have little immediacy compared to illicit drugs, AIDS, inadequate housing, unemployment, and violent crime. If the issue is cut properly, however, it may well attract both constituencies. In some low-income communities, for example, people of color have recognized self-interest in opposing the heavy targeting of their communities by tobacco advertisers and have mobilized around this issue (Ellis et al. 1995). Even in a low-income neighborhood with severe housing problems, an organizer might have little success in recruiting people to a housing meeting. The general problem is too broad to organize around. Specific issues must be cut to appeal to particular constituencies: rent control to tenants, low-interest home improvement loans to homeowners, a lead paint program to renters with young children.

Of course, the better the chances for success are, the greater is the likelihood that people will make a commitment to get involved. Thus, a campaign to raise welfare benefits by 25 percent in the face of drastic cuts in state expenditures certainly would be met with skepticism, if not laughter. But an effort to stop an ill-conceived, highly criticized workfare program from being implemented might be attractive to many people. Before getting involved, people need to have some clear sense that a victory is possible. The rough outlines of the campaign will have to be laid out before general recruitment is done.

To predict a campaign's potential constituency, it is important that the organizer analyze both the breadth and depth of the issue's self-interest draw. Some issues may be mildly attractive to a broad range of people, whereas others may appeal very strongly to a narrower segment. For instance, there might be more people who would express an interest in establishing new recreation programs than would seek action on an abandoned building. But the smaller number affected by the abandoned building might feel much more deeply about that issue than those interested in recreation.

The depth of an issue's appeal is partly a function of the emotional response it triggers. Frequently, defensive fights (such as "stop the cutbacks") seem to arouse more passion than do efforts to win a positive reform or program. Often, positive efforts are actually phrased in the negative. Thus, a campaign to bring in more city services adopts the slogan "Save the neighborhood," whereas an effort to win a traffic light is conducted under the banner of "Stop endangering our kids." The famous ACORN chant "We're fed up, won't take it no more!" captures the essence of the defensive fight; it is an active response to an intolerable situation. Like the proverbial straw that breaks the camel's back, such issues may be able to move people into action who have never moved before. Not surprisingly, most spontaneous organizing efforts have grown out of defensive situations.

Campaigns to bring about a positive change do, of course, often generate plenty of emotion and anger. Issues such as HIV/AIDS, drugs, abortion, and day care have moved large numbers of people on both the right and the left into action during the past few years. Furthermore, any organization that seeks to empower people must move beyond the realm of defensive responses to the proactive campaigns that change power relationships. But it is critical to generate sufficient passion to move lots of people in these positive efforts. Only if an organization involves many people who care deeply about an immediate, compelling issue can it be won.

## GOALS

The goals of a constituency are whatever people want done to solve the problem they have identified—removal of lead paint or asbestos from a local school, prevention of threatened cutbacks in medical care access for the poor, establishment of smoke-free workplaces. The goals of an issue campaign have to be clear, concrete, and compelling. It does little good to have realizable goals that no one really supports.

Possible solutions to the problem at hand should be tested with a number of people as part of the issue-cutting process. It is important to start by finding out which options people really want. This should be a true bottom-up process, not merely a ratification of the goals of leaders, organizers, planners, politicians, or various interested parties. The process of testing different alternatives helps people develop ownership of both the issue and the strategy, which is essential if the campaign is to be truly broad-based and participatory.

Once an organization develops a general sense of preferred solutions, it must determine what is realistic. This is an area in which research plays a key role. Good research is essential for predicting what might be won from an opponent and what levels of organization and effort will be necessary to achieve success. As information is learned, it should be shared. Similarly, when drastic cuts in federal funding or local tax revenues make a proposed solution totally unrealistic, group members should discuss the obstacles rather than avoid the subject. The formulation of goals is a dynamic process that evolves as more information is gathered and viable options are presented.

The specific objectives will continue to be shaped and refined as more factors are weighed and analyzed. At this point, when the issue is first cut, it is sufficient to draw the broad outline of what is wanted. Again, the demands will be a function of who the constituency is, who the target will be, and how the organization can find points of leverage to bring pressure to bear.

## TARGETS

The language of social services is replete with references to target groups, areas, and populations. Invariably, the people who are defined as having the problem are targeted for some sort of program, service, or other form of assistance. Organizing looks outside the affected constituency and targets those who cause the problem or those who have the power, directly or indirectly, to bring about a change. Thus, in organizing, the people with an interest in a particular issue take collective action on their own behalf against external targets that have the ability to meet their demands. Those targets arise from an analysis of potential (or actual) opposition, what is needed to overcome it, and who has the power to make the decisions necessary to produce an organizational victory. It is important to distinguish between opposition and targets because they are not always the same. James Katz (1980) phrases the distinction nicely:

> The opposition is anyone who is opposed to you and capable of acting against you; the targets are the persons and institutions you act against. Not everyone in the opposition is a worthwhile target; some may be too inaccessible, too powerless, or too peripheral to the resolution of the issue. However, there might be other players who are not necessarily opposed to your campaign—they might even be neutral or favorable— but who may influence the outcome in your favor. These are known as "indirect targets." (4)

Targets typically are straightforward and direct. Aside from vulnerability, a good target should have the power to make concrete, specific decisions about the organization's demands. Alinsky's (1972) famous dictum says it all: "Pick the target, freeze it, personalize it, and polarize it" (130). Thus, when community organizations are targeting an institution, it is important to understand the decision-making process thoroughly and then accurately fix responsibility with the key individuals who have the relevant power. Organizers and the community groups they work with must distinguish between formal and informal decision-making processes, remembering that those who wield the most power may not always occupy the most visible positions. The organization may have to move first on those who are officially responsible, thereby smoking out the real powers that be. In other instances, the best strategy will be to move directly on the hidden powers.

Here again, good research is a must. It is impossible to fight a whole bureaucracy; individuals who can make the necessary decisions should be singled out as targets and not allowed off the hook. It is critical that the right target be chosen in the first place. Clearly fixing responsibility on the proper person helps focus the organization's energy and brings the issue to life for people. There is nothing like a villain to energize a campaign. Thus, during a winter when Boston cut off service for unprecedented numbers of hard-pressed customers, Massachusetts Fair Share's campaign for rate reform gathered new momentum as the company's president was singled out as "Shutoff King of the Year." From small landlords to presidents of multinational corporations, from city councilors to U.S. senators, the best targets will generate anger and emotion in organization members.

Accessibility, vulnerability, and ability to meet the organization's demands will help determine the best targets. At times, indirect targets will have to be chosen, whereas in other instances multiple targets will work best. As more is learned about the opposition, many options will become clearer, and wise decisions will be easier to make.

### HANDLES

A door cannot be opened without some form of handle; neither can an organizing issue. Handles can be laws, regulatory processes, or bureaucratic rules and procedures that may be open to interpretation in ways than could benefit the local organization or community.

Handles can also be precedents, broken promises, or conflicts of interest, each of which provides a natural opportunity for a community group to apply pressure backed by some historical or moral justification. When the prestigious Hastings Law School in San Francisco reneged on promised internal security patrols for low-income residents of four apartment buildings it owned, residents tried without success to convey their concerns to management. The law school's broken promise was then used by the Tenderloin Senior Organizing Project as the basis for helping concerned residents organize a tenants' association. The latter won an out-of-court settlement from the law school and was able to establish a system whereby the property manager met regularly with the tenants' group to explore and address their concerns (see chapter 15).

Finally, incidents, events, and situations (such as an upcoming election) can provide political handles or hooks and have the added virtue of often lending themselves to media coverage. When a Hawaii chapter of Mothers against Drunk

Driving (MADD) learned of a planned substantial weakening of the state's drunk driving law, the organization kicked off a campaign on Memorial Day, in front of the state's eternal-flame war monument, and urged people to remember their highway dead along with their war fatalities. A large sign in front of the podium bore the phone numbers of the governor and the senate president, who received a record number of calls and letters in response to this well-publicized event (Wallack et al. 1993). The choice of a good and media-worthy handle—the symbolic linking of a MADD campaign with Memorial Day—set the stage for subsequent and effective organizing to defeat the proposed policy change.

Whatever form handles may take, they help explain how the organization can win and why its position is justifiable. Thus, the concept entails both a tool that the organization can use to maximize its power on the issue and a rationale that underscores the legitimacy of the campaign. Once again, however, the goal in organizing is to involve as many people as possible, not simply to win on an issue and solve the problem. The best handles will maximize participation and emphasize the organization's direct-action focus.

These four factors—constituency, goals, targets, and handles—are essentials that must be considered when cutting the issue. As I have pointed out, all four are interrelated and should not be considered separately and sequentially. Indeed, cutting an issue can start with any of these factors and then move forward to integrate the others.

## Issue Selection and Strategic Analysis: A Final Note

This chapter has focused on the criteria that groups and communities should consider in the issue selection process. It has then examined the factors that make up the process of cutting the issue, a vital part of strategic development. Although a discussion of all the parameters of a strategic analysis is beyond the scope of this chapter (see Staples 1984), a few key points are worthy of mention.

First, a strategic analysis is a straightforward, useful way of examining the helping and hindering forces that will affect any change effort. A SWOT analysis (Barry 1997; see appendix 4) in which one lays out the strengths and weaknesses internal to a case or an organization and the opportunities and threats in the external environment provides an excellent tool for such work. The approach enables organizers and the communities they work with to think about the various factors working for and against a change and to consider a variety of change strategies that take these forces into account.

Second, Roland Warren's (1983) three major types of change strategies should be considered, with attention to the conditions under which each is most appropriate. Collaborative strategies are effective when there is broad agreement among all parties on the goals of the change effort. Campaign strategies are used when there are differences among the parties that could be resolved by consensus. Finally, contest strategies are used when there are significant differences among the parties and little hope of achieving consensus.

Third, although the mechanics of a strategic analysis are quite simple, the depth of the analysis is what really counts. Assumptions should not be made quickly or superficially, and nothing should be taken for granted. Most important, the various factors should be viewed dynamically rather than statically. Action and change are the goal, not just analysis of the status quo for the sake of analysis. Too often, when done by academicians, such studies lead to explanations and rationalizations for why no change is possible. Organizers and leaders must avoid such analysis paralysis and concentrate on how action can alter the various forces to achieve victory.

Finally, several key factors should be part of any strategic analysis. These are *opposition, objective conditions, organizational capacity,* and *support.* Analysis of these four factors answers several basic questions. Who is against you? What is beyond your control? What is your group capable of doing? What is the possibility for help via coalitions and other mechanisms? Whether done formally through a strategic analysis or more informally, analysis of these factors, in conjunction with the process of cutting the issue, should give a reasonably accurate picture of the level of organizational action and clout necessary to achieve success.

In sum, an organization must weigh a tremendous number of factors and consider many variables when choosing and cutting issues and developing strategies. But the group should be careful not to analyze and strategize to the point where no campaign can materialize. It is impossible to figure out every single possibility. There is a time to act!

## Acknowledgments

Adapted from "Analyze and Strategize: Issues and Strategies," in *Roots to Power: A Manual of Grassroots Organizing*, pp. 53–92, by Lee Staples. Copyright © 1984 by Praeger Publishers. Reproduced with permission of Greenwood Publishing Group, Inc., Westport, Conn.

## References

Alinsky, S. D. 1972. *Rules for Radicals*. New York: Random House.

Barry, B. W. 1997. *Strategic Planning Workbook for Non-Profit Organizations*. St. Paul, Minn.: Wilder Foundation.

Cortes, E., Jr. 1993. "No Permanent Friends, No Permanent Enemies." *Shelterforce* (January–February): 3.

Dewey, J. 1946. *The Public and Its Problems: An Essay in Political Inquiry*. Chicago: Gateway.

Ellis, G., D. F. Reed, and H. Scheider. 1995. "Mobilizing a Low-Income African-American Community around Tobacco Control: A Force Field Analysis." *Health Education Quarterly* 22, no. 4: 443–57.

Katz, J. 1980. *Action Research*. Washington, D.C.: Institute for Social Justice.

Miller, M. 1993. "Community Organizing." In *A Journey to Justice*. Louisville, Ky.: Presbyterian Committee on the Self-Development of People.

Staples, L. 1984. *Roots to Power*. New York: Praeger.

Wallack, L., L. Dorfman, D. Jernigan, and M. Themba. 1993. *Media Advocacy and Public Health: Power for Prevention*. Newbury Park, Calif.: Sage.

Wallack, L., K. Woodruff, L. Dorfman, and I. Diaz. 1999. *News for a Change: An Advocate's Guide to Working with the Media*. Thousand Oaks, Calif.: Sage.

Warren, R. 1983. "Types of Purposive Social Change at the Community Level." In *Readings in Community Organization Practice*, edited by R. M. Kramer and H. S. Specht. 3d ed. Englewood Cliffs, N.J.: Prentice Hall.

# Part IV

# Alternative Community Organizing Models

## Alinsky-Based, Women-Centered, and Freirian Approaches

ALTHOUGH the term *community organizing* often is used in the United States in reference to the social action philosophy and methods typified by the work of people like the late Saul Alinsky and Caesar Chavez, the term in fact embraces a broad array of alternative approaches. In chapter 11, Susan Stall and Randy Stoecker explore and contrast two ideal types along the organizing continuum: social action organizing in the Alinsky tradition and what they call the women-centered organizing model. To conduct this critical analysis, the authors use both the lens of gender, with its attention to concepts such as public and private spheres, and the notion of community as a liminal space, or border area, where separate cultures or structures (such as the public-private spaces) may cross over. The starkly different approaches to domains such as leadership, participation, and task versus process orientation in the Alinsky and women-centered organizing models are discussed and illustrated in part through relevant case examples. The sociohistorical contexts of the two traditions also are illuminated, as are the circumstances in which one model might be more effective than the other. Yet by invoking the concepts of gender and liminality, the authors make a powerful case for moving beyond historic dichotomies between public and private spheres and hence between Alinsky-influenced and women-centered models. Instead, they build on the strengths of each tradition, with the goal of forging synergistic new approaches that ultimately may be best suited for the complex times (and the complex and overlapping communities) in which we now live.

In contrast to Alinsky-based and women-centered organizing models, each of which is at least sixty years old, community organizing applications of the philosophy and methods of adult educator Paulo Freire, particularly in the developed world, are considerably more recent. To date, in fact, textbooks on community organizing seldom give more than passing mention to Freire's (1973, 1994) approach and its potential and actual applications in community building and community organizing. The devotion of an entire chapter (chapter 12) to Freire's pedagogy and its application in an innovative and nationally recognized social action program with adolescents reflects editor Meredith Minkler's belief that this approach represents one of the most important contributions to community organizing and community building theory and practice in the past thirty years. By emphasizing equality and mutual respect between group members and facilitators and using problem-posing dialogue and action based on critical reflection, Freire's approach takes traditional community organizing in important new directions. It further complements and extends the approaches to community building described by John L. McKnight, Cheryl L. Walter, and others in previous chapters.

Although a number of promising applications of the Freire approach now can be found in health education, social work, and related fields (Carroll and Minkler 2000), Nina Wallerstein and her colleagues have probably received the greatest acclaim and visibility for their Adolescent Social Action Program (ASAP) in New Mexico. Chapter 12 begins with a description of this unique university-community partnership, whose goals were to reduce morbidity and mortality among youths in nearly thirty public schools, encourage students to make healthier choices in their own lives, and facilitate (through the use of Freirian praxis) active engagement in their communities through political and social action. The chapter then explores the program's conceptual grounding in both Freirian philosophy and Ronald Rogers's (Rogers et al. 1978) protection-motivation theory, with attention to how these two very different change approaches can in fact complement and enhance each other. The authors detail three steps in a Freirian approach—receptive listening, dialogue, and action—and consider their applications in the case example. They examine the program's research processes and outcomes, candidly discuss the difficulties of evaluation, and introduce a current CDC-funded project that builds in part on the ASAP model. The authors end the chapter with a discussion of the special challenges of community building and organizing with adolescents and implications for others interested in adapting this model in their own work.

### References

Carroll, J., and M. Minkler. 2000. "Freire's Message for Social Workers: Looking Back, Looking Ahead." *Journal of Community Practice* 8, no. 1: 21–36.

Freire, P. 1973. *Education for Critical Consciousness*. New York: Seabury.
———. 1994. *Pedagogy of Hope*. New York: Continuum.
Rogers, R. W., C. W. Deckner, and C. R. Mewborn. 1978. "An Expectancy-Value Theory Approach to the Long-Term Modification of Smoking Behavior." *Journal of Clinical Psychology* 34, no. 2: 562–66.

SUSAN STALL
RANDY STOECKER

# Chapter 11

# Toward a Gender Analysis of Community Organizing Models

## Liminality and the Intersection of Spheres

WHEN WE SPEAK of community organizing, we need to consider just what we mean by *community*. In this chapter, we begin our thinking of community informed by a gender analysis that emphasizes the historical division of American culture into public and private spheres that split the public work done mostly by men in the formal economy and government from the private work done mostly by women in the community and home (Tilly and Scott 1978). That historical split has also separated notions of family and politics-economics. Community, as it exists between family and politics-economics, plays a unique dynamic role in the separation of private and public spheres.

To the many preexisting definitions of community, we add the idea of community as a liminal space. Rooted in ethnography and anthropology (Turner 1974), *liminal spaces* were originally defined as cultural crossover points. More recently, they have been described as either cultural or physical; in either case, however, they are marked as border zones: a space where two social structures or two cultures cross over into each other (Dear 2001, Zukin 1991). In liminal spaces, multiple structures or cultures coexist, intersect, or transform each other (Lie 2002).

We see community, be it geographical (a neighborhood) or cultural (an identity community), as a liminal space in which the structures of private and public spheres and cultural beliefs that maintain the separation of spheres come together. On the one hand, community often occurs as an extension of the private sphere, creating a space where social reproduction activities are shared beyond the boundaries of nuclear families. Women of color and low-income

196

women, who were not afforded access to the nineteenth-century cult of domesticity that isolated white middle-class and wealthy women at home (Cott 1977, Glenn et al. 1994), expanded the boundaries of mothering and the private sphere beyond the private household as they raised and nurtured children in extended family networks within communities struggling for survival (Collins 2000, Stack 1974). Central to the institution of black motherhood, for example, are women-centered networks of blood mothers and "othermothers"—"women who assist blood-mothers by sharing mothering responsibilities" (Collins 2000, 178).

On the other hand, community is also often an extension of the public sphere. Formal neighborhood associations, local school parent-teacher associations, community-based political action groups, and community development organizations are all extensions of community relationships that interact directly with the public sphere. In contrast to the primary relationships more characteristic of private-sphere extensions of community, public-sphere extensions are more likely to involve secondary relationships. Public-sphere organizations are also more likely to work on government policy issues, public school concerns, and local financial lending and with other political and economic players in the public sphere. In many cases, they present the community's public face, sometimes even hiding the private-sphere aspects of community—for example, as in the case of a midwestern urban gay community that represents itself in the public sphere though a neighborhood improvement organization rather than through a gay rights organization (Niswander 1996).

The reality of community as a liminal space where ideas and structures of public and private spheres cross over corresponds to what we see as two distinct styles of community organizing. One derives from the practice of community as an extension of the private sphere, and the other derives from the practice of community as an extension of the public sphere.

In this chapter we examine how gender structures and identities play out in community organizing. After examining the basic traits of each tradition, we explore some key differences between the two approaches. We then return to the concept of community as a liminal space, looking at the difficulties that arise when each model is practiced separately and offering examples that use the liminality of community to greatest advantage in combining community organizing practices across the separation of spheres.

By way of setting the stage for the comparison of organizing models, we underscore that the public and private spheres central to a gender analysis have always influenced each other (through routes such as the economic impact of women's unpaid domestic labor or the impact of economic policy changes on family quality of life) but have been organized around different logics with different cultures. The separation of spheres has also led to important differences between men and women and to two different community organizing styles. The community organizing model that we believe most exemplifies the public-sphere approach has been associated primarily with Saul Alinsky, widely regarded as the father of social action organizing (see chapter 3). The community organizing model that we believe best exemplifies the private-sphere approach has been developed by a wide variety of women.

The Alinsky model begins with *community organizing*—the public sphere battles between the haves and the have-nots. The women-centered model begins by *organizing community*—building expanded private-sphere relationships and empowering individuals through those relationships.

The Alinsky model is based on a conception of separate public and private spheres. Community organizing was not a job for family types, a position Alinsky reinforced through his own marital conflicts, his demands on his trainees, and his poverty. In fact, if anything, the main role of the private sphere was to support the organizer's public-sphere work (Alinsky 1971). His attitude toward which issues were important also illustrates his emphasis on the public sphere. Although problems began in the private sphere, it was important to move the community to understand how those problems were connected to larger issues outside of the community. Thus, problems could not be solved within the community but by the community's better representation in the public sphere (Reitzes and Reitzes 1987a, 27–28). This is not to say that Alinsky ignored private-sphere issues. His first successful organizing attempt, in a working-class neighborhood in Chicago known as Back of the Yards, produced a well-baby clinic, a credit union, and a hot lunch program (Finks 1984, 21). But these programs were accomplished through public-sphere strategizing, not through private relationships. By establishing and maintaining the hot lunch program, Alinsky pushed the Back of the Yards Neighborhood Council (BYNC) to understand its relationship to the national hot lunch program, including the notion that "in order to fight for their own Hot Lunch project they would have to fight for every Hot Lunch project in every part of the United States" (Alinsky 1969, 168).

The women-centered organizing model has a long history but has only recently received much attention (Ackelsberg 1988, Barnett 1995, ECCO 1989, Gutierrez and Lewis 1998, Haywoode 1991, Naples 1998, Weil 1995, West and Blumberg 1990; see also chapter 13). Although organizing efforts are rooted in private-sphere issues or relationships, the organizing process of the women-centered model problematizes the split between public and private because it includes "activities which do not fall smoothly into either category" (Tiano 1984, 21), thus illustrating the liminal qualities of the community. Women-centered organizing extends "the boundaries of the household to include the neighborhood" and, as its efforts move ever further out, ultimately tries to "dissolve the boundaries between public and private life, between household and civil society" (Haywoode 1991, 175). Women-centered organizing also often requires bridging a gap between the community's needs and its resources, mobilizing to demand necessary state resources or to engage in institutional transformation (Collins 2000, Pardo 1998a). For African American women who are raising families in a deteriorating inner-city neighborhood, good mothering may require struggling for better schools, improved housing conditions, or a safer neighborhood (Naples 1992) and demonstrates the liminality of community and the importance of the connections between the spheres (Ackelsberg 1988). This type of organizing emphasizes community building, collectivism, caring, mutual respect, and self-transformation (Barnett 1995).

It is important to note that we use these models as ideal constructs and recognize that they may not be mutually exclusive in the real world. Indeed, many Alinsky organizations have been reluctant to engage in public conflict (Bailey 1972, Lancourt 1979); and Alinsky followers such as Fred Ross, Cesar Chavez, and Ed Chambers have increasingly emphasized private sphere issues and family and community relationship building (IAF 1978, Reitzes and Reitzes 1987a). Because we want to understand gender influences on the two models, we focus on the more traditional Alinsky-style organizing rather than recent adaptations by groups such as the Industrial Areas Foundation (IAF) (1978). Likewise, the women-centered model has to date seldom been portrayed as a model (see Bradshaw et al. 1994 for an exception); and thus its practitioners, many of whom are trained in Alinsky-style organizing, are diverse. Nevertheless, the Alinsky-based and women-centered models are distinct strains of influence on community organizing.

## Comparing the Models

### HUMAN NATURE AND CONFLICT

The Alinsky and women-centered models begin from different starting points—the rough-and-tumble world of aggressive public-sphere confrontation and the more relational world of private-sphere personal and community development. Consequently, they have very different views of human nature and conflict.

Among all the tenets of the Alinsky model, the assumption of self-interest continues to have the strongest sway (Beckwith n.d.) and is greatly influenced by the centrality of the public sphere. Modern society, from Alinsky's perspective, is created out of compromise between self-interested individuals operating in the public sphere. This makes sense when we consider that the public sphere has been structured to emphasize competition between men, forcing a separation and the ever-present potential for conflict between competitors (Brittan 1989, Illich 1982, Sherrod 1987). In addition, Nancy Chodorow (1978) has effectively shown how young boys learn to separate themselves from others, while girls learn to connect with others, under the conditions of separated spheres in which parenting is solely the mother's responsibility. Although the applicability of Chodorow's analysis to communities of color has been questioned (the work was based on all white samples; see Collins 2000), her perspective is intriguing and, together with previously mentioned notions about a private (female) and public (male) split, suggests how self-interest is structured in the public sphere and socialized into its mostly male participants.

From a perspective that emphasizes the importance of the public sphere, the process of organizing people requires an appeal to their self-interest. The assumption is that people become involved because they think there is something in it for them (Alinsky 1969; 1971). Alinsky's emphasis on self-interest was connected to his wariness of ideology. In his view, organizing people around abstract ideology leads to boredom at best and ideological disputes at worst. He did hope that, as the community became organized, the process would bring out innate altruism and affective commitment. But even that level of commitment was based on building victories through conflict with targets (Lancourt 1979; Reitzes and Reitzes 1987a; 1987b).

Because Alinsky saw society as a compromise between competing self-interested individuals in the public sphere, conflict was inevitable; and a pluralist polity was the means through which compromise was reached. Since poor people are at an initial disadvantage in that polity, the organizer's job is to prepare citizens to engage in the level of public conflict necessary for them to be included in the compromise process (Reitzes and Reitzes 1987a). Reflecting the conflict orientation that is necessary for working in the masculine, competitive, public sphere, Alinsky contended that the only way to overcome the inertia that exists in most communities (Reitzes and Reitzes 1987a, 70) is to "rub raw the resentments of the people in the community" (Alinsky 1971, 116), relying on symbols and images that reinforce a "successful forceful masculinity" (Reitzes and Reitzes 1987a, 70). The male-dominated world of sports and the military provided images and metaphors for building teamwork and igniting competition and antagonism against opponents to win a particular movement campaign (Acker 1990). In order to engage in the level of battle necessary to win, "the rank and file and the smaller leaders of the organizations must be whipped up to a fighting pitch" (Alinsky 1969, 151). Alinsky treated the neighborhood as a public-sphere arena, engaging small-scale conflicts within communities against unscrupulous merchants, realtors, and even entrenched community organizations to build military-like victories and a sense of power (Reitzes and Reitzes 1987a). For example, consider Alinsky's 1960s involvement in Rochester, New York, with the organization FIGHT, where he pressured Kodak to support an affirmative hiring and jobs program. FIGHT began with a drawn-out negotiation process, and then Alinsky escalated to confrontational rhetoric and pickets. When Kodak reneged on a signed agreement, Alinsky and FIGHT organized a proxy campaign for Kodak's annual meeting. Forty members of FIGHT and Friends of FIGHT attended the meeting, demanded that Kodak reinstate its original agreement by 2 P.M., and walked out to eight hundred supporters in the street. They came back at 2 P.M. and were told that Kodak would not reverse its position. Applying a military metaphor, the FIGHT leadership came out and told the crowd: "Racial War has been declared on Black communities by Kodak. If it's war they want, war they'll get." Threats of a major demonstration in July and further escalation of the conflict produced a behind-the-scenes agreement at the eleventh hour (Finks 1984, 213–21).

Unlike the Alinsky model, women-centered organizing defines human nature from an ethic of care. This ethic is built on years of caretaking work in the family and the expanded private sphere, particularly in community associations (Stall 1991). The women-centered model begins with women's traditional roles in mothering, not inherently linked to biological sex but derived from a "socially constructed set of activities and relationships involved in nurturing and caring for people" (Glenn et al. 1994). These activities and relationships become transformed by community othermothers in the black community, who build community institutions and fight for the welfare of their neighbors (Collins 2000). Building on Patricia Hill Collins's work, which first appeared in 1991, Nancy A. Naples (1992) describes "activist mothering" as a broadened understanding of mothering practices "to comprise all actions, including social activism, that addressed the needs of their children and the community" (448).

Rather than a morality of individual rights, women develop a collectivist orientation (Robnett 1997) and learn a morality of responsibility connected to relationships (Gilligan 1977). Their activism is often a response to the needs of their own children and of other children in the community (Gilkes 1980). As Collins (2000) explains, "Community othermothers' participation in activist mothering demonstrates a clear rejection of separateness and individual interest as the basis of either community organization or individual self-actualization. Instead, the connectedness with others and common interest expressed by community othermothers models a very different value system" (192). Women-centered organizers view justice not as a compromise between self-interested individuals but as practical reciprocity in the network of relationships that make up the community (Ackelsberg 1988, Haywoode 1991, Stall 1991). In her study of the group Mothers of East Los Angeles (MELA), Mary Pardo (1990, 1998b) reported that the core women activists were long-time community residents who had a history of working on issues that grew out of their responsibilities as parents (such as education). These Mexican American activists garnered their years of experience and their local networks to organize against state-supported projects such as a prison and an incinerator, which they believed would negatively affect their children's safety and health. Through their organizing efforts, these activists expanded the traditional definition of *mother* to include militant political activism. One MELA activist explained, "You know if one of your children's safety is jeopardized, the mother turns into a lioness. . . . We have to have a well-organized, strong group of mothers to protect the community and oppose things that are detrimental for us" (Pardo 1990, 4).

In the women-centered model, the maintenance and development of personal connections that provide a safe environment for people to develop, change, and grow is more immediately important than conflict to gain institutional power (Kaplan 1982). For women, community relationships include the social fabric created through routine activities related to the expanded private sphere, such as child care, housekeeping, and shopping (DeVault 1991), as well as through social arrangements they make to protect, enhance, and preserve the cultural experience of community members (Feldman and Stall in press). These communities of relationships serve as free spaces—arenas outside of the family where women can develop a "growing sense that they [have] the right to work—first in behalf of others, then in behalf of themselves" (Evans and Boyte 1981, 61; 1986).

For women of the Wentworth Gardens public housing development in Chicago, the basement laundromat is a free space. In 1968, a group of women resident activists created and now continue to manage their own laundromat, providing both on-site laundry facilities and a community space that serves as a primary recruitment ground for community activists. The ongoing volunteer work of women residents over three decades has assured the laundromat's continued success. In addition, the women have gained skills and self-confidence to develop the community further, leading them to open an on-site grocery store and obtain other housing improvements. A resident service committee made up of laundromat volunteers meets when necessary to resolve problems and allocate laundromat profits to annual community festivals, scholarship funds, and other activities. (Feldman and Stall 1994, in press). Free spaces such as these exist between the residents' individual private lives and large-scale institutions and are grounded in the fabric of community life (Evans and Boyte 1986).

## POWER AND POLITICS

Both models appear to have internally inconsistent understandings of power and politics. These inconsistencies are rooted partly in how each thinks about human nature but are also affected by how they deal with the public-private split. The Alinsky model sees power as zero-sum but the polity as pluralist. The women-centered model sees power as infinitely expanding but the polity as structurally biased. Understanding both the differences between the models and their seeming inconsistencies requires us to look at how each deals with the public-private split.

For the Alinsky model, "organizing and power are almost synonymous" (see chapter 2), and both power and politics occur in the public sphere. When power is zero-sum, the only way to get more is to take it from someone else—a necessity in a masculinized public sphere structured around competition and exploitation. Alinsky was adamant that real power could not be given but only taken. This view of power as zero-sum, modeled after predominantly male political and economic elites, means that one is either advantaged or disadvantaged, either exploiting or exploited (Acker 1990). Thus, poor communities can gain power through public-sphere action: picking a single, elite target; isolating it from other elites; personalizing it; and polarizing it (Alinsky 1971). In the 1960s, the Woodlawn Organization (TWO), one of Alinsky's most famous organizing projects, was based in an African American neighborhood on Chicago's South Side. When TWO was shut out of urban renewal planning in the neighborhood, group members commissioned their own plan and threatened to occupy Lake Shore Drive during rush hour. Not only did they get agreement on a number of their plan proposals, they also controlled a new committee to approve all future plans for their neighborhood, shifting control of urban planning from city hall to the neighborhood (Finks 1984, 153; Reitzes and Reitzes 1987).

In women-centered organizing, power begins in the private sphere of social relationships and thus is not conceptualized as zero-sum but as limitless and collective. Co-active power is based on human interdependence and the collaborative development of all in the group or the community (Follett 1940, Hartsock 1974; see also Bradshaw et al. 1994). The goal of a women-centered organizing process is empowerment, a developmental process that includes building skills through repetitive cycles of action and reflection that evoke new skills and understandings and in turn provoke new and more effective actions (ECCO 1989, Kieffer 1984). Empowerment includes developing a more positive self-concept and self-confidence as well as a more critical world view; it also involves cultivation of individual and collective skills and resources for social and political action (Rappaport 1986, Van Den Bergh and Cooper 1986, Weil 1995; see also chapter 2). In the case of the Cedar Riverside Project Area Committee, an organization dedicated to planning resident-controlled redevelopment of a counter-culture Minneapolis neighborhood, tensions developed in the 1980s between those who emphasized building power as an outcome and those who saw empowering residents as a process. One woman organizer compared her approach to that of the lead organizer: "I disagree with Tim, but he's a very empowering person. Tim is more Alinsky. For me, the process, not the outcome, is the most important. . . . The empowerment of individuals is why I became involved. . . . I was a single mother looking for income, and was hired as a block worker for the dispute resolution board, and gained a real sense of empowerment" (Stall and Stoecker 1998, 741). Power, for this organizer, was gained not through winning a public sphere battle but by bringing residents together to resolve disputes and build relationships within their own community.

In practice, both models must eventually operate in the public sphere. But the public-private split still influences how each relates to politics. The Alinsky model sees community organizations as already located in the public sphere and consequently already part of the political system. The problem is not gaining access; the rules of politics already grant access. Rather, the problem is effectively organizing to make the most of that access. Alinsky believed that poor people could form their own interest group and access the polity just like any other interest group. They may have to act up to be recognized initially, but once recognized, their interests would be represented just like anyone else's. Because Alinsky did not question the masculine competitive structure of the public sphere and the self-interested personalities required of its participants, he did not see a need for dramatic structural adjustments in the political system. The system was, in fact, so good that it would protect and support the have-nots in organizing against those elites who had been taking unfair advantage (Alinsky 1969, Lancourt 1979, Reitzes and Reitzes 1987a). When the IAF-trained Ernesto Cortez returned to San Antonio, Texas, to help found Communities Organized for Public Service (COPS) in 1973, he began with the traditional strategy of escalating from negotiations to protests to achieve better city services for Latino communities. Soon after its initial successes, COPS turned to voter mobilization, winning a close vote to change San Antonio's council from at-large to district representation. From there group members were able to control half of the council's seats, bringing more than half of the city's federal community development block grant funds to COPS projects from 1974 to 1981. Eventually COPS found that its political lobbying and voter mobilization tactics outpaced the effectiveness of confrontation and protest (Reitzes and Reitzes 1987a, 121–23). Chicago-based civil rights organizer turned community organizer Heather Booth took this pluralist organizing approach to its logical extreme when her Chicago-based Citizen Action Project focused its energies entirely on voter mobilization in cities and states around the country (Reitzes and Reitzes 1987a).

The women-centered model approaches politics from the experience and consciousness of the exclusionary qualities of the public-private sphere split, which becomes embedded in a matrix of domination along structural axes of gender, race, and social class and hides the significance of women's work in local settings. This matrix has historically excluded women from public-sphere politics and restricted them through the sexual division of labor to social reproduction activities centered in the home (Cockburn 1977; Kaplan 1982; see also chapter 13). As a consequence, women have politicized the expanded private sphere as a means to combat exclusion from the public agenda (Kaplan 1982). Cynthia Hamilton (1991), a community organizer in south-central Los Angeles, described a primarily women-directed organizing campaign in the late 1980s to stop the construction of a solid waste incinerator planned for their community. These low-income women, primarily African

American and with no prior political experience, were motivated by the health threat to their homes and children. They built a loose but effective organization, the Concerned Citizens of South Central Los Angeles, and were gradually joined by white, middle-class, and professional women from across the city. The activists began to recognize their shared gender oppression as they confronted the sarcasm and contempt of male political officials and industry representatives, who dismissed the women's human concerns as "irrational, uninformed, and disruptive" (Hamilton 1991, 44), and restrictions on their organizing created by family needs. Eventually they forced incinerator industry representatives to compromise and helped their families accept a new division of labor in the home to accommodate activists' increased public political participation.

## LEADERSHIP DEVELOPMENT

Leadership is another characteristic of these models that shows the influence of the public-private split and the importance of community as a liminal space. The Alinsky model maintains an explicit distinction between public-sphere leaders (called organizers) and private-sphere community leaders. One goal of the Alinsky model is to develop the ability of those private-sphere community leaders to occupy positions in formal organizations that can extend their leadership beyond the community into the public sphere. For Alinsky, the organizer is a paid professional consultant from outside the community whose job is to get people to adopt a delegitimizing frame (Ferree and Miller 1985, Gamson et al. 1982) that breaks the power structure's hold over them (Bailey 1972). Advocates of the Alinsky approach contend that organizing is a complex task requiring professional-level training and experience (Bailey 1972; Reitzes and Reitzes 1987a; see also chapter 3). The Alinsky model also maintains a strict role separation between outside organizers and the indigenous leaders whom organizers are responsible for locating and supporting (Lancourt 1979, Reitzes and Reitzes 1987b). New leaders have to be developed, often outside of the community's institutionally appointed leadership structure. The primary focus is not on empowering those individuals, however, but on building a strong organization and getting material concessions from elites.

Organizers have influence but only through their relationships with indigenous leaders (Lancourt 1979). It may appear curious that Alinsky did not emphasize building indigenous organizers, especially since the lack of indigenous organizing expertise often led to organizational decline after the pros left (Lancourt 1979). Tom Gaudette, an Alinsky-trained organizer who helped build the Organization for a Better Austin (OBA) in Chicago, explicitly discouraged his organizers from living in the neighborhood, arguing they had to be able to view the community dispassionately in order to be effective at their job (Bailey 1972, 80). But when viewed through the lens of the public-private split, it is clear that the organizers are leaders who remain in the public sphere, always separate from the expanded private sphere of community. Because the organizers remain in the public sphere, they are the link that pulls private-sphere leaders and their communities into public action. Both the location of the organizer outside the local community and the elevation of rational, dispassionate role-playing contribute to the gendering of this role.

There is less separation between organizers and leaders in the women-centered model because women-centered organizers, rather than being outsiders, are often rooted in local networks. They are closely linked to those with whom they work and organize, and they act as mentors or facilitators of the empowerment process. Felix Rivera and John Erlich (1995) describe this as primary contact appropriate for indigenous community organizers (see also chapter 13). Private-sphere issues seem paramount to these organizers. They find they need to deal with women's sense of powerlessness and low self-esteem (Miller 1986) before involving them in sustained organizing efforts. Mentoring others as they learn the organizing process is premised on the belief that all have the capacity to be leaders and organizers. Rather than focusing on or elevating individual leaders, women-centered organizers seek to model and develop group-centered leadership (Payne 1989) that "embraces the participation of many as opposed to creating competition over the elevation of only a few" (ECCO 1989, 16). Instead of moving people and directing events, this approach conceives of leadership as teaching (Payne 1989). Analyses of women-centered organizing and leadership development efforts also underline the importance of centerwomen, or bridge leaders. Using existing local networks to develop social groups and activities that create a sense of familial-community consciousness, these leaders connect people with similar concerns and heighten awareness of shared issues (Robnett 1996, 1997; Sacks 1988). Women-centered leaders can transform social networks into a political force and help translate the skills that women learn in their families and communities (such as interpersonal skills, planning and coordination, conflict mediation) into effective public-sphere leadership. Belinda Robnett (1996) argues, "The activities of African-American women in the civil rights movement provided the bridges necessary to cross boundaries between the personal lives of potential constituents and adherents and the political life of civil rights movement organizations" (1664). Thus, ironically, gender as a "construct of exclusion . . . helped to develop a strong grassroots tier of leadership. . . . women who served as 'bridge leaders' who were central to the development of identity, collective consciousness, and solidarity within the civil rights movement" (Robnett 1996, 1667). Although the bridge leaders she observed were not exclusively women, this intermediate layer of leadership was the only one available to women at that time (Robnett 1996).

Since the late 1950s, Mrs. Hallie Amey, a bridge leader now in her seventies, has been a key activist and a centerperson in nearly all of the Wentworth Gardens organizing efforts. Mrs. Beatrice Harris, another woman resident activist, provides some insight into the dynamics of Mrs. Amey's leadership role:

> She's the type of person who can bring a lot of good ideas to the
> community. . . . And she's always there to help. And she's always here;
> she's always doing things. And she's always pulling you, she's pushing
> you, and she's calling you, "We've got to do this!" She makes sure you
> don't forget what you have to do. Early in the morning she's on the
> phone, "Mrs. Harris, what time you coming out?" That was to say,
> "You gonna do it without me having to ask, or you giving me an
> excuse." (Feldman and Stall in press)

By closely examining the work of women-centered leaders such as Mrs. Amey, we can learn how potential constituents are persuaded to act, how consensus and trust are formed, and how action is mobilized (Robnett 1997).

### THE ORGANIZING PROCESS

Finally, the Alinsky and the women-centered models adopt organizing processes that reflect the influence and different conceptualizations of the public-private split. Within the Alinsky model the organizing process centers on identifying and confronting public issues to be addressed in the public sphere. Consequently, the organization needs to be publicly visible and traditionally masculine—big, tough, and confrontational. Door knocking often is the initial strategy for identifying issues. Those issues then become the means of recruitment to the organizing effort. The organization bills itself as the best, if not the only, means of resolving those issues. The mass meeting is the means for framing issues and celebrating gains. Cumulative victories are important to the process of building up to the mass meeting, beginning with an easily winnable issue and using the energy it generates to build to bigger issues. The public activities of the mass march, public rally, explicit confrontation, and celebrated win are all part of building a strong organization that can publicly represent the community's interests. The annual convention is the culmination of the Alinsky organizing process. The first convention of the East Toledo [Ohio] Community Organization (ETCO) in 1979 was preceded by flyers emphasizing the city's neglect of the east side of Toledo, broken promises from officials, the victories of initial organizing, and growing unity in the community. ETCO mailed packets across East Toledo that produced five hundred registrants for the meeting. At the meeting itself, the 500 to 1,000 people gathered passed thirteen resolutions covering dangerous rail crossings, park maintenance, utility complaints, service shortages, truck traffic, and many other issues (Stoecker 1991).

In the Alinsky model, the organizer isn't there just to win a few issues but to build an enduring formal organization that can continue to claim power and resources for the community—to represent the community in a competitive public-sphere pluralist polity. These organizations typically have traditional decision-making structures that mirror the male-dominated public-sphere structures they confront. The organizer is supposed to build the organization from the community's pre-existing formalized organizational base of churches, service organizations, clubs, and so on. In many cases, the community organizations created also spawn community-based services such as credit unions and daycare centers. This is not a process to be undertaken lightly or with few resources. Alinsky often insisted that, before he would work with a community, it had to raise $150,000 to cover three years of expenses (Lancourt 1979). When Ed Chambers took over the IAF from Alinsky, he required $160,000 just to cover startup costs for a serious organizing project (IAF 1978). For Alinsky, the organization itself was part of the tactical repertoire of community organizing. Dave Beckwith, an Alinsky-influenced organizer with the Center for Community Change, also argues for the centrality of the organization:

> If an organization doesn't grow, it will die. . . . People naturally fade in and out of involvement as their own life's rhythms dictate—people move, kids take on baseball for the spring, they get involved with Lamaze classes, whatever. If there are not new people coming in, the shrinkage can be fatal. New issues and continuous outreach are the only protection against this natural process.          (Beckwith with Lopez 1997, 13)

This emphasis on building a formal organization reflects, and can be attributed to, the public-sphere emphasis and the gendered assumptions of the Alinsky model. Operating within the rules of the existing masculine competitive structure, where there are only winners and losers, means valuing competition even within the organization, a separation between leaders and followers, and a gendered distinction between maintaining relationships and achieving goals.

The presence and partial restriction of women in the private sphere leads the women-centered organizing model to emphasize a very different organizing process. Rather than a large public-sphere organization, the process begins by creating a safe and nurturing space where women can identify and discuss issues immediately affecting the private sphere (Gutierrez and Lewis 1998). This model uses the small group to establish trust and build "informality, respect, [and] tolerance of spontaneity" (Hamilton 1991, 44). Civil rights organizer Ella Baker was dubious about the long-term value of mass meetings, lobbying, and demonstrations. Instead, she advocated for organizing people in small groups so that they could understand their potential power and how best to use it, which had a powerful influence on the Student Nonviolent Coordinating Committee (Britton 1968, Payne 1989). Small groups create an atmosphere that affirms each participant's contribution, provides time for individuals to share, and helps participants listen carefully to each other. Gutierrez and Lewis affirm, "The small group provides the ideal environment for exploring the social and political aspects of personal problems and developing strategies for work toward social change" (chapter 13). Moreover, smaller group settings create and sustain the relationship building and sense of significance and solidarity so integral to community. Women in Organizing (WIO), a 1990s urban-based project in Chicago, organized low-income, African American teenage mothers to gain self-sufficiency and political empowerment. One of the organizing staff members described the effort of this Young Moms Program:

> Our work is about connecting women with each other, about
> transforming their experience in terms of working with mixed groups
> of people of different races, about building the confidence of individual
> women and building the strengths of groups. . . . All of our work is really
> about leadership development of women, of learning more of
> how consciousness develops, of how we can collectively change the
> world. (Stall and Stoecker 1998, 747)

While WIO did help these young women organize an advocacy meeting with public officials, the meeting was preceded by nearly five months of trainings that addressed less traditional issues such as personal growth and challenges in parenting as well as more traditional organizing issues (Stall 1993). Engagement in practices of storytelling, potluck meals, and instructional round tables helped the teenaged moms begin to redefine their relationship to power and advocate for the societal supports they needed to succeed.

Because the women-centered model focuses less on immediate public-sphere action, a continuing organization is not as central as it is in initial organizing. In place of the focus on organization building are "modest struggles"—"small, fragmented, and sometimes contradictory efforts by people to change their lives" (Krauss 1983, 54). These short-lived collective actions (such as planting a community garden, opening a daycare, organizing a public meeting) are often begun by loosely organized groups. The organizing efforts of African American women in south-central Los Angeles against the incinerator siting functioned for a year and a half without any formal leadership structure. Their model depended on a rotating chair, which stymied the media's hunger for a spokesperson (Hamilton 1991, 44). If empowerment is "a process aimed at consolidating, maintaining, or changing the nature and distribution of power in a particular cultural context" (Bookman and Morgen 1988, 4), modest struggles become a significant factor in this process. Engagement in modest resistance focused on the expanded private sphere allows women to use community as a liminal space, bridging the spheres, influencing their community, and gaining a sense of control over their lives.

Attention to modest struggles is necessary to understand the more elusive process of resistance that takes place beneath the surface and outside of what have conventionally been defined as community organizing, social protest, or social movements. Research on New York City co-op apartment tenants in the 1980s found that the tenant leaders were almost always women, the majority of them African American and long-time residents of their building and their community (Leavitt and Saegert 1990). These women leaders used skills learned when sustaining their own families in the larger sphere of the building. For example, women tenants often met around kitchen tables and, by preparing and sharing food with neighbors, fostered social ties that extended the practical solidarity of family caretaking to the entire building. Women residents "equated sharing their dish with the recognition of their role," and trust was nurtured in the context of personal relationships. "[T]hey made building-wide decisions with the same ethic of personal care that they applied to friends and family." Members of tenant associations discussed rent payment and eviction issues in terms of the situations of each tenant involved and searched for alternatives that supported residents' overall lives as well as ensured that good decisions were made for the whole building (Clark 1994, 943). In a time of shrinking resources, the formation of low-income tenant cooperatives is a form of modest resistance. In this case, strong tenant associations, rooted in rich social networks and on a gender-based response to home and community, were essential to making co-op ownership possible.

## Conclusion: Gender, Liminality, and the Separation of Spheres

This chapter has elaborated two models of community organizing that have developed both from the gendered positions of their founders and their consequent experientially derived conceptualizations of the public and private spheres. The Alinsky model sees the community as part of the market-driven, exchange-based public sphere needing to be organized to compete effectively with other public-sphere interests. The model emphasizes self-interest, confrontation, professional organizers, and formal organizations. The women-centered model, developed by women and primarily engaged in by women for other women and children (increasingly women in female-headed households), mirrors the traditional pattern of gender differentiation found in American families in which women generally have the primary responsibility for caring for families, neighbors, and friends. This model views the community as an extension of the private sphere, which needs to be organized to build and maintain its own relationships and resources. It thus emphasizes relationship building, co-active power, indigenous organizers, and informal organizational structures.

What are the implications of these two models for the future of community organizing? The women-centered organizing model has had enormous impact on the field of community organizing and has, in fact, dissolved some of the boundary between the public and private spheres. Within the field, women-centered organizing has transformed the traditional organizing agenda so that issues formerly considered private—violence against women (Park 1998, Wittner 1998), toxic waste disposal (Krauss 1998), and postpartum depression (Taylor 1996)—have been moved from the realm of private troubles to public issues, in many cases transforming the agendas, the constituents, and the strategies of traditional organizing. Community organizing is committed to democratic goals and supports humane ends. With the greater influx of women into the Alinsky model of community organizing and the popularization of feminist goals among men and women, there is evidence that the inclusion of sexuality, emotionality, and procreation in community organizing is slowly transforming its gendered logic and practice, the sexual division of labor among community organizers, and the issues that community organizations are willing to address (Stall 1986).

Nevertheless, there is still a pronounced difference between the logics of the public and private spheres in society. The corporate and government sectors show no signs of becoming less competitive, and there are constant cries to preserve a private sphere protected from the brutalities of public life. In this context, the weaknesses of one model are the strengths of the other (see chapter 3). The masculine confrontational style of the Alinsky model, which must assume prior community bonds so it can move immediately into public-sphere action, may be disabling for certain grassroots organizing efforts, "particularly in domains where women are a necessary constituency" (Lawson and Barton 1990, 49). Imagine trying to employ the Alinsky model when organizing young moms who are socially isolated and exhausted from the daily grind of trying to make ends meet. The Alinsky model's lack of emphasis on relationship building means that, when neighborhoods are less and less communities and the people in them less and less empowered, the community can engage in the battle but not sustain it.

The strengths of the women-centered model are centered in building relationships that can sustain a struggle over the long haul. The social role of motherhood is still important for women's activism: "Women essentially remain responsible for much of the 'emotional work' of family and community life" (Taylor 1996, 170). And while we have argued that the women-centered model can span the boundaries between the public and private spheres—making personal issues into public issues—we are concerned that the model cannot, by itself, transform the public sphere. One criticism of consciousness raising in the women's movement is that it hasn't translated very effectively into action (Cassell 1989, Ferree and Hess 1985, Rosen 2000) Women-centered organizing can move private-sphere issues such as health, housing, and sanitation into the public sphere. But once they are so placed, their resolution is subject to the competitive, masculine, zero-sum processes of that sphere.

Thus, the women-centered model, and community organizing in general, faces a paradox of empowerment: the need to organize simultaneously at the personal and structural levels (Rappaport 1981). To us, this means making use of the idea of the community as a liminal space. If community is the space where private and public spheres intersect and mingle, and to the extent that women-centered organizing emphasizes the private-sphere qualities of community while the Alinsky model emphasizes its public-sphere qualities, then the most effective form of community organizing may well be the one that uses liminality to greatest advantage. Such a model would build primary relationship bonds around social reproduction issues (Stoecker 1992) while also using public-sphere tactics to press for broader social changes. (See Bradshaw et al. 1994 for further discussion of a hybrid organizing model that mixes both feminist and Alinsky approaches.)

There are examples of such models operating today. Perhaps one of the most well-known examples began with a group of women in the Love Canal community of New York. Lois Gibbs was "just a housewife" when she became concerned about the frequency and severity of illnesses among children in the community. As the women who maintained community relationships shared their concerns with each other, they also learned that their community was sitting on a toxic dump. In the early days of their efforts, however, their organizing model was primarily women-centered. It was not until they started playing hardball, using Alinsky-style politics of identifying and targeting officials for public actions, including temporarily holding two Environmental Protection Agency officials hostage, that they began to make headway on getting the local school closed and community members relocated (Gibbs 1998).

Another interesting case of bridging the public and private spheres through the liminality of community comes from the Kensington Welfare Rights Union (KWRU). The union formed in the North Philadelphia neighborhood of Kensington through the efforts of a group of women threatened by welfare "reform" in 1991. The most famous of the women, Cheri Honkala, had raised her son while homeless, at times sleeping in cars. Like many women in poverty, members of the group practiced a women-centered organizing model, mostly providing each other with shared social reproduction support and informal sharing sessions to bolster their self-esteem. But the severity of the Pennsylvania governor's welfare cuts forced them to extend their model into the public sphere. Today KWRU is known as one of the most confrontational poverty groups in the country, organizing around hunger and poverty issues with the same tenacity as war and peace issues, all the while continuing to maintain women-centered organizing activities that build relationships in order to meet basic food, clothing, shelter, and medical care needs (KWRU 2003).

The importance of thinking more deeply about community organizing and organizing community in liminal spaces such as poor neighborhoods cannot be overstated. For it is in liminal spaces that new ideas, new strategies, new identities, and new possibilities form that can reverberate throughout the cultures and structures that cross over in such spaces. This is the case with the Alinsky and women-centered organizing models and the separation of spheres. While individual women's rights efforts such as access to education, employment, and competitive athletics have transformed the lives of individual women, they have not transformed the separation between private and public spheres because they have not focused on social transformation through such liminal spaces. Consequently, women can become corporate managers, but they are forced to manage the same male-dominated corporate model as men do and suffer the same child-care dilemmas as poor employed women do. Those same struggles, if fought through the liminal space of community, linking women-centered and Alinsky organizing models, provide an opportunity for change that can transform both private- and public-sphere culture and practice.

At this early stage of thinking about the role of the liminal space of community in social change, we can offer no easy road maps, only suggestions of ways to continue to explore the possibilities. First, there may be times when the liminality of community may extend into one sphere more than the other. Robert Fisher (1984) showed a see-sawing between more militant and more community-building periods of community organizing, which seems to correspond to progressive and reactionary periods in history. Reactionary periods such as the 1980s also force social movements into abeyance (Taylor 1989); at these times, maintaining community bonds and providing emotional support become paramount because public-sphere action seems ineffectual. In such periods, the women-centered model sustains the possibility for future public-sphere action.

Second, we need to learn whether certain circumstances might call for certain organizing models. Will the women-centered model be more effective in communities whose social relationships have been destroyed by disinvestment, where the targets are far away, and where government is ineffectual? In such circumstances, the Alinsky model may be impractical because it depends on preexisting relationships; its success depends on not just confronting the enemy but being able to extract real concessions. Conversely, will the Alinsky model be more effective in relatively stable communities confronted with an immediate threat perpetrated by an identifiable villain where the community's public-sphere connections are strong? In these cases, the ability to confront the villain and make believable threats of consequences is crucial.

Linking the concepts of community, liminality, Alinsky-style organizing, and women-centered organizing is more than an intellectual endeavor. It is a very practical task with implications for social change strategies and tactics. Our past strategic thinking about community organizing has been split too much between private-sphere concerns and public-sphere strategies. Understanding not only how but why to cross the public-private sphere divide is crucial to winning age-old battles in both spheres.

## Acknowledgments

This chapter was fully cowritten, and names are listed alphabetically. It is a revised version of Susan Stall and Randy Stoecker, 1998, "Community Organizing or Organizing Community: Gender and the Crafts of Empowerment," *Gender and Society* 12, no. 6: 729–56. Copyright © 1998 by Sociologists for Women in Society. Reprinted by permission of Sage Publications, Inc.

## References

Ackelsberg, M. 1988. "Communities, Resistance, and Women's Activism: Some Implications for a Democratic Policy." In *Women and the Politics of Empowerment*, edited by A. Bookman and S. Morgen, 279–313. Philadelphia: Temple University Press.

Acker, J. 1990. "Hierarchies, Jobs, Bodies: A Theory of Gendered Organizations." *Gender and Society* 4, no. 2: 139–58.

Alinsky, S. 1969. *Reveille for Radicals*. New York: Vintage.

———. 1971. *Rules for Radicals*. New York: Vintage.

Bailey, R., Jr. 1972. *Radicals in Urban Politics: The Alinsky Approach*. Chicago: University of Chicago Press.

Barnett, B. M. 1995. "Black Women's Collectivist Movement Organizations: Their Struggles during the 'Doldrums.'" In *Feminist Organizations: Harvest of the New Women's Movement*, edited by M. M. Ferree and P. Y. Martin, 199–219. Philadelphia: Temple University Press.

Beckwith, D. No date. *Introduction to Organizing*. Toledo, Ohio: University of Toledo, Urban Affairs Center.

Beckwith, D., with C. Lopez. 1997. "Community Organizing: People Power from the Grassroots." Paper presented on COMM-ORG: The Online Conference on Community Organizing and Development. http://comm-org.utoledo.edu/papers.htm.

Bookman, A., and S. Morgen, eds. 1988. *Women and the Politics of Empowerment*. Philadelphia: Temple University Press.

Bradshaw, C., S. Soifer, and L. Gutierrez. 1994. "Toward a Hybrid Model for Effective Organizing in Communities of Color." *Journal of Community Practice* 1, no. 1: 25–41.

Brittan, A. 1989. *Masculinity and Power*. New York: Blackwell.

Britton, J. 1968. "Interview with Ella Baker: June 19, 1968." Transcript. Moorland-Springarn Collection, Howard University.

Cassell, J. 1989. *A Group Called Women: Sisterhood and Symbolism in the Feminist Movement*. Prospect Heights, Ill.: Waveland.

Chodorow, N. 1978. *The Reproduction of Mothering*. Berkeley: University of California Press.

Clark, H. 1994. "Taking up Space: Redefining Political Legitimacy in New York City." *Environment and Planning* 26, no. 6: 937–55.

Cockburn, C. 1977. "When Women Get Involved in Community Action." In *Women in the Community*, edited by M. Mayo, 61–70. London: Routledge and Kegan Paul.

Collins, P. H. 2000. *Black Feminist Thought: Knowledge, Consciousness, and the Politics of Empowerment*. New York: Routledge.

Cott, N. F. 1977. *The Bonds of Womanhood: "Woman's Sphere" in New England, 1780–1835*. New Haven, Conn.: Yale University Press.

Dear, M. 2001. *The Postmodern Urban Condition*. New York: Blackwell.

DeVault, M. L. 1991. *Feeding the Family: The Social Organization of Caring As Gender Work*. Chicago: University of Chicago Press.

Education Center for Community Organizing (ECCO). 1989. *Women on the Advance: Highlights of a National Conference on Women and Organizing*. Stony Point, N.Y.: ECCO.

Evans, S. M., and H. C. Boyte. 1981. "Schools for Action: Radical Uses of Social Space." *Democracy*, pp. 55–65.

————. 1986. *Free Spaces: The Sources of Democratic Change in America*. New York: Harper and Row.

Feldman, R. M., and S. Stall. 1994. "The Politics of Space Appropriation: A Case Study of Women's Struggles for Homeplace in Chicago Public Housing." In *Women and the Environment*, edited by I. Altman and A. Churchman, 167–99. Human Behavior and Environment Series, no. 13. New York: Plenum.

————. In press. *The Dignity of Resistance: Women Residents' Activism in Chicago Public Housing*. New York: Cambridge University Press.

Ferree, M. M., and B. B. Hess. 1985. *Controversy and Coalition: The New Feminist Movement*. Boston: Hall.

Ferree, M. M., and F. Miller. 1985. "Mobilization and Meaning: Toward an Integration of Social Psychological and Resource Perspectives on Social Movements." *Sociological Inquiry* 55, no. 1: 38–61.

Finks, P. D. 1984. *The Radical Vision of Saul Alinsky*. New York: Paulist Press.

Fisher, R. 1984. *Let the People Decide: Neighborhood Organizing in America*. Boston: Twayne.

Follett, M. P. 1940. *Dynamic Administration*. New York: Harper and Row.

Gamson, W. A., B. Fireman, and S. Rytina. 1982. *Encounters with Unjust Authority*. Homewood, Ill.: Dorsey.

Gibbs, L. 1998. *Love Canal: The Story Continues*. Stony Creek, Conn.: New Society.

Gilkes, C. T. 1980. "Holding Back the Ocean with a Broom: Black Women and Community Work." In *The Black Woman*, edited by L. Rodgers-Rose, 217–32. Beverly Hills, Calif.: Sage.

Gilligan, C. 1977. "In a Different Voice: Women's Conceptions of Self and Morality." *Harvard Educational Review* 47, no. 4: 481–517.

Glenn, E. N., G. Chang, and L. R. Forcey. 1994. *Mothering: Ideology, Experience, and Agency*. New York: Routledge.

Gutierrez, L. M., and E. A. Lewis. 1998. "A Feminist Perspective on Organizing with Women of Color." In *Community Organizing in a Diverse Society*, edited by F. G. Rivera and J. L. Erlich, 97–116. 3d ed. Boston: Allyn and Bacon.

Hamilton, C. 1991. "Women, Home, and Community." *Women of Power* (spring): 42–45.

Hartsock, N. 1974. "Political Change: Two Perspectives on Power." *Quest* 1, no. 1: 10–25.

Haywoode, T. L. 1991. "Working Class Feminism: Creating a Politics of Community, Connection, and Concern." Ph.D. diss., City University of New York.

Illich, I. 1982. *Gender*. New York: Pantheon.

Industrial Areas Foundation (IAF). 1978. *Organizing for Family and Congregation*. Franklin Square, N.Y.: IAF.

Kaplan, T. 1982. "Female Consciousness and Collective Action: The Case of Barcelona, 1910–1913." *Signs* 7, no. 3: 545–66.

Kensington Welfare Rights Union (KWRU). 2003. "KWRU: Frequently Asked Questions." http://www.kwru.org/kwru/kwrufaq.html.

Kieffer, C. H. 1984. "Citizen Empowerment: A Developmental Perspective." In *Studies in Empowerment: Steps toward Understanding Action*, edited by J. Rappaport, C. Swift, and R. Hess, 9–36. New York: Haworth.

Krauss, C. 1983. "The Elusive Process of Citizen Activism." *Social Policy* (fall): 50–55.

————. 1998. "Challenging Power: Toxic Waste Protests and the Politicization of White, Working-Class Women." In *Community Activism and Feminist Politics*, edited by N. A. Naples, 129–50. New York: Routledge.

Lancourt, J. I. 1979. *Confront or Concede: The Alinsky Citizen-Action Organizations*. Lexington, Mass.: Lexington Books.

Lawson, R., and S. E. Barton. 1990. "Sex Roles in Social Movements: A Case Study of the Tenant Movement in New York City." In *Women and Social Protest*, edited by G. West and R. Blumberg, 41–56. New York: Oxford University Press.

Leavitt, J., and S. Saegert. 1990. *From Abandonment to Hope: Community-Households in Harlem.* New York: Columbia University Press.

Lie, R. 2002. "Spaces of Intercultural Communication." Paper presented at the twenty-third annual conference of the International Association for Media and Communication Research, Barcelona, July 21–26. http://www.portalcomunicacion.com/forumv/forum3/pdf/f3_eng.pdf.

Miller, J. B. 1986. *Toward a New Psychology of Women.* Boston: Beacon.

Naples, N. A. 1991. "Contradictions in the Gender Subtext of the War on Poverty: The Community Work and Resistance of Women from Low Income Communities." *Social Problems* 38, no. 3: 316–32.

———. 1992. "Activist Mothering: Cross-Generational Continuity in the Community Work of Women from Low-Income Urban Neighborhoods." *Gender and Society* 6, no. 3: 441–63.

———, ed. 1998. *Community Activism and Feminist Politics.* New York: Routledge.

Niswander, S. C. 1996. "Neighborhood Pride and Politics: Understanding a Depoliticized Gay and Lesbian Neighborhood Community, a Case Study of the Old West End Neighborhood, Toledo, Ohio." Unpublished paper.

Pardo, M. 1990. "Mexican American Women Grassroots Community Activists: 'Mothers of East Los Angeles.'" *Frontiers* 11, no. 1: 1–7.

———. 1998a. "Creating Community: Mexican American Women in Eastside Los Angeles." In *Community Activism and Feminist Politics,* edited by N. A. Naples, 275–300. New York: Routledge.

———. 1998b. *Mexican American Women Activists: Identity and Resistance in Two Los Angeles Communities.* Philadelphia: Temple University Press.

Park, L.S.H. 1998. "Navigating the Anti-Immigrant Wave: The Korean Women's Hotline and the Politics of Community." In *Community Activism and Feminist Politics,* edited by N. A. Naples, 175–98. New York: Routledge.

Payne, C. 1989. "Ella Baker and Models of Social Change." *Signs* 14, no. 4: 885–99.

Rappaport, J. 1981. "In Praise of a Paradox: A Social Policy of Empowerment over Prevention." *American Journal of Community Psychology* 9, no. 1: 1–26.

———. 1986. "Terms of Empowerment/Exemplars of Prevention: Toward a Theory for Community Psychology." Paper presented at the annual meeting of the American Psychological Association, Washington, D.C.

Reitzes, D. C., and D. C. Reitzes. 1987a. *The Alinsky Legacy: Alive and Kicking.* Greenwich, Conn.: JAI.

———. 1987b. "Alinsky in the 1980s: Two Contemporary Community Organizations." *Sociological Quarterly* 28, no. 2: 265–84.

Rivera, F., and Erlich, J., eds. 1995 *Community Organizing in a Diverse Society.* 2d ed. Boston: Allyn and Bacon.

Robnett, B. 1996. "African-American Women in the Civil Rights Movement, 1954–1965: Gender, Leadership, and Micromobilization." *American Journal of Sociology* 101, no. 2: 1661–93.

———. 1997. *How Long? How Long?* New York: Oxford University Press.

Rosen, R. 2000. *The World Split Open: How the Modern Women's Movement Changed America.* New York: Viking Penguin.

Sacks, K. B. 1988. *Caring by the Hour.* Urbana: University of Illinois Press.

Sherrod, D. 1987. "The Bonds of Men: Problems and Possibilities in Close Male Relationships." In *The Making of Masculinities: The New Men's Studies,* edited by H. Brod, 213–39. Winchester, Mass.: Allen and Unwin.

Stack, C. 1974. *All Our Kin: Strategies for Survival in a Black Community.* New York: Harper and Row.

Stall, S. 1986. "Women Organizing to Create Safe Shelter." *Neighborhood Works* (September–October, November–December).

————. 1991. "'The Women Are Just Back of Everything . . . :' Power and Politics Revisited in Small Town America." Ph.D. diss., Iowa State University, Ames.

————. 1993. "Women in Organizing Project Evaluation." Unpublished report prepared for Women United for a Better Chicago.

Stall, S., and R. Stoecker. 1998. "Community Organizing or Organizing Community? Gender and the Crafts of Empowerment." *Gender and Society* 12, no. 6: 729–56.

Stoecker, R. 1991. "Community Organizing and Community Development: The Life and Times of the East Toledo Community Organization." Unpublished paper.

————. 1992. "Who Takes Out the Garbage? Social Reproduction and Social Movement Research." In *Perspectives on Social Problems*, edited by G. Miller and J. A. Holstein, 239–64. Greenwich, Conn.: JAI.

Taylor, V. 1989. "Social Movement Continuity: The Women's Movement in Abeyance." *American Sociological Review* 54, no. 5: 761–75

————. 1996. *Rock-a-By Baby: Feminism, Self-Help, and Postpartum Depression*. New York: Routledge.

Tiano, S. 1984. "The Public-Private Dichotomy: Theoretical Perspectives on Women in Development." *Social Science* 21, no. 4: 11–28.

Tilly, L. A., and J. W. Scott. 1978. *Women, Work, and Family*. New York: Holt, Rinehart, and Winston.

Turner, V. 1974. *Dramas, Fields and Metaphors: Symbolic Action in Human Society*. Ithaca, N.Y.: Cornell University Press.

Van Den Bergh, N., and L. B. Cooper. 1986. *Feminist Visions for Social Work*. Silver Spring, Md.: National Association of Social Workers.

Weil, M. 1995. "Women, Community, and Organizing." In *Tactics and Techniques of Community Interventions*, edited by J. E. Tropman, J. L. Erlich, and J. Rothman, 118–33. Itasca, Ill.: Peacock.

West, G., and R. L. Blumberg. 1990. *Women and Social Protest*. New York: Oxford University Press.

Wittner, J. 1998. "Reconceptualizing Agency in Domestic Violence Court." In *Community Activism and Feminist Politics*, edited by N. A. Naples, 81–104. New York: Routledge.

Zukin, S. 1991. *Landscapes of Power: From Detroit to Disney World*. Berkeley: University of California Press.

NINA WALLERSTEIN
VICTORIA SANCHEZ
LILY VELARDE

Freirian Praxis in
Health Education and
*Chapter 12*    Community Organizing

A Case Study of an
Adolescent Prevention Program

Today's ADOLESCENTS are confronted by many risks, including fears about the future, lack of employment opportunities, media targeting by the alcohol and tobacco industries, family and community violence, and social norms of peer pressure to engage in risky behaviors. In addition, young people are bombarded with the "don't" messages of health professionals and prevention specialists, such as "Don't drink and drive," "Don't have sex," and "Don't use drugs." Implicitly, adolescents are asked to assume full individual responsibility for their behavior in the face of social conditions that foster powerlessness and alienation. For adolescents in low-income communities of color, real and perceived powerlessness is often particularly profound.

This chapter illustrates how a university and community partnership has worked with youths to address the interconnectedness of personal choices and social conditions through a mix of empowerment education and community organizing strategies. In New Mexico, a group of interdisciplinary university faculty, staff, and graduate students in collaboration with school administrators, teachers, and middle and high school students have sought to understand and address the interplay between individual and social change in one health education intervention, the Adolescent Social Action Program (ASAP). The intervention incorporated Paulo Freire's (1970) empowerment education theory of dialogue and praxis with community organizing strategies and Ronald Rogers's (1984) protection-motivation behavior change theory.

After offering an overview of ASAP and its theoretical framework and processes, we summarize evaluation results from qualitative and quantitative studies. We conclude by discussing a new youth empowerment intervention, based in part on the ASAP experience, and then discuss the implications for health educators and community organizers of using a Freirian approach with youth.

## The Adolescent Social Action Program

ASAP was a youth-centered, intergenerational, and experiential prevention program initiated in 1982 among schools, both on and off reservations, and serving predominantly Native American, Hispanic, and low-income Anglo communities. Funded over time by multiple grants from the U.S. Department of Education, the New Mexico Department of Health, and a large National Institute on Alcohol Abuse and Alcoholism (NIAAA) (1994–99) research grant, ASAP staff recently decided to close down the program due to lack of funding for institutionalizing the prevention services rather than the research. Consultation still continues about the ASAP experience, research design, and Freirian methodology (see Wilson et al. in press).

ASAP was a collaborative effort among the University of New Mexico, University Hospital, the county detention center, and more than thirty multiethnic schools and communities throughout New Mexico. Formerly known as the Alcohol and Substance Abuse Prevention Program, ASAP's goals were to reduce morbidity and mortality among adolescents who lived in high-risk environments; encourage them to make healthier choices in their own lives; and facilitate, via empowerment education, their active engagement in political and social action in their communities.

ASAP consisted of a seven-week experience for small groups of youths brought into the hospital or the detention center to interview and interact with patients and jail residents who had problems related to drug, tobacco, and alcohol abuse; interpersonal violence; HIV infection; and other risky behaviors (Wallerstein and Bernstein 1988). The ASAP facilitators (trained university graduate students from the health professions and social sciences) followed an extensive curriculum (still available) that included structured dialogue about the patients' and jail residents' stories and exercises in decision making, conflict mediation, communication, problem posing, and resistance to peer pressure. In each session, facilitators helped youths develop questions for the interviews, construct role plays, and address specific anxieties or fears that were arising in the hospital and jail settings.

At the heart of the program was Freire's educational empowerment approach (Wallerstein and Sanchez-Merki 1994). With the guidance of the ASAP facilitators, adolescents applied and practiced the Freirian model—that is, a listening-dialogue-action-reflection cycle with the patients and jail residents. The youths listened to the patients' and residents' life stories. After the interviews, the youths engaged in dialogue about the issues they had heard about; exchanged personal experiences about their lives; and analyzed the social, medical, and legal consequences of risky behaviors. The debriefing component of the program took the participants beyond a "scared straight" model, which has proved to be ineffective (Rogers and Mewborn 1976, Job 1988), and allowed them to practice critical thinking skills. At this juncture, the adolescents began to explore action strategies to make healthier choices for themselves and their communities.

ASAP incorporated protection-motivation theory directed at increasing students' threat appraisal and coping self-efficacy for behavior change (Rogers 1984, Stainback and Rogers 1983). The integration of behavior and social change is especially important for youths of color who face poverty, racism, and unemployment and are therefore overrepresented in injury and mortality statistics.

At the end of the seven-week curriculum, ASAP typically offered the adolescents two options: to participate in a peer education component or to work on a social action project. The peer education program allowed the adolescents to continue the Freirian model with elementary school students. They practiced the craft of conducting empowerment education and acted as role models for younger children. The social action model, however, extended into community organizing. Adolescent participants were encouraged to devise their own social or health projects for their schools and neighborhoods. This approach encouraged the youths to explore existing social-legal policies and community resources, evaluate prevention strategies for risky behaviors, and participate in actions to transform alcohol and tobacco norms in their communities.

## Philosophical and Theoretical Bases of ASAP

The underlying theory and philosophical framework for ASAP come from Brazilian educator Paulo Freire (1970, 1973). He originally developed his ideas in the 1950s, through highly successful literacy programs for slum dwellers and peasants in Brazil. Choosing emotionally and socially charged words and pictures of students' problems, he generated discussion about how to improve their lives. During the past three decades, Freire's educational ideas have been a catalyst for worldwide programs in literacy (Unda 2002, Fiore and Elsasser 1982), English as a second language (Wallerstein 1983, Auerbach and Wallerstein in press), health education (Minkler 1992, Werner and Bower 1982, Wallerstein and Bernstein 1994), worker health and safety and union education (Delp et al. 2002, Burke et al. 2002, Wallerstein and Weinger 1992), youth programs (Alschuler 1980, Reed 1981), college courses (Shor 1980, 1987; Shor and Freire 1987), grassroots organizing with populations including the homeless (Yeich 1996), and community development (Hope et al. 1984; Barndt 1989; Vella 1994, 1995; Arnold et al. 1995).

To Freire, the purpose of education was human liberation, meaning that people are subjects of their own learning, not empty vessels filled by teachers' knowledge. To promote the learner as subject, Freire proposed a structured dialogue approach in which everyone participates as co-learners to create a jointly understood reality. Through dialogue, individuals engage in critical reflection, or conscientization, to analyze the societal context for personal problems and their own role in working on the problems. The goal of dialogue is praxis, or the ongoing interaction between reflection and the actions that people take to promote individual and community change. In health education, social work, and community organizing, there has been growing interest in the role of Freirian theory in health enhancement, with the goal of helping people collectively move beyond feelings of powerlessness and assume control over their lives (Wallerstein 1992, Carroll and Minkler 2000, Yeich 1996).

ASAP also incorporated protection-motivation theory, an attitudinal change theory that assumes that intention to act is an indicator or a predictor of behavior change. Protection-motivation theory proposes that decisions to act are initiated through a variety of informational sources and mediated through a nonlinear cognitive perceptual process (Rogers 1984, Rogers et al. 1978, Floyd et al. 2000), resulting in either an adaptive or a maladaptive response. Variables in Rogers's model include personal vulnerability, severity, response, and self-efficacy and a set of beliefs that centers around rewards and costs. Rogers's model purports that a positive, adaptive response occurs when exposure to a stimulus increases one's threat appraisal and coping appraisal and when rewards decrease for engaging in a maladaptive behavior (Rippetoe and Rogers 1987).

The coping appraisal variables of self-efficacy (the belief that one has the ability to complete a task successfully) and response efficacy (the belief that one's actions will make the desired difference) improve the likelihood of self-protective behavior. Socially responsible behaviors can increase through enhanced self-efficacy to help others, strengthened collective efficacy (the belief that the group can make a difference), and political efficacy (the belief that one can make a difference in the political arena).

## The Integration of Freire and Protection-Motivation

Through the Freirian model, ASAP linked educational processes to individual changes and community organizing. During the hospital-detention center sessions, the predominant model was the cultivation of decision making, critical consciousness, leadership skills, and community building. Starting from the youths' emotional responses as they listened to the patients' and jail residents' stories (their threat appraisal), Freirian dialogue helped create a cognitive awareness of precursors to and consequences of alcohol problems that lead participants to increased coping appraisal to protect themselves. Empathy with each other and critical analysis of societal forces in a safe group context created a bridge between one-dimensional behavioral change and group efforts for social change. The youths were encouraged to engage in dialogue about their own lives and their relationships to their communities and to develop an awareness of school and neighborhood resources in order to build socially responsible behaviors. Active participation was a key tenet of ASAP in the issues that adolescents bring to the dialogue and their choice of follow-up activities.

To implement the Freirian structured dialogue model, which integrates threat and coping appraisals, ASAP used a listening-dialogue-action methodology. This three-part process encompasses a participatory orientation to learning rather than a passive mode of receiving information. ASAP participants entered the program at the listening stage and, upon completion of the curriculum, left in an action mode. Yet listening, dialogue, and action are not linear processes; rather, they are overlapping, cyclical components of learning and change. For example, listening continued throughout the program as students interviewed patients, discussed issues with facilitators, selected an action project, evaluated and relistened to their own analysis of the impact of their actions, and chose other actions. This cyclical process embodies the Freirian concept of praxis and also reflects a cognitive-perceptual process that encourages attitudinal and behavior change. Figure 12.1 illustrates the interaction between protection-motivation variables and the Freirian listening-dialogue-action model.

## LISTENING

The ASAP methodology begins in the receptive listening stage. Students interviewed individuals who had experienced medical, social, or legal consequences related to their alcohol use, other drug problems, or interpersonal violence. The small-group context of seven students and two facilitators created a supportive environment, essential for promoting the active participation of youths. Key to this environment was facilitators' ability, as co-learners, to model and promote empathy, reinforce active listening skills, and encourage participatory discussion.

Students immediately adopted an action stance as they engaged in the role of questioner versus passive recipient of information. For students from high-risk environments in particular, this process gave them an opportunity to adopt a new activist role in the dominant-culture hospital environment. Not only did they interview the patients, but they also had the opportunity to interview the hospital personnel who cared for the patients: helicopter flight crews, paramedics, technicians, nurses, and physicians.

The motivation to explore the meaning of the interviewees' stories came from the development of empathy—often spurred by curiosity and wonder about

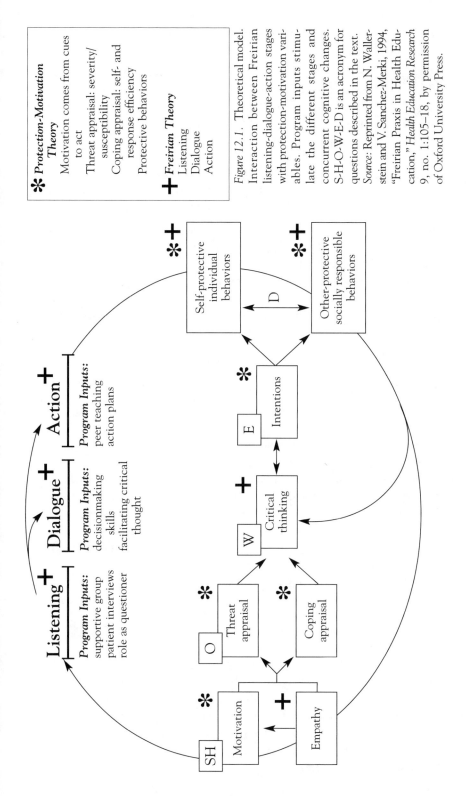

**Protection-Motivation Theory**
Motivation comes from cues to act
Threat appraisal: severity/susceptibility
Coping appraisal: self- and response efficiency
Protective behaviors

**Freirian Theory**
Listening
Dialogue
Action

*Figure 12.1.* Theoretical model. Interaction between Freirian listening-dialogue-action stages with protection-motivation variables. Program inputs stimulate the different stages and concurrent cognitive changes. S-H-O-W-E-D is an acronym for questions described in the text. *Source:* Reprinted from N. Wallerstein and V. Sanchez-Merki, 1994, "Freirian Praxis in Health Education," *Health Education Research* 9, no. 1:105–18, by permission of Oxford University Press.

people in the hospital or in jail but kept alive by facilitators through guided discussion. Motivation to continue also came from personal identification (the initial step toward increased susceptibility) with the patients or inmates. Students wondered, "Could I be here? Or could my father, mother, or friend?"

## DIALOGUE

Once the key issues are elicited in the listening stage, the Freirian process uses discussion catalysts, or triggers, to pull together the issues into a concrete example so that people can interpret and project meaning onto the reality they see. A good trigger is a creation from the listening process that captures the emotional meaning of key problematic issues and the social context of these issues in participants' lives yet does not present solutions.

In ASAP, the patients' and jail residents' stories were the major triggers for discussion. These stories portrayed the consequences of risky behaviors and the rich complexities of problems and solutions. Other triggers in the curriculum were role plays, student stories about their own lives, videotapes, collages, and photographs. Although triggers present open-ended situations, critical thinking does not occur spontaneously. To promote different levels of critical thinking, the facilitators used an inductive questioning guide, S-H-O-W-E-D (Shaffer 1983, Dow-Velarde et al. 2002). Sample questions for the acronym might include the following:

> What do we *see*, or how do we name this problem?
> What's really *happening* to this individual in his or her life?
> How does this story relate to *our* lives, and how do we feel about it?
> *Why* has this person experienced these problems as an individual or a family member? *Why* do we face these problems on a community or societal level?
> How might we become *empowered* now that we better understand the collective nature or the problem?
> What can we *do* about these problems?

The questions asked the youths to describe the problem, consider how it affected their personal lives, develop a critical analysis of the context of the problem, and strategize social actions.

As an immediate emotional reaction to the patients' and jail residents' stories, the youths began to personalize the stories and life experiences of the interviewees. The youths' protection-motivation's variables of personal susceptibility and severity had increased: "This could happen to me," and "This is serious." Almost without prompting from the facilitator, youths were asking themselves, "What do we see, what is really happening here, and how does this relate to our lives? Our families? Our communities?"

To move the youths toward an adaptive coping response, facilitators at this juncture needed to acknowledge the feelings elicited by the interviews yet help participants move past their emotions to a cognitive understanding of what happened in these peoples' lives to create their medical, legal, or social problems. In particular, facilitators needed to push youths to think beyond their peers and their families to a societal analysis. To do so, facilitators asked questions such as "Why does the homeless person in the emergency room feel helpless? Why does he drink? Does he have the support or resources to go into treatment?"

It is this component of critical thinking leading to action (or conscientization, in Freire's terms) that separates ASAP from most other health education programs, which appeal primarily to individual behavior change. Through the dialogue, students acquired beliefs in their ability to help themselves and others. A belief in personal power and skill may be important for low-income or minority youths who have heightened vulnerabilities and powerlessness.

As students discussed their own lives through the dialogic model, they brought in their personal experiences, cultural backgrounds, and norms. ASAP students were encouraged to draw on their strengths (such as pride in their family and culture) to help them address the problems they face in their lives.

## ACTION

Although the action stage is the last step we discuss, it is not the final step, merely a component of the reflection-action-reflection cycle, or praxis. Group actions that emerge during the dialogue process are reflected upon and in turn promote further actions that address problems in participants' communities.

Youths were asked to take an action stance from the beginning of the program (for example, by assuming the role of interviewer for patients and medical personnel); but by the fourth week, the action stage became prominent. Students had completed their work with patients and inmates, worked through many of the emotions elicited by the interactions, and were now engaging in a community action project.

In the first years of the program, ASAP students often defined their actions solely in the arena of presentations and peer teaching. In the latter years of the program, however, the social action approach facilitated greater organizing opportunities within their schools and larger communities. These opportunities included neighborhood organizing and community-based research in the production of their own curriculum, community murals, and ethnic-cultural institutes that reflected their community, culture, and the voice of local youths. ASAP adolescents have conceptualized, written, and produced several ASAP videos and fotonovellas (short "picture novels" that use stories, photographs, or comic-strip characters to communicate messages and reach a wider audience). These videos and fotonovellas have then been used as aids for other educational and organizing efforts in local schools and community centers (Dow-Velarde et al. 2002).

As a result of increasing interest in youth issues statewide, ASAP youths began participating in larger endeavors. At the New Mexico State Fair in 1994, for example, they helped plan and participate in "A Day without Alcohol Is Fair." In Albuquerque's Civic Plaza, adolescents took part in "A Day without Colors" by directing activities and running the ASAP booth. They linked with Street Reach, a gang prevention project, in which ASAP adolescents shared the health information and coping strategies they had learned. ASAP adolescents have been involved in a local youth-produced series of television programs on teenage life in New Mexico. Service has often been a part of ASAP social actions, with youths from Laguna-Acoma Pueblos, for example, helping senior citizens with house cleaning and repair and engaging in environmental cleanup campaigns.

In the policy arena, ASAP youths have played an active role in the New Mexico Peer Leadership Conference, which produced policy recommendations on tobacco use for the legislature and the governor's office. They have joined Youth Link, a statewide endeavor that seeks to engage young people in statewide policy development (see chapter 22).

Thus, Freirian action emphasizes the importance of youths becoming advocates for healthier schools and communities. By taking the emphasis off the individual as lone actor, Freirian action places individuals within their social and political context. This is particularly important for health educators who work in nondominant cultures (for example, with the Native American and Hispanic youths in ASAP), where communal decision making and traditional community responsibility are highly valued (Spector 1979).

## Summary of ASAP Research Process and Outcomes

Although there are many Freirian-inspired programs throughout the world, few efforts have been made to research the processes created by these programs or to evaluate their health and social outcomes. Research into Freirian programs poses special difficulties because, like most community organizing efforts, change targets evolve over time as people become engaged in their community. Community-level change requires long-term commitment, with both intended and unintended results. In essence, there are several major research questions that require careful investigation:

What are the major processes of this type of intervention?
What are the potential outcomes at different levels (that is,
	individual, school, policy, community norms), and the interactive
	relationships between individual- and community-level changes?

More specifically, how do youth leadership and empowerment
strategies promote increased community capacity to create
organizational and community changes?

A qualitative exploratory study undertaken by Nina Wallerstein in the late
1980s sought to answer these questions. (See Wallerstein and Sanchez-Merki
1994 for a complete review of the research methodology and findings.) Two ASAP
sites were selected: a large Albuquerque high school, with 1,700 students, 39
percent from low-income families, and almost 70 percent Hispanic; and a
reservation middle-high school (sixth through twelfth grades), an hour outside
of Albuquerque, with 450 students. More than 90 percent of the students in
the latter school were Native Americans from the Laguna and Acoma reservations, and unemployment on the reservations at the time ranged from 50 to
75 percent.

The study population consisted of two groups of high school students from
each site who were observed and interviewed throughout their participation in
ASAP. Questions focused on several areas: perceptions of and satisfaction with
the program, teenagers' concerns, beliefs in control and feelings about the future,
individual substance use behaviors, relationships with friends and family, participation in groups, perception of community strengths and problems, and actions
related to community change.

To deepen the study of the program's context and the cultural differences at
each site, researchers also undertook a limited multisite case study approach (Yin
1994). Two subunits were chosen within each site: the individual participating
students to assess individual change possibilities, and the school and community
context and implementation of the intervention to assess community change
possibilities.

Although the initial research questions focused to a great extent on how a
Freirian program could promote community change, the continuing data analysis pointed toward a refocus on individual actors and how they engage in a larger
change process. In the final data analysis, five major themes emerged: (1) the changes
in youths' abilities to engage in dialogue, (2) youths' emotional changes related
to connectedness with others and self-disclosure, (3) youths' critical thinking ability to perceive the social nature of the problems and their personal link to society, (4) youths' level of actions to promote changes, and, most important, (5) youths'
own perception of how they could be involved in change.

A three-stage model of change that combined the five processes into one
central pattern of change surfaced. That pattern concerned the youths' perception of their changing self-identity, the fifth process just mentioned (see figure 12.2).
Participatory dialogue from the program appeared to start a three-stage process of
self-identity change: action orientation of caring, individual responsibility to

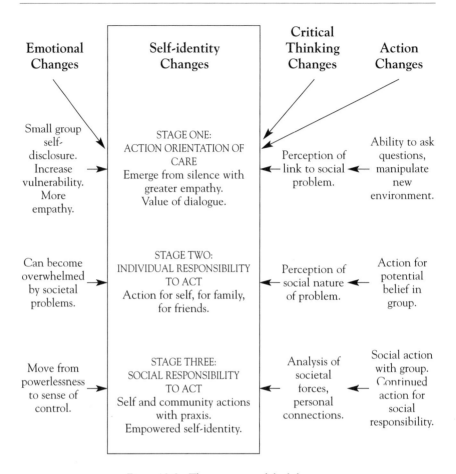

*Figure 12.2.* Three-stage model of change.
*Source:* Reprinted from N. Wallerstein and V. Sanchez-Merki, 1994, "Freirian Praxis in Health Education," *Health Education Research* 9, no. 1:105–18, by permission of Oxford University Press.

act, and social responsibility to act within each stage. The youths experienced changes on emotional, critical thinking, and action levels (Wallerstein 1989).

In the first stage, the youths developed an action orientation of caring about the problem, each other, and their ability to act in the world. The key processes involved in this stage were the recognition (emotionally and cognitively) of one's personal connection and susceptibility to the problem and the nonjudgmental small-group environment, which enabled dialogue and self-disclosure, the development of empathy for others, and the new active role of question asker. In the words of one Laguna student, "It's scary at times to talk about feelings . . . but once feelings got out, it wasn't so hard. Everyone could share. . . . If you want to cry, cry."

In the second stage, the youths began to act for individual changes, expressing an ability to help others who were close to them. This second stage, individual responsibility, evolved naturally as individuals attempted to fulfill their new ethic of care. The motivation for action was significant in that it arose directly out of the participatory and caring dialogue in the hospital-jail experience. The students' increased self-efficacy to talk and help others and their own self-articulated behavior changes reinforced their self-confidence and their own recognition of their personal changes in self-perception and in perception of others. As one student commented, "Talking to these people at the hospital, they really got me to think, wow, just think, some of these people around my neighborhood might want to just talk. Maybe if we just talk to them and tell them I did care about you, maybe that would make an impression in their life."

In the third stage, the youths reached a level of understanding about the need for social responsibility and the possibility for larger social actions. This third stage, social responsibility, requires critical thinking and ongoing support to maintain the commitment to work on problems over the long term, despite having an appreciation for the difficulties of both personal and social change.

Many students from both schools suggested that group actions could be more effective than individual actions. In the words of one student, "Probably anyone can do something, if you get enough people against it. [You] need more people to change the community, working together that are informed. . . . Alone, [you] can't make the ideal community happen."

Interesting cultural differences also emerged from the data. For example, although both the Native American and the Hispanic students expressed a belief that groups could make a difference, the Hispanic students saw an important role for individuals: "Groups can have a bigger influence, [but] maybe individuals can help set up groups." "[It's] people working together, one person has to stand up and say something. A group is easier; you have support."

The Native American students expressed the opposite point of view: "Individuals can do nothing, maybe talk to officials, but I don't think they'll do anything. . . . I went to the tribal council and said bars just make people go bad. The first lieutenant agreed, but the governor didn't want to close the bars because the tribe gets half the profit."

Nevertheless, these latter comments of hopelessness were not congruent with the students' actions: all but two of the ten Laguna-Acoma students were involved in peer education and tribal council presentations, for example. Whether their comments reflected a cultural belief that figures of authority are the ones to make the changes, an accurate appraisal of the situation, or some combination of these and other factors is not known. Such findings point up the need for far greater attention to the interaction of social and cultural factors in community organizing and interventions research.

In addition to identifying three stages of change, research results from this study underscored the role of many of the individual change processes as intermediate variables to community empowerment outcomes or as psychological empowerment outcomes (Zimmerman 2000). Variables identified within this qualitative study included the protection-motivation variables for self- and other protection, empathy, critical thinking, belief in group action, and group behaviors, such as extent of participation in social actions.

In the 1990s, ASAP received funding from NIAAA (R01 AA08943-01A3) to conduct a randomized school trial of the program, using a questionnaire that incorporated the newly identified cognitive protection-motivation and empowerment variables. Eight hundred seventh-grade students (half intervention and half control schools) were followed from pre-test until the year-and-a-half follow-up post-test. While in-depth analysis of the results is available from the authors, the program showed intervention youth developing a number of statistically significant increases of other-protective socially responsible efficacies that had previously not been reported in the protection-motivation or empowerment literature and are relatively new for adolescent prevention research. These included response and self-efficacies around protecting families and friends, empathy, and social influence–perceived control. One of the program benefits was the improved attitudes of intervention males; it is possible that the hospital-detention center environment is more attractive to male adolescents, who tend to take greater risks and require higher levels of stimulation.

On the whole, program effectiveness was modest, which poses interesting questions for intervention research. In this case, standardized implementation of ASAP proved difficult because of the open-ended character of the Freirian-based curriculum and the uneven abilities of college-student facilitators to deliver the program consistently (Helitzer et al. 2000). Moreover, measurement for interventions based on empowerment and protection-motivation is still under development. Although ASAP scales for "other-protective" and "self-protective" cognitive domains reflected good internal reliability, additional cognitive measures have been proposed beyond what was available when we started the NIAAA research: youth sense of community, collective efficacy, political efficacy, belief in effectiveness of group action, self-attitudes of leadership, as well as behavioral measures of community participation and advocacy.

Finally, although individual outcomes of psychological empowerment may interact with community empowerment, community outcomes are more problematic to assess and require complementary qualitative data gathering. Direct impact on the school and community is hard to gauge, even when ASAP has concentrated on community action. One example of a community change was that ASAP students from Laguna-Acoma were asked to make presentations at the tribal council and at several village meetings. Although girls normally are not permitted to attend village meetings, the ASAP girl students were given their first opportunity to participate in the political system of their tribal villages.

Community empowerment research within community psychology and public health has supported further interest in the measurement of psychological, organizational, and community changes and the use of research processes to strengthen community organizing (Zimmerman and Rappaport 1988, Zimmerman 2000, Israel et al. 1994, Wallerstein and Bernstein 1994, Fetterman et al. 1996). But research still needs to be undertaken to link individual changes in self-efficacy, participation, and action orientation with indicators of community capacity or empowerment—that is, communities with the capacity for solving problems, developing support structures, and increasing access to resources (Cottrell 1976, Wallerstein 1992, Eng and Parker 1994, Parker et al. 2001).

Even with instruments that measure change with the community as the unit of analysis, assessment of the impact of Freirian interventions, like all open-ended community organizing efforts, must largely be a discovery process. Community researchers have argued that empowerment is a dynamic construct that may vary across time, across domains (such as school or family), and across contexts; as such, empowerment cannot be measured through a universal or global measurement tool (Zimmerman 2000). Qualitative research should therefore accompany any measurement instruments to take into account the preconditions for change—that is, the existence of other viable community groups; the barriers imposed from inside and outside the community; and the particular culture, power dynamics, and history of the community undergoing the change. Part of the evaluation will always be a case study that provides a detailed account from which others can learn.

## ASAP as Inspiration for Intervention Research

ASAP has made a major contribution to the conceptual and methodological base of an ambitious new CDC-funded, community-based participatory research (CBPR) project in several diverse, low-income neighborhoods in Contra Costa County, California. Youth Empowerment Strategies (YES!) is a three-year, after-school program and research project modeled on the principles of individual and community capacity building and CBPR (Wilson et al. in press). Through the project, high school and college graduate-student pairs receive extensive training to work with children entering the developmental transition into adolescence and the social transition into middle school. In small, co-facilitated groups at local elementary schools, children in the YES! program take part in a variety of participatory and empowerment approaches designed to facilitate critical thinking skills and both self- and collective efficacy.

Although YES! differs from ASAP in several important ways (for example, working with younger children and adding as a centerpiece a photovoice process in which youth use cameras to document and then discuss and act on their concerns; see chapter 19), it also replicates many of ASAP's key features. As in ASAP, for example, participants in YES! engage in social action projects. They focus in year 1 (fifth grade) on their school community, in year 2 (sixth grade) on their local neighborhood, and in year 3 (seventh grade) on the broader community level. Freirian problem posing and the S-H-O-W-E-D acronym are used as tools for looking critically at visual depictions of the themes discussed in each group (Wilson et al. in press).

The YES! project will ultimately involve 160 students and 160 controls who will be followed over three years to determine the impacts of the program on multilevel empowerment and sense of social responsibility as well as on children's health attitudes and behaviors. In providing ongoing consultation to the YES! project team as well as assistance in training and other areas, ASAP co-developer Nina Wallerstein is helping adapt the lessons from ASAP to this new project, which researchers hope will yield valuable information about the process of empowerment, including whether an intervention with this young a population can positively influence children's health outcomes (Wilson et al. in press).

## Implications for Community Organizing within Health Education Practice

Some core issues exist about the limits and benefits of community organizing within a program such as ASAP or YES! First, we must consider the ability of youths to assume responsibility for organizing. Adolescents' acquisition of skills while co-learning with adults is a primary step for community organizing. They learn to work across age and ethnic-cultural borders; yet in the end, due to the many financial, ethical, legal, and mechanistic issues, youths still depend on adults. Their organizing strategies may go only as far as the alliance formed with supportive adults. For example, resources such as transportation, materials, supplies, money, and personal contacts exist within adult supporters. Even if youths have access to these resources, they also depend on family support. They need parental or legal guardian consent to remain involved or to conduct the organizing events. The hope is, however, that after having participated in ASAP or YES!, youths will develop decision-making skills, a belief in group action, awareness and self-efficacy toward social responsible action, and a belief and confidence in themselves as leaders who can make a difference.

Second, the school as the starting place for the program raises questions of community as an organizing base. Unfortunately, many youths identify with their school, their neighborhood, their ethnic culture, or their gang and will not work across these boundaries. Broader organizing would have to take these polarized subcommunities into account to help bridge the differences and build a community of youths who could have citywide policy impact.

Third, most funding for programs like ASAP is categorical—for alcohol and other drug prevention. Since alcohol and drugs have been a prominent concern for teenagers, and adolescents can choose projects within the broad range of adolescent risky behaviors, categorical funding may not be a major obstacle. As discussed in chapter 7, however, in a situation where a community's or group's perceived needs or concerns do not correspond to those of the funding source, the ethical and practical use of a model like this one would be hampered.

Fourth, we must consider the challenge of integrating Freirian listening-dialogue-action educational methods into health education programs and community organizing strategies. This challenge is important for established health education programs such as ASAP and for other organizing efforts that depend on group processes. The Freirian education skills of listening, structured dialogue, and responsiveness to emotions that emerge in the dialogue require practice and a commitment to communities over time, which is especially important in building trust with youths. Actions that yield results need to be built in from the beginning of any effort to sustain youth commitment. Continual reflection on actions, or praxis, is critical for movement from stage 2, or individual responsibility to act, to stage 3, or social responsibility to act. Without critical awareness, participants who may be motivated to become actors for change can redevelop feelings of hopelessness and powerlessness.

Finally, Freirian facilitators are challenged to be co-learners and to honor youths as full decision-making partners in a health education or organizing effort. In reality, power dynamics permeate most relationships between adults and youths, whether because adults bring expectations or because adult facilitators often come from a class or ethnic group that differs from that of their target population (Labonte 1994). Although a focus on disfranchised communities may inadvertently perpetuate power dynamics and racism (Pinderhughes 1990), a Freirian approach enables both sides (adult facilitators and youths) to analyze social problems and learn how to challenge the hierarchies together. Organizers themselves would find it useful to engage in self-reflection and self-renewal as they seek to understand their role in community change and how actions they take with the group may either challenge the status quo or promote further dependency.

## Conclusion

This chapter has presented a comprehensive model that combines Freirian empowerment education, critical consciousness, and praxis with community organizing principles such as leadership development, community building, high-level participation, and advocacy. Although direct community organizing is not the starting place, the ASAP model illustrates how young people are introduced to the skills required to participate in community organizing and to explore the processes of working with the barriers and resources presented to them. The process engages them in learning to combine many of the principles with an over-arching social change agenda.

As demonstrated throughout this chapter, a Freirian approach can be inte-grated with individual cognitive change theories to create programs directed at both individual and community change. The three-stage model of change suggests that people engaged in Freirian programs can evolve beyond powerlessness to cre-ate a sense of empowerment—that they can make a difference in their worlds.

Because a Freirian approach presupposes an interactive model of behavior and social change, it acknowledges that individuals can best develop a sense of self-direction and empowerment in the context of transforming community power-lessness. With praxis, health educators and organizers can model and promote their own growth as they promote the growth of the youths with whom they work.

## Acknowledgments

This chapter was adapted from N. Wallerstein and V. Sanchez-Merki, 1994, "Freirian Praxis in Health Education," *Health Education and Research* 9, no. 1: 105–18, by permission of Oxford University Press.

## References

Alschuler, A. S. 1980. *School Discipline: A Socially Literate Solution*. New York: McGraw-Hill.

Arnold, R., B. Burke, C. James, D. Martin, and B. Thomas. 1995. *Educating for a Change*. Toronto: Doris Marshall Institute.

Auerbach, E., and N. Wallerstein. In press. *ESL for Action: Problem-Posing at Work*. 2d ed. Edmonton, Alberta: Grassroots.

Barndt, D. 1989. *Naming the Moment: Political Analysis for Action*. Toronto: Jesuit Centre for Social Faith and Justice.

Burke, B., J. Geronimo, D. Martin, B. Thomas, and C. Wall. 2002. *Education for Chang-ing Unions*. Toronto: Between the Lines.

Carroll, J., and M. Minkler. 2000. "Freire's Message for Social Workers: Looking Back, Look-ing Ahead." *Journal of Community Practice* 8, no. 1: 21–36.

Cottrell, L. S., Jr. 1976. "The Competent Community." In *Further Explorations in Social Psy-chiatry*, edited by B. H. Kaplan, R. N. Wilson, and A. A. Leighton, 195–209. New York: Basic Books.

Delp, L., M. Outman-Kramer, S. Schurman, and K. Wong. 2002. *Teaching for Change: Pop-ular Education and the Labor Movement*. Los Angeles: UCLA, Center for Labor Research and Education.

Dow-Velarde, L., R. Starling, and N. Wallerstein. 2002. "Identity in Early Adolescence via Social Change Activities: Experience of the Adolescent Social Action Program." In *Understanding Early Adolescent Self and Identity*, edited by T. M. Brinthaupt and R. P. Lipka, 276–91. Albany: State University of New York Press.

Eng, E., and E. Parker. 1994. "Measuring Community Competence in the Mississippi Delta: The Interface between Program Evaluation and Empowerment." *Health Education Quarterly* 21, no. 2: 199–220.

Fetterman, D., S. Kaftarian, and A. Wandersman. 1996. *Empowerment Evaluation: Knowledge and Tools for Self-Assessment and Accountability*. Thousand Oaks, Calif.: Sage.

Fiore, K., and N. Elsasser. 1982. "Strangers No More: A Liberatory Literacy Curriculum." *College English* 44, no. 2: 115–28.

Floyd, D. L., S. Prentice-Dunn, and R. W. Rogers. 2000. "A Meta-Analysis on Protection Motivation Theory." *Journal of Applied Social Psychology* 30, no. 2: 407–29.

Freire, P. 1970. *Pedagogy of the Oppressed*, translated by M. B. Ramos. New York: Seabury.

———. 1973. *Education for Critical Consciousness*. New York: Seabury.

Helitzer, D., S. J. Yoon, N. Wallerstein, and L. Dow y Garcia-Velarde. 2000. "The Role of Process Evaluation in the Training of Facilitators of an Adolescent Health Education Program." *Journal of School Health* 70, no. 4: 141–47.

Hope, A., S. Timmel, and C. Hodzi. 1984. *Training for Transformation: A Handbook for Community Workers*. Vols. 1–3. Gweru, Zimbabwe: Mambo.

Israel, B., B. Checkoway, A. Schulz, and M. Zimmerman. 1994. "Health Education and Community Empowerment: Conceptualizing and Measuring Perceptions of Individual, Organizational, and Community Control." *Health Education Quarterly* 21, no. 2: 149–70.

Job, R. F. 1988. "Effective and Ineffective Use of Fear in Health Promotion Campaigns." *American Journal of Public Health* 78, no. 2: 163–67.

Labonte, R. 1994. "Health Promotion and Empowerment: Reflections on Professional Practice." *Health Education Quarterly* 21, no. 2: 253–68.

Minkler, M. 1992. "Community Organizing among the Elderly Poor in the United States: A Case Study." *International Journal of Health Services* 22, no. 2: 303–16.

Parker, E. A., R. L. Lichtenstein, A. J. Schultz, B. A. Israel, M. Schork, K. J. Steinman, and S. A. James. 2001. "Disentangling Measures of Individual Perceptions of Community Social Dynamics: Results of a Community Survey." *Health Education and Behavior* 28, no. 4: 462–86.

Pinderhughes, D. 1990. *Understanding Race, Ethnicity, and Power: The Key to Efficacy in Clinical Practice*. New York: Free Press.

Reed, D. 1981. *Education for Building a People's Movement*. Boston: South End.

Rippetoe, P., and R. W. Rogers. 1987. "Effects of Components of Protection-Motivation Theory on Adaptive and Maladaptive Coping with a Health Threat." *Journal of Personality and Social Psychology* 52, no. 3: 596–604.

Rogers, R. W. 1984. "Changing Health-Related Attitudes and Behavior: The Role of Preventive Health Psychology." In *Interfaces in Psychology*, edited by R. McGlyn, J. Maddox, C. Stoltenberg, and R. J. Harvey. Lubbock: Texas Tech University Press.

Rogers, R. W., C. W. Deckner, and C. R. Mewborn. 1978. "An Expectancy-Value Theory Approach to the Long-Term Modification of Smoking Behavior." *Journal of Clinical Psychology* 34, no. 2: 562–66.

Rogers, R. W., and C. R. Mewborn. 1976. "Fear Appeals and Attitude Change: Effects of a Threat's Noxiousness, Probability of Occurrence, and the Efficacy of Coping Responses." *Journal of Personality and Social Psychology* 34, no. 1: 54–61.

Shaffer, R. 1983. *Beyond the Dispensary*. Nairobi, Kenya: Amref.

Shor, I. 1980. *Critical Teaching and Everyday Life*. Boston: South End.

———, ed. 1987. *Freire for the Classroom: A Sourcebook for Liberatory Teaching*. New Haven, Conn.: Boynton/Cook.

Shor, I., and P. Freire. 1987. *A Pedagogy for Liberation*. South Hadley, Mass.: Bergin and Garvey.

Spector, R. E. 1979. *Cultural Diversity in Health and Illness*. New York: Appleton-Century-Crofts.

Stainback, R., and R. Rogers. 1983. "Identifying Effective Components of Alcohol Abuse Prevention Programs: Effects of Fear Appeals, Message Style, and Source Expertise." *International Journal of Addictions* 18, no. 3: 393–405.

Unda, J. 2002. *Seeds for Change: A Curriculum Guide for Worker-Centered Literacy.* Ottawa: Canadian Labour Congress.

Vella, J. 1994. *Learning to Listen, Learning to Teach: The Power of Dialogue in Educating Adults.* San Francisco: Jossey-Bass.

———. 1995. *Training through Dialogue: Promoting Effective Learning and Change with Adults.* San Francisco: Jossey-Bass.

Wallerstein, N. 1983. *Language and Culture in Conflict: Problem Posing in the ESL Classroom.* Reading, Mass.: Addison-Wesley.

———. 1989. *Empowerment Education: Freire's Theories Applied to Health: A Case Study of Alcohol Prevention for Indian and Hispanic youth.* Ann Arbor, Mich.: UMI Dissertation Information Service.

———. 1992. "Powerlessness, Empowerment, and Health: Implications for Health Promotion Programs." *American Journal of Health Promotion* 6, no. 3: 197–205.

Wallerstein, N., and E. Bernstein. 1988. "Empowerment Education: Freire's Ideas Adapted to Health Education." *Health Education Quarterly* 15, no. 4: 379–94.

———, eds. 1994. Special issue. *Health Education Quarterly* 21, nos. 2–3.

Wallerstein, N., and V. Sanchez-Merki. 1994. "Freirian Praxis in Health Education: Research Results from an Adolescent Prevention Program." *Health Education Research* 9, no. 1: 105–18.

Wallerstein, N., and M. Weinger, eds. 1992. "Empowerment Approaches to Worker Health and Safety Education." *American Journal of Industrial Medicine* 22, no. 5: 619–784.

Werner, D., and B. Bower. 1982. *Helping Health Workers Learn.* Palo Alto, Calif.: Hesperian Foundation.

Wilson, N., M. Minkler, S. Dasho, R. Carrillo, N. Wallerstein, and D. Garcia. In press. "Training Students As Partners in Community Based Participatory Research: The Youth Empowerment Strategies (YES!) Project." *Journal of Community Practice.*

Yeich, S. 1996. "Grassroots Organizing with Homeless People: A Participatory Research Approach." *Journal of Social Issues* 52, no. 1: 111–21.

Yin, R. K. 1994. *Case Study Research Design Methods.* 2d ed. Newbury Park, Calif.: Sage.

Zimmerman, M. A. 2000. "Empowerment Theory: Psychological, Organizational and Community Levels of Analysis." In *Handbook of Community Psychology,* edited by J. Rappaport and E. Seidman, 43–63. New York: Academic/Plenum.

Zimmerman, M., and J. Rappaport. 1988. "Citizen Participation, Perceived Control, and Psychological Empowerment." *American Journal of Community Psychology* 16, no. 5: 725–50.

# Community Organizing and Community Building within and across Diverse Groups

# Part V and Cultures

THE PAST TWO DECADES have witnessed a growing appreciation of the community organizing and community building efforts taking place among and with women; people of color; people with disabilities; lesbian, gay, bisexual, and transgendered people; and other diverse groups. For the most part, however, this wealth of experience has not been well represented in the literature. Furthermore, what literature does exist suggests that traditional models of community organizing are often ill-suited to work with disfranchised groups, whose reality tends to differ markedly from that of the architects of many of these models.

Part 5 begins, in chapter 13, with Lorraine M. Gutierrez and Edith A. Lewis's thoughtful approach to organizing with women of color, which stresses the utility of feminist perspectives for developing a culture- and gender-relevant model of practice. Although the reader will see important parallels between some aspects of Gutierrez and Lewis's model and the women-centered organizing model presented in chapter 11, Gutierrez and Lewis accent both theory development and the lived experience of women of color. Using a framework composed of interrelated principles of education, participation, and capacity building, the authors draw on the literature and a wealth of personal experience in social work to develop an approach that acknowledges and confronts the combined effects of racism, classism, and sexism. Building in part on the work of Felix Rivera and John Erlich (1995), Gutierrez and Lewis see varying roles for organizers that depend, in part, on their degree of oneness and identification with the community in question. Regardless of the role organizers play, however, the authors argue that a number of precepts are critical to effective organizing with women of color, among them learning actively, recognizing and embracing the conflict inherent in cross-cultural work, involving women of color early on in leadership roles, and in other ways contributing to community capacity.

The theme of community organizing by and with women of color is further developed in chapter 14, where Galen El-Askari and Sheryl Walton share a case study of lessons in cultural humility and the need for broader systems change. Their example concerns two local health departments' attempt to create a partnership with local communities in ambitious community building and organizing projects. Using a strengths-based approach, and acknowledging from the outset numerous opportunities for cultural misunderstandings and miscommunications, the authors offer a deeply personal account of the genesis and evolution of the Healthy Neighborhoods Project in West Contra Costa County, California, and its successful replication in the neighboring city of Berkeley. This chapter grapples with a number of difficult issues, among them the particular challenges posed by community distrust of health departments and universities, cultural misunderstanding on multiple levels, clashes between community and bureaucratic needs and ways of doing things, and professional discomfort over true sharing of power and control with community residents. The particular difficulties faced by one of the authors as an "outsider within" also are candidly shared, as are the accomplishments of these two inspiring projects and the lessons learned on all sides about collaborative community building and organizing efforts.

Like the Healthy Neighborhoods Project, the case study presented in chapter 15 is set in a low-income community in northern California plagued by high rates of violent crime, substance abuse, HIV/AIDS, and other problems related in part to persistent poverty and neglect. But this case study involves a very different population—the elderly residents of San Francisco's Tenderloin hotels, whose high rates of social isolation, depression, and other mental disabilities had characterized them as an unorganizable population. Chapter 15 chronicles the birth, evolution, and closure of the Tenderloin Senior Organizing Project (TSOP), an outreach and organizing effort that was largely successful in proving this characterization false. Grounded in the philosophy and methods of Saul Alinsky, (1972), Paulo Freire (1973), and John McKnight (1987), the project differs from more traditional health and social programs serving the elderly by emphasizing individual and community empowerment and resident determination of needs and goals.

The transformation of TSOP over time from an outreach to a true organizing project is discussed, as are its efforts in areas such as leadership building, coalition formation around issues, and the creation of social support networks and tenants' organizations as vehicles for grassroots organizing. Factors contributing to the demise of the project after sixteen years are explored, as are efforts and challenges in the area of evaluating or measuring project outcomes and tracking replication efforts. Although this chapter illustrates the often impressive changes that disfranchised and oppressed communities can achieve by identifying and building on their strengths, it also points up the impossibility of large-scale change without a deep societal-level commitment to the reduction of social inequalities.

## References

Alinsky, S. D. 1972. *Rules for Radicals*. New York: Random House.

Freire, P. 1973. *Education for Critical Consciousness*. New York: Seabury.

McKnight, J. 1987. "Regenerating Community." *Social Policy* 17 no. 3: 54–58.

Rivera, F., and J. Erlich, eds. 1995. *Community Organizing in a Diverse Society*. 2d ed. Boston: Allyn and Bacon.

LORRAINE M. GUTIERREZ
EDITH A. LEWIS

Chapter 13

# Education, Participation, and Capacity Building in Community Organizing with Women of Color

THE FIELD of community organizing has only recently begun to address the need for an approach to practice that respects and builds on the special challenges posed by our increasingly diverse society. Although much community organizing has taken place among women and communities of color, for example, surprisingly little attention has been paid to the ways in which race, gender, ethnicity, or social class will affect the organizing effort. This oversight has often prevented organizers from working effectively with women or communities of color (Bradshaw et al. 1994, Burghardt 1982, Rivera and Erlich 1995). By failing to recognize and take into account the many ways in which issues of oppression affect organizing work, organizers can perpetuate the objectification and exploitation of these groups (Burghardt 1982). Organizers whose own racial or ethnic stereotypes distort their view of communities of color, for example, will be ineffective in building leadership or working in partnership (Bradshaw et al. 1994, Rivera and Erlich 1995). In this way, community organizing efforts can perpetuate the very problems they were designed to solve.

This chapter begins by examining several recent contributions to our thinking about organizing with women of color, with special attention to the contributions of feminist perspectives on organizing. An empowerment framework stressing education, participation, and capacity building is then developed and used to explore different dimensions of effective community organizing with women of color. Examples of organizing both within and across racial-ethical groups illustrate many of the points made and offer lessons for social change professionals in their roles as organizers.

## Multicultural Perspectives on Community Organizing

Much of the literature that does exist on multicultural organizing emphasizes the ways in which organizers can develop cultural competence for working in part-

240

nership with communities. In particular, this literature has stressed the ways in which organizers can use their own self-awareness to build bridges for work within communities. Organizers are encouraged to take the role of the learner in approaching a community and discovering its problems and strengths (Burghardt 1982, Bradshaw et al. 1994, Rivera and Erlich 1995).

A critical contribution to organizing with communities of color may be found in Felix Rivera and John Erlich's (1995) approach to identifying the appropriate roles for the organizer in light of his or her relationship to the community. If the organizer is a member of the community, these analysts argue, then primary contact is appropriate. Primary contact involves immediate and personal grassroots work with the community. In contrast, an organizer who has a similar ethnic or racial background but is not part of the community should instead be involved on the secondary level. This level involves participation as a liaison between the community and the larger society. The tertiary level of contact is most appropriate for those who are not members of the group. They can provide valuable contributions to the community through consultation and the sharing of technical knowledge. For example, outside professionals interested in participating in community work with a local African American neighborhood could first establish relationships with key individuals in the community. The professional as organizer's responsibilities would be those defined by the community, no matter how insignificant those tasks might seem on the surface. Efforts to learn the strengths of the community as they are exemplified in daily learning activities within the community would be a primary activity for the organizer. In this way, residents would, in time, recognize the organizer's willingness to use the culturally competent perspective of noninterference, and more opportunities for work with that community might be revealed (Lewis 1993).

In work on organizing with communities of color, Catherine Bradshaw, Steven Soifer, and Lorraine Gutierrez (1994) propose a hybrid model of organizing that integrates aspects of Saul Alinsky's (1972) approach to social action organizing with relevant perspectives from feminist organizing. Flexibility, leadership identification and training, the appropriate use of both collaborative and confrontational tactics, and the role of the organizer as a learner and facilitator are among the characteristics of this hybrid model. Of particular importance in this model are skills for developing cultural competence that enable the outside organizer to better understand, respect, and learn from the community. These skills involve (1) cultivating awareness of one's own understanding of the community, (2) finding ways to learn more about the local community through key informants, (3) working as partners to develop local leadership, and (4) focusing on ways to build cohesiveness within and between ethnic communities. As is by now clear, the most critical role of the organizer is that of a learner who approaches the community to understand and facilitate change.

## Contributions from Feminism

Much of the conceptual and practice-based literature on organizing with women has been written from a feminist perspective (Gutierrez and Lewis 1995; Hyde 1986, 1994; Weil 1995). Feminist approaches can contribute to organizing with women of color because they emphasize integrating personal and political issues through dialogue. Feminist organizing assumes that sexism is a significant force in the experiences of all women and one that lies at the root of many of the problems they face. Therefore, a major focus for organizing with women of color is to identify ways in which sexism, racism, and other forms of oppression are affecting their lives (Bricker-Jenkins and Hooyman 1986; Gould 1987; Hyde 1986, 1994; Faulkner and Kopacsi 1988; Morell 1987; Zavella 1986). Common methods for feminist organizing include the development of consciousness-raising groups, creation of alternative services, and social action that incorporates street theater and other holistic methods (Hyde 1986, 1994).

An important focus of feminist approaches is reflected in their concern about developing ways to work across differences. All women are thought to be a part of a community of women as well as members of their own specific communities. Therefore, organizers need to work to bridge differences between women based on factors such as race, class, physical ability, and sexual orientation on the principle that diversity is strength. According to this perspective, "Feminist practitioners will not only strive to eliminate racism, classism, heterosexism, anti-Semitism, ableism, and other systems of oppression and exploitation, but will affirm the need for diversity by actively reaching out to achieve it" (Bricker-Jenkins and Hooyman 1986). This goal for feminist organizing has been most effective when carried out from a multicultural perspective (Gutierrez and Lewis 1994).

## Organizing with Women of Color

Very little literature has looked specifically at methods for organizing women of color. Yet as we have discussed elsewhere (Gutierrez and Lewis 1994, 1995), organizing by women within ethnic communities in the United States has a rich and diverse history. For example, a century ago, leaders such as Ida B. Wells Barnett organized the Black Women's Clubs, which were instrumental in developing nursing homes, daycare centers, and orphanages in African American communities. These clubs also organized for social change, particularly on anti-lynching and antirape campaigns and in the foundation of organizations such as the National Urban League (Collins 2000, Gutierrez and Lewis 1995, Macht and Quam 1986, Smith 1986).

Women of color have always worked to improve conditions within their communities and in society in general and have been more likely than European American middle-class women to see community activism as a natural outgrowth of their gender role (Ackelsberg and Diamond 1987, Gilkes 1980). During the mid- to late twentieth century, for example, women played important roles in the movement for equality and civil rights in ethnic minority communities (Evans 1980, Muñoz 1989, West 1990, Withorn 1984). Neighborhood violence, economic issues, and environmental concerns are just a few of the areas on which women of color in urban communities have organized ("Fighting Back" 1988, Hirsch 1991, "Mothers' Group" 1989).

Effective community organizing efforts will build upon these traditions. By looking at these historical and contemporary efforts, we can identify ways to draw upon their strengths and learn from and adapt the strategies that already exist. As already noted, the role of the organizer can and should vary according to her relationship to the community or the issue being addressed (Rivera and Erlich 1995). To determine the appropriate role, we must involve the community in defining the issues it wishes to address and the strategies it feels will be most effective and culturally appropriate in attempting to achieve collectively set goals. For example, a Native American woman may be able to use her role as a member of the community and a designated leader to work on the primary level with her community to bring about change. A very different role in relation to the community would be taken by a Latina or Japanese American organizer, who could provide important technical assistance or research skills but would not work on this primary level. Although we emphasize the necessity of participation by community members in primary roles, the important roles that can be played by nonmembers of the community on the secondary and tertiary levels should not be overlooked.

## Education, Participation, and Capacity Building

What does this analysis suggest about community organizing with women of color? Using an empowerment framework that stresses the core concepts of education, participation, and capacity building, we can develop sensitive and effective methods for community practice. Many of the methods described here are equally relevant to organizers and community members; and the processes of education, participation, and capacity building should take place within the organizer as well as with community members. These reciprocal process methods can be summarized as follows:

### Education
1. Learn about, understand, and participate in the women's ethnic community
2. Recognize and build upon ways in which women of color have worked effectively within their own communities; build upon existing structures

3. Serve as a facilitator, and view the situation through the lens or vision of women of color

*Participation*

4. Use the process of praxis to understand the historical, political, and social context of the organizing effort
5. Begin with the formation of small groups
6. Recognize and embrace the conflict that characterizes cross-cultural work

*Capacity building*

7. Involve women of color in leadership roles
8. Understand and support the need that women of color may have for their own separate programs and organizations

## EDUCATION

Educational efforts toward community organizing and change need to be grounded in the ways in which women of color share similarities and differences with European American women and men of color. Community organizers have often recognized the impact of powerlessness on women of color who are suffering under institutional racism. Frequently overlooked in this process, however, is the role of gender inequity in influencing the life chances of women of color. The history of community participation by women of color has often been ignored by the field. When women of color are viewed solely as members of their racial or ethnic group and gender is not taken into account, community organizers may alienate women of color and reinforce ways in which sexism, both in the larger society and within ethnic minority communities, is a form of oppression (Aragon de Valdez 1980, Collins 2000, Weil 1995, Zavella 1986).

As suggested in previous chapters, an important first step in effective community organizing involves defining *community*. The fact that women of color can be members of multiple communities and hold multiple identities based on race, gender, geography, and other factors presents both a challenge and an opportunity for organizers. From an organizing perspective, however, the central issue for organizing often defines the community. For example, if the issue is toxic waste dumping in a community, then the neighborhood or city may be an appropriate level for work. If the issue is sterilization abuse and reproductive rights, then gender may be the focus. Awareness of these memberships in multiple communities can be helpful when an organizer is building coalitions or alliances among different groups.

An organizer who is from a different racial, ethnic, or class background than the women she works with must recognize how her life experience has colored her perceptions and how her status has affected her power relative to the political structure. Her beliefs and perceptions should not dominate the organizing effort. She must work toward serving as a facilitator and view the situation through the lens or vision of women of color. In part, this requires allowing that vision to alter how the organizer views her own work and sharing that new information with others who hope to organize and work in communities of color.

When organizing with low-income women in a housing project, one of the authors of this chapter initially attempted to separate individual from community concerns. She believed at first that group members would work on individual problem resolution for eight weeks and then, having established a pattern of interaction within the group, would be able to work cooperatively on analysis and resolution of community concerns. It became clear within the first two meetings that the group could not separate and sequentially work with individual and community concerns. As one participant put it, "My individual problems are the community's problems." The flexibility to alter the design based on the realities of the community allowed the group to continue working toward resolution of its identified goals, not those of the facilitator-researcher. This example illustrates the importance of understanding the community's vision of reality and the process of praxis, or action based on critical reflection, to unravel and address the salient historical, social, and political forces at work. In the preceding example, had the outside organizer insisted on separating the individual from the community problem, she would have alienated and probably lost committed community activists for whom this separation was artificial and inappropriate. By respecting the community's vision of the intimate interdependence of these levels, however, she was able to facilitate a process through which participants proceeded to make change on both the individual and community levels (Lewis and Ford 1990).

Organizers should also use the process of praxis to understand and address the historical, political, and social contexts of the organizing effort. This means that the organizing process as well as the outcome will inform both the organized community and the community of the organizer. As organizers and community groups analyze the process and outcome of organizing efforts, the outcome of a tactic often emerges as less important than what the community and organizer learn about the nature of the problem being addressed. In this way, community issues are often redefined (Freire 1970, Lewis 1993).

The involvement of women of color in the battered women's movement nicely illustrates this principle. When many feminist shelters observed that they were unsuccessful in reaching women of color, they defined the problem as inadequate outreach. When this outreach was unsuccessful, women of color in some localities informed many shelter programs that their approach was alienating and foreign to communities of color. They often identified the lack of women of color in administrative or permanent staff positions as one way in which the program indicated a lack of commitment to their community. Programs that have been most successful with women of color have been those that addressed their own racism, classism, and ethnocentrism in the development of alternative programs (Schechter 1982).

## PARTICIPATION

Participating in the women's ethnic community is an important step for educating the organizer and building bridges for future work. This participation can result in an analysis of societal institutions, including the one represented by the organizer, and how they might ultimately benefit or hurt the community. Churches, community centers, schools, and social clubs can be avenues for reaching women of color and effecting change within the community. Knowledge can also be gained about specific communities of color through reading and participation in community events (Faulkner and Kopacsi 1988). Particularly for an organizer who is not an ongoing member of the community of women with whom she will be working, developing an understanding of the community's cultural context is vital.

In an effort to become involved in the community, one organizer participated in activities sponsored by the local community center. She worked for several months in enrichment programming for the children of the community before proceeding to work with the women. During this time, she became aware of community members' patterns of interaction, their relationships with agencies in the city, and other potential issues in the community. Community members and group participants had the opportunity to meet and talk with the community worker and watch her interact with their children. Many of the initial participants in subsequent organizing efforts later mentioned that their decision to participate in the work was directly related to their approval of the facilitator's work with their children and the nature of her presence in the community (Lewis and Ford 1990).

Effective organizing often begins with the formation of small groups. The small group provides the ideal environment for exploring the social and political aspects of personal problems and developing strategies for work toward social change (Gutierrez 1990, Hyde 1994, Pernell 1985, Schechter et al. 1985). It can also be a forum for identifying common goals among diverse groups of women.

The latter strategy involves organizing small groups of individuals to work on specific problems and later coordinating these small groups so that they can work in coalition with others on joint issues. On the community level, the small group, or house meeting strategy, has been the primary way in which women of color have been organizing movements to improve conditions in ghettos and barrios (Hirsch 1991, "Mothers' Group" 1989, "Fighting Back" 1988). For example, Clementine Barfield's work with Save Our Sons and Daughters in Detroit began with discussions among a small group of mothers who had experienced the loss of a child through a violent death in the inner city (Bates-Rudd 2001).

Building these alliances to develop community efforts can be particularly challenging when they involve more than one ethnic or other group. This is particularly true because the United States remains a highly segregated society in which many people experience little meaningful interaction with those outside their own race, class, ethnic group, or sexual orientation. Effective organizing across diverse groups requires breaking down societal boundaries to build alliances. Furthermore, it necessitates recognizing and embracing the conflict that characterizes cross-cultural work. Conflicts will inevitably arise both within those organizations that have been successful in reaching a diverse group and between the organization and a larger community that may be threatened by the absence of expected boundaries. In some respects, the emergence of conflict indicates that meaningful cross-cultural work is taking place. But the sources and resolution of conflict will affect the outcomes of the organizing effort. The extent to which the organizer anticipates conflict related to group interaction, the effects of internalized oppression, wider political strategies to hinder or destroy the community change effort, and similar factors often determines whether or not organizing efforts are successful (Ristock 1990, West 1990).

Conflict includes the discomfort many organizers feel when they find themselves the sole person from a different ethnic or class background in a group of women of color or when they attempt to participate for the first time in a community event that has previously been attended solely by persons from the community. It is important for organizers to recognize that they will be tested by community members to determine whether they, like others who came before, are present only to "take." Giving on the community's terms, as illustrated in the previous example of the organizer's work with children, is one example of the testing process.

In our experience, European American organizers are often less comfortable than women of color with the conflict engendered by the development of a multicultural organization. Conflicts are a part of our everyday lives. They reflect choices about fact, value, and strategy alternatives that we face intra- or interpersonally (Lewis 1988). Too often, women have been socialized into conflict-avoidance behaviors. These behaviors only temporarily delay conflicts, which will resurface when issues are not addressed directly. Addressing a conflict has often been misconstrued as synonymous with confrontation, another conflict resolution strategy. They are, however, quite different. Confrontation often means minimizing or attack on a party with which there is conflict. This minimization, either at the personal or political level, can easily be perceived as a threat, which inevitably escalates the conflict rather than creates a dialogue about its nature.

Addressing conflict directly means employing interpersonal skills such as engagement, active listening, and consensus building. It means viewing the situation through various lenses in the presence of all who are involved in the conflict and then managing to reach some consensus about how to proceed. The process of reaching consensus often involves being open about our differing conflict styles and managing to hear the content, rather than just the affect, of the messages being presented. To do so also requires taking a strengths approach—in this case, acknowledging the capacity or strengths in the conflict style of the group—with those who have only been privy to one way of handling conflicts. In this way, conflict-avoidance techniques may be valued for their ability to offset the attack, whereas confrontation approaches may be valued for their ability to focus immediate attention on the conflict.

Conflict resolution that results in genuine dialogue and analysis of the basis of difference will have a direct effect on the outcome of an organizing effort. For example, only after European Americans involved women of color in their organizations did many European American women encounter a different view of gender roles and how they translate into different strategies and goals. Once women of color were included in such organizations, work concerning sexual assault had to recognize and deal with the fears of many European American women concerning men of color. In one organization, it was only after the group began a campaign confronting the myth of the black rapist that women of color in the organization and the larger community came to believe that the organization represented their needs.

Dealing with such conflict is difficult but valuable. If we are to work toward a more equitable society, this vision must be integral to the work of our organizations. We must know ourselves and be open to knowing others. Dealing with community backlash and conflict also requires taking risks to speak out in support of our vision. The inability to resolve these conflicts has resulted in the death of some organizations and minimized our ability to work in coalition.

### CAPACITY BUILDING

Contemporary organizing by women of color has often taken a grassroots approach based upon existing networks of family, friends, or informal and formal ethnic community institutions. In this way, individual, family, and community interests are viewed as compatible and integrated with one another. Many African American women, Latinas, and other women of color describe themselves as motivated to engage in activism because of their commitment to their communities and ethnic groups (Collins 2000; Gilkes 1980, 1983; Lacayo 1989). Women also have often been active in the mutual aid societies in ethnic communities, such as the Hui among the Chinese, the Ko among the Japanese, and the tribal councils among Native Americans (Gutierrez and Lewis 1995). Each of these organizations has served as a vehicle for assisting individual ethnic group members, families, and entire communities in the establishment of business loans, funerals, and community programs.

Organizers must recognize and build upon these networks and the myriad ways in which women of color have worked effectively in their own communities. Outside organizers, regardless of their own race or ethnicity, need to work with community leaders and learn from them the most effective ways of working in particular communities. Working with existing leaders may involve organizers in activities that are different from those in which they usually engage. For example, to provide survival services, existing community leaders may be active in church-related activities or with municipal agencies (Bookman and Morgan 1986). Organizers can learn from these women ways that they have found to survive and leverage political power.

Organizers also need to recognize how women of color have been involved in advocating for women's rights since the beginning of the feminist movement. For example, many of the first shelters for battered women were founded by women of color who were responding to the needs in their communities (Schechter 1982). Recognition of the contributions of women of color to feminist causes can help to break down some of the barriers and difficulties that exist in this work.

As already suggested, however, community organizing with women of color may involve a broader perspective than the one initially envisioned by the organizer. This broader perspective recognizes the many ways in which race, gender, class, and ethnicity are intertwined. Consequently, it underscores the impossibility of separating the needs of women from those of their families and communities (Gutierrez and Lewis 1994). The role of women in the civil rights movements of the 1950s and 1960s certainly illustrates the importance of gender in mobilization efforts. The successful Montgomery, Alabama, bus boycott, for example, is usually credited to African American male ministers who were in public leadership positions. But the impetus for the boycott was a group of African American women who impressed on the ministers that the cause was just and that they would launch the boycott themselves if the ministers did not take a public stance. The women raised the consciousness of the ministers and in this way contributed significantly to social action. Nevertheless, they were willing to work behind the scenes rather than spearhead the boycott themselves because they thought it was imperative that African American men's leadership be supported. This delicate interaction of race, ethnicity, class, and gender must be in the forefront of the organizer's praxis perspective.

All too often, organizing with women of color has taken the unidirectional outreach approach in which communities of color are targets of change rather than active participants and collaborators. When the former approach is used, women of color often resist organizing efforts and, in some cases, undermine them (Schechter 1982, Faulkner and Kopacsi 1988). It is crucial, therefore, to involve women of color in leadership roles from the onset. Predominantly European American organizations wishing to collaborate with women of color will need to incorporate women of color as leaders and active participants before taking on this kind of work. Such collaboration may require redefining the kind of work the organization does as well as looking critically at members' attitudes toward institutions such as the church and family. The history of attempts at collaboration suggests that cross-cultural work requires identifying how racism may exclude women of color from leadership roles (Burghardt 1982, Schechter 1982). Successful collaboration requires European American organizers to change their interactions with women of color and become capable of sharing power and control of their programs. This type of organizational work embraces a tenet of feminist organizing: diversity is strength.

Issues of perceived or actual social class differences must be taken into account, even when the organizer is from the same ethnic or gender background as the community in which she is working. As noted, the definition of community may be psychological as well as geographic. Those entering or reentering communities need to recognize that their economic or educational backgrounds may seem to make them somehow different from other community members. They must anticipate suspicion or backlash as a possible consequence. As in other conflict situations, a process of dialogue and action can be used to work through this problem so that the organizer can then participate in the community on its own terms. One of the chapter authors received a high compliment during a community meeting, when she was introduced to others as "not an educated fool."

One method for building effective coalitions is the incorporation of informal debriefing groups for community workers. These groups include all members of the community and provide opportunities for input and clarification of the organizing process. Those in key leadership positions model their ongoing praxis experiences by being open about the choices made in the organizing effort and the assumptions upon which these choices rest. Debriefing sessions allow community members who are not an integral part of the organizing effort to share additional strategies and evaluate the impact of the design on the community to date. Some groups have used the house meeting strategy to provide debriefing opportunities, whereas others have relied on formal written materials such as community newsletters to keep community members informed. Consistent ongoing debriefing efforts need to be built into the organizing design and expanded as needed.

Within the realm of organizing, there is room for multiethnic organizations and cross-ethnic coalitions but also for organizations developed by and for women of color. In the latter regard, organizers need to understand and support the need that women of color may have for their own separate programs and organizations. For women of color, a separate group or organization in which we can explore who we are in relation to the communities in which we live often creates a vision for future work. A separate organization is one means for building on strengths and nurturing capacity within a community. For example, in work with women of color in an educational setting, the formation of a women of color caucus had positive impact on the ability of a women's studies program to hire more faculty of color and develop courses that were more racially and ethnically inclusive. Although the formation was initially viewed by some as divisive, all participants in the program ultimately recognized that the caucus was a critical element in the empowerment of women of color and their capacity to work for positive change for all.

## Conclusion

This chapter has used a framework of education, participation, and capacity building to explore empowering strategies and approaches for community organizing with women of color. Borrowing in part from Rivera and Erlich (1995), we have argued that different roles are appropriate for an organizer depending upon her relationship to the community (for example, whether she is a member, a nonmember with a similar racial or ethnic background, or a person of a different racial or ethnic group).

Regardless of the role played, however, several principles are critical in effective organizing with women of color. These include being an active learner and facilitator who can view a given situation through the lens of women of color, recognizing and embracing the conflict that characterizes cross-cultural work, involving women of color in leadership roles, and in other ways contributing to the building of community capacity. Both feminist perspectives and cultural perspectives on organizing in communities of color offer valuable lessons for organizers who cross race, ethnic, gender, class, and other lines in their organizing efforts.

### References

Ackelsberg, M., and I. Diamond. 1987. "Gender and Political Life: New Directions in Political Science." In *Analyzing Gender: A Handbook of Social Science*, edited by B. Hess and M. Feree, 504–25. Newbury Park, Calif.: Sage.

Alinsky, S. D. 1972. *Rules for Radicals*. New York: Random House.

Aragon de Valdez, T. 1980. "Organizing As a Political Tool for the Chicana." *Frontiers* 5, no. 2: 7–13.

Bates-Rudd, R. 2001. "Her Crusade Continues." *Detroit News*, January 24.

Bookman, A., and S. Morgan, eds. 1986. *Women and the Politics of Empowerment*. Philadelphia: Temple University Press.

Bradshaw, C., S. Soifer, and L. Gutierrez. 1994. "Toward a Hybrid Model for Effective Organizing with Women of Color." *Journal of Community Practice* 1, no. 1: 25–41.

Bricker-Jenkins, M., and N. Hooyman. 1986. *Not for Women Only: Social Work Practice for a Feminist Future*. Silver Spring, Md.: National Association of Social Workers.

Burghardt, S. 1982. *The Other Side of Organizing*. Cambridge, Mass.: Schenkman.

Collins, P. 2000. *Black Feminist Thought: Knowledge, Consciousness, and the Politics of Empowerment*. 2d ed. New York: Routledge.

Evans, S. 1980. *Personal Politics*. New York: Vintage.

Faulkner, A., and R. Kopacsi. 1988. "The Powers That Might Be: The Unity of White and Black Feminists." *Affilia* 3, no. 2: 33–50.

"Fighting Back: Frances Sandoval and Her Mother's Crusade Take Aim at Gangs." 1988. *Chicago Tribune Magazine*, October 16, pp. 10–24.

Freire, P. 1970. "Cultural Action for Freedom." *Harvard Educational Review* 40: 205–25, 452–77.
Gilkes, C. 1980. "Holding Back the Ocean with a Broom: Black Women and Community Work." In *The Black Woman*, edited by L. F. Rodgers-Rose, 217–32. Beverly Hills, Calif.: Sage.
———. 1983. "Going up for the Oppressed: The Career Mobility of Black Women Community Workers." *Journal of Social Issues* 39, no. 3: 115–39.
Gould, K. 1987. "Feminist Principles and Minority Concerns: Contributions, Problems, and Solutions." *Affilia* 2, no. 3: 6–19.
Gutierrez, L. 1990. "Working with Women of Color: An Empowerment Perspective." *Social Work* 35, no. 2: 149–54.
Gutierrez, L., and E. Lewis. 1994. "Community Organizing with Women of Color: A Feminist Approach." *Journal of Community Practice* 1, no. 2: 23–43.
———. 1995. "A Feminist Perspective on Organizing with Women of Color." In *Community Organizing in a Diverse Society*, edited by F. Rivera and J. Erlich, 97–116. 2d ed. Boston: Allyn and Bacon.
Hirsch, K. 1991. "Clementine Barfield Takes on the Mean Streets of Detroit." *Ms.* 1, no. 4: 54–58.
Hyde, C. 1986. "Experiences of Women Activists: Implications for Community Organizing Theory and Practice." *Journal of Sociology and Social Welfare* 13, no. 3: 545–62.
———. 1994. "Committed to Social Change: Voices from the Feminist Movement." *Journal of Community Practice* 1, no. 2: 45–64.
Lacayo, R. 1989. "On the Front Lines." *Time*, September 11, pp. 14–19.
Lewis, E. 1988. "The Single Door: Social Work with the Families of Disabled Children." *Social Casework* 69, no. 1: 61–63.
———. 1993. "Continuing the Legacy: On the Importance of Praxis in the Education of Social Work Students and Teachers." In *Multicultural Teaching in the University*, edited by D. Schoem, L. Frankel, X. Zuniga, and E. Lewis, 26–36. New York: Praeger.
Lewis, E., and B. Ford. 1990. "The Network Utilization Project: Incorporating Traditional Strengths of African Americans into Group Work Practice." *Social Work with Groups* 13, no. 3: 7–22.
Macht, M., and J. Quam. 1986. *Social Work: An Introduction*. Columbus, Ohio: Merrill.
Morell, C. 1987. "Cause Is Function: Toward a Feminist Model of Integration for Social Work." *Social Science Review* 61, no. 1: 144–55.
"Mothers' Group Fights Back in Los Angeles." 1989. *New York Times*, December 5, p. A32.
Muñoz, C. 1989. *Youth, Identity, and Power: The Chicano Movement*. London: Verso.
Pernell, R. 1985. "Empowerment and Social Group Work." In *Innovations in Social Group Work: Feedback from Practice to Theory*, edited by M. Parenes, 107–17. New York: Hawthorn.
Ristock, J. 1990. "Canadian Feminist Social Service Collectives: Caring and Contradictions." In *Bridges of Power: Women's Multicultural Alliances*, edited by L. Albrecht and R. Brewer. Philadelphia: New Society.
Rivera, F., and J. Erlich, eds. 1995. *Community Organizing in a Diverse Society*. 2d ed. Boston: Allyn and Bacon.
Schechter, S. 1982. *Women and Male Violence: The Visions and Struggles of the Battered Women's Movement*. Boston: South End.
Schechter, S., S. Szymanski, and M. Cahill. 1985. *Violence against Women: A Curriculum for Empowerment*. New York: Women's Education Institute.
Smith, A. 1986. "Positive Marginality: The Experience of Black Women Leaders." In *Redefining Social Problems*, edited by E. Seidman and J. Rappaport, 101–13. New York: Plenum.

Weil, M. 1995. "Women, Community, and Organizing." In *Tactics and Techniques of Community Intervention*, edited by J. E. Tropman, J. L. Erlich, and J. Rothman, 118–34. 3d ed. Itasca, Ill.: Peacock.

West, G. 1990. "Cooperation and Conflict among Women in the Welfare Rights Movement." In *Bridges of Power: Women's Multicultural Alliances*, edited by L. Albrecht and R. Brewer, 149–71. Philadelphia: New Society.

Withorn, A. 1984. *Serving the People: Social Services and Social Change*. New York: Columbia University Press.

Zavella, P. 1986. "The Politics of Race and Gender: Organizing Chicana Cannery Workers in Northern California." In *Women and the Politics of Empowerment*, edited by A. Bookman and S. Morgan. Philadelphia: Temple University Press.

GALEN EL-ASKARI
SHERYL WALTON

| Chapter 14 | Local Government and Resident Collaboration to Improve Health |
|---|---|

## A Case Study in Capacity Building and Cultural Humility

THE PATH TOWARD effective partnerships between local health departments and communities is fraught with obstacles and sometimes seemingly insurmountable challenges. A journey on this path requires great perseverance, flexibility, humility, and caring. Success depends on the ability of organizations and individual staff members to commit to deeply examining their own personal and professional beliefs, behaviors, and assumptions about culture and relationships. There also is a critical need to document and disseminate findings about the outcomes of such efforts because hard evidence of the effectiveness of such partnerships for health improvement and enhanced community problem solving has been difficult to uncover (Kreuter et al. 2000, Shortell et al. 2002).

This chapter describes and critically analyzes the Healthy Neighborhoods Project (HNP) in Contra Costa County, California, and its subsequent replication in a neighboring health department. We begin by reviewing the background and context in which this model was developed, using as a conceptual framework John L. McKnight and John P. Kretzmann's (1990) asset-based community development (ABCD) model; Roz Lasker, Elisa Weiss, and Rebecca Miller's (2001) newer concept of partnership synergy; and Melanie Tervalon and Jane Murray-Garcia's (1998) concept of cultural humility. Following the case study presentations, we then draw on experiences from both partnerships to highlight lessons learned and key concepts, principles, and practices that can help us address the challenges and build on opportunities afforded by other city and county health department–initiated partnerships with residents.

## Conceptual Framework

*Let's put aside our preconceived notions of each other and instead each of us—the residents, the community agencies, and the health department—come to the table and offer up our varied gifts that we can pool to transform our community.*

　　—Joyce White, resident activist, city of Richmond, California,
　　in a conversation with Galen El-Askari (health department
　　program manager) in Joyce's kitchen, 1994

This statement captures the philosophical base and value orientation of the Healthy Neighborhoods Project. It also reflects the project's grounding in McKnight and Kretzmann's (1990) ABCD model (see also chapter 9), which provides a critical component of the conceptual framework for understanding the HNP and its subsequent replication. Briefly, these community development theorists propose moving away from the deficit mentality at the base of much human services work to identify instead and build on individual and community assets. Whereas the traditional needs-oriented assessment approach teaches people to see themselves as having special problems to be addressed by outsiders, the asset-based community development approach encourages community members to recognize, actively develop, and mobilize their own assets. According to McKnight (1995), each person can be imagined as a half-glass of water—partly empty (has deficiencies) but also partly full (possesses capacities): "For those whose 'emptiness' cannot be filled by human services, the most obvious 'need' is the opportunity to express and share their gifts, skills, capacities, and abilities with friends, neighbors, and fellow citizens" (103–4).

The HNP also reflects Roz Lasker and her colleagues' (2001) notion of partnership synergy. Building on definitions of *synergy* as "the power to combine the perspectives, resources, and skills of a group of people and organizations," Lasker et al. (2001) suggest that "the synergy that partners seek to achieve through collaboration is more than a mere exchange of resources. By combining the individual perspectives, resources, and skills of the partners, the group creates something new and valuable together—something that is greater than the sum of its parts" (184).

They further argue that increased creativity, comprehensive thinking, practicality, and transformative potential are unique advantages of collaboration. Without using the term, resident activist Joyce White clearly was describing the power of partnership synergy in her statement about pooling gifts to "transform our community."

A final component of the HNP's conceptual framework lies in the concept of cultural humility. As noted in chapter 1, physician Melanie Tervalon and her colleagues (Tervalon and Murray-Garcia 1998) originally coined the term primarily in reference to race and ethnicity, remarking that although we can never become truly competent in another's culture, we can engage openly, acknowledge the limitations of our understanding, and seek to broaden it. Building on this approach, we describe cultural humility as the ability to listen both to persons from other cultures and to our own internal dialogue. In this way, we discover how easily we discount another's truth when it passes through our own cultural lens.

Cultural humility also involves the ability to recognize and understand the effects of privilege, including, importantly, "white privilege" and "the power from unearned privilege" that it entails (McIntosh 1989, 11). Finally, cultural humility includes understanding and addressing the impact of professional cultures, which tend to be highly influenced by white, western, patriarchal belief systems, as they help shape interactions between health departments and local communities. As suggested in this and other chapters, sharing power can be an important outcome of having and demonstrating cultural humility in such contexts.

Linking the concepts of cultural humility, asset-based community development and partnership synergy form an overarching hypothesis that partnerships will be improved and longer-term health and social outcomes more easily achieved in low-income communities of color when (1) residents are engaged in and driving community development; (2) critical public health capacities of government staff are increased, particularly with respect to cultural humility; and (3) public agencies and their staffs undergo cultural and systems change. Each of these dimensions, along with the asset building and partnership synergy models, is illustrated in the case study that follows.

## The Healthy Neighborhoods Project and Its Evolution

### LAUNCHING THE HNP IN THE COMMUNITY

Contra Costa County, located on the eastern shores of San Francisco Bay in northern California, features considerable geographic, sociological, and economic diversity. Like other Bay Area counties, Contra Costa is becoming increasingly heterogeneous both ethnically and culturally, and in the West County area where this case study takes place, the great majority of residents are now people of color. Declining agricultural production and expanded industrial and residential development have resulted in a more diversified economic base, transforming Contra Costa from a primarily suburban into a more complex and varied urban area. The urban areas include the city of Richmond in the western region of the county and the city of Pittsburg in the eastern region. As in many counties, most of Contra Costa County's urban areas have large pockets of extreme poverty.

In 1994, the Healthy Neighborhoods Project began as a pilot project in a public housing community in Pittsburg. Soon afterward, it was replicated in five other neighborhoods. In each of these neighborhoods, the health department had been frustrated by attempts to engage communities in public health projects. The department's attempts to mobilize the community around tobacco control in the early 1990s, in the wake of several tobacco control policy victories and an influx of cigarette tax dollars, was emblematic of the frustrations experienced (Ellis et al. 1995). A long history of failed efforts and mistrust among the department, the nearby University of California at Berkeley (which often used this community for its own research purposes), and community-based organizations made dialogue with grassroots local leaders difficult at best, particularly since the tobacco control initiative did not address a real community-identified need (Ellis et al. 1996).

As illustration, imagine a community fraught with economic stress and gang violence. Enter the professional health educator (making a good salary with benefits) with her antismoking program. She understands that community involvement is critical to public health and seeks a buy-in from key leaders. What she may not understand, whether she is new to the department or not, is the following:

- The community leaders she is approaching have probably already been tapped for other categorical programs that the health department has rolled out into the community. Furthermore, the local university has probably sought to involve them in community surveys and other research efforts.
- Every community needs assessment, every research study, and nearly every intervention has focused on community deficits and thereby directly or indirectly reinforced the view that these neighborhoods are cesspools of problems, undermining community self-esteem.
- In many communities, an influx of resources for one health program or another seldom has resulted in outcomes that residents can tangibly see or feel. Instead, many residents have concluded that the primary benefits of such programs are salaries for outside professionals and publications for faculty members.
- There may be a select group of community-based organizations (CBOs) that have well-established relationships with the health departments and are eager to accept contracts and other resources to work as a partner on a health program. As suggested in chapter 5, however, these CBOs don't always have a good track record of engaging residents on the grassroots level and may represent particular interest groups rather than the larger community.

After several years' worth of good intentions had been met with anger, mistrust, or, at best, passive indulgence, Contra Costa Health Department staff members did two things. First, despite having their time paid for by categorical dollars for tobacco control, they spent long hours in the community, with the blessing of the public health director, supporting local efforts to address two areas that were of great concern to residents: substance abuse and gang violence. Second, they decided to broaden outreach beyond the traditional CBOs and ask residents in the community, who were respected by their neighbors, how to proceed. And this is how the conversation with Joyce in her kitchen came about.

In collaboration with community leaders and leadership in the health department, one of the authors of this chapter (Galen El-Askari), who was then a program manager with the health department, launched the Healthy Neighborhoods Project. Consistent with McKnight and Kretzmann's (1990) ABCD approach (see chapter 9), the project was based on the assumption that although low-income neighborhoods have obvious problems that affect health and well-being, they also have tremendous assets and capacities that often remain untapped. The HNP was designed to help residents identify and build on assets by stimulating community involvement and developing and implementing a resident-driven action plan to address neighborhood issues and concerns.

At the heart of the HNP were six trained resident community organizers, a project coordinator, and 120 neighborhood health advocates (NHAs) who made up neighborhood action teams in each participating neighborhood. Local teams were recruited by the project coordinator and the organizers. Criteria for participation included living in the neighborhood, reflecting the diversity of the community, having a sincere interest in improving the neighborhood, and being willing to commit to participating for one year. All team members participated in two to three days of initial training in areas such as community organizing, asset mapping, participatory evaluation, and team building. An initial training activity, which introduced them to the model of capacity building, also inventoried their own strengths and skills, which later were mobilized in their neighborhoods.

The community organizers and NHAs also participated in biweekly inservice sessions throughout the year on topics such as recruitment, meeting facilitation, public speaking, and media advocacy, or the strategic use of media to frame issues from a community or health perspective (see chapter 23). Hands-on technical assistance was provided by the project coordinator (chapter co-author Sheryl Walton), who worked closely with each neighborhood team on a weekly basis and assisted individual organizers and advocates with personal and professional skill development. With the assistance of health education staff members, residents conducted community asset mapping (see chapter 9) and planned and facilitated community forums. Similarly, a health department evaluator helped the NHAs design a community assessment instrument, which they then used to conduct door-to-door surveys in approximately five hundred homes to learn what people liked about their neighborhood and what they'd like to see changed. Following the survey, health advocates were again trained to help in data analysis and interpretation, and their analysis later was described by the evaluator as demonstrating a sophisticated understanding of their community (Minkler 2000).

In keeping with the HNP's accent on cultural humility, and with a growing body of evidence that resident participation, control, and increased social capital can have substantial health and social benefits (Eng et al. 1990, Sanders-Phillips 1996, James et al. 2001, Kawachi et al. 1997, Wallerstein 2002), service providers and local elected officials also received some training to enable them to make a critical paradigm shift. Because even the best-meaning providers and professional staff members can inadvertently create dependency by relating to community members as recipients of services, the staff, along with elected officials and other policymakers were oriented to the project by learning how to avoid jargon and how to step back and allow residents to voice their opinions in their own time on their own terms. At resident training sessions and community meetings, for example, providers and elected leaders were asked to observe and be available as resources but to refrain from advocating or voting when decisions were being made.

### CHALLENGES AND DILEMMAS

The grounding of the HNP in an asset-based and culturally humble approach, and its inclusion of staff as well as resident training, proved to be an effective model for synergistic partnership and one that helped generate a number of impressive outcomes (outlined later in this chapter). At the same time, however, participants faced many obstacles and challenges at each stage of the process that had to be carefully addressed.

When the HNP was first being conceived, for example, a key community member walked out of a planning meeting angry and in tears. Later organizers discovered that their good intentions about gaining resident input and plotting it on flipcharts felt to her like a situation in which outsiders were trying to control the process. HNP staff had to find the humility to hear her truth, despite their strong belief that they were facilitating a participatory process. The tendency is to defend and blame; the essential capacity is to suspend beliefs long enough to hear and accept the truth of another.

Particular difficulties also sometimes arose for staff members of color, who often found themselves in the position of the "outsider within." Although the socialization process in professions crosses racial and ethnic lines, many professionals of color feel as if they live in two worlds (Chavez et al. 2003). From a capacities point of view, they are bicultural. Yet from a personal point of view, meeting professional demands while effectively translating and brokering for the community can be extremely stressful. In the HNP, staff members of color also sometimes expressed the feeling that they were doing twice the work of fellow staff members who were not culturally identified with the community and therefore did not play dual roles.

Regardless of one's race or ethnicity, the process of authentic community building can be painful and sometimes frightening to staff members who are used to the predictability of the dominant professional culture (see chapter 5). Health department workers who are comfortable with their professional role of being people who value "caring for" and "providing service," for instance, may not as easily accept the necessity in community building of being engaged fully, authentically, and truthfully with community members. Not to reveal our pain, our limitations, our mistakes, and our own process of opening and evolving itself is a barrier to the kinds of connections that must be made to build community. As Jean Vanier (1989) has remarked, "in all of us and in every community, there is the fear of challenge; and the danger of covering up tensions and the things that are not going well, or at least refusing to look at them and to confront them" (135).

### CHALLENGES INTERNAL TO THE HEALTH DEPARTMENT

While the HNP was unfolding in the community, a parallel process was taking place inside the walls of the health department, which similarly involved confronting and addressing challenges. An initial challenge, for example, involved facilitating the new notion of braided funding streams through which categorical money from tobacco, maternal-child health, and other areas was combined to support the new project. This process itself sometimes led to turf issues, which were exacerbated when tobacco prevention staff developed a project to which no identifiable health issue was attached. Because the HNP supported neighborhood priorities whatever they were, personnel in other health department arenas often were concerned that HNP staff might be moving in on their territory.

Additionally, some public health staff members questioned the HNP philosophy, believing that health departments are most effective in addressing large, county-wide policy issues through work with agencies and institutions. Others felt it was more appropriate for government to obtain large grants and subcontract to CBOs to work directly with residents rather than working on the grassroots level themselves. In other parts of the health department, direct service staff members had trouble abandoning the problem-solving focus of categorical programs and sought to evolve the role of neighborhood teams into outreach workers to promote pre-defined health goals.

Recognizing the importance of having other relevant health department programs on board before the project commenced, HNP staff members convened several meetings in hopes of addressing staff concerns. Although some people remained skeptical, the project eventually went forward with strong support from the department's director, who recognized that strong and authentic resident involvement was essential to creating a healthy community.

Along with the larger challenges of securing systems change in health department personnel's acceptance of such a project were numerous bureaucratic obstacles that had to be overcome if the project were to succeed. For example, paying wages to nontraditional employees such as community organizers may present a significant hurdle if those employees do not fit existing job classifications.

Similarly, kitchen-table organizing wouldn't live up to its name without food. Yet many expenses essential to the project's success, such as for food, child care, translation, gifts or incentives, and stipends or resident travel, may be disallowed by public agencies and traditional funders. HNP staff members had to learn to plan in advance for rigidities in the organizational structure that could become stumbling blocks. Alternative mechanisms such as finding a fiscal agent to handle petty cash funds or special bank accounts for discretionary expenses were established during the early days of the HNP to help overcome such obstacles. But community residents also had to be prepared for the numerous frustrations that result from dealing with a large bureaucracy.

Organizational culture and systems change also were needed with respect to normal working hours. Because residents typically were more available to meet during evenings, weekends, and some holidays, flex-hours and incentives (for example, allowing some health department staff members to work from noon to 9:00 P.M.) were important accommodations. Partly as a result of such flexibility within the department, a solid resident team consistently appeared for meetings with staff; and when residents were eventually invited during work hours to attend quarterly meetings with health department programs, they often would make arrangements to attend.

Ironically, the very success of the HNP led to particularly difficult challenges as the project reached maturity. A goal of the project, for example, was to provide county jobs for residents. Many members of the strong cadre of community organizers and NHAs trained through the project could have been major assets to the county health department in regular paid-staff capacities. But the civil service system requirements for such jobs, which often included college degrees, tended to be above the qualifications of even the most exceptional and best-trained resident team members. As we will suggest later in this chapter, substantial cultural and system change are necessary in public agency bureaucracies to help overcome such obstacles.

### PROJECT ACCOMPLISHMENTS
### AND CONTINUED CHALLENGES

Despite many challenges and dilemmas, residents involved in Contra Costa's HNP have successfully applied their skills to advocate for neighborhood services and environmental modifications to improve health and quality of life in each neighborhood. These accomplishments have included advocating for and bringing about changes on multiple levels and in many diverse areas:

- Installation of speed bumps
- Removal of a tobacco billboard targeting youth
- Successful competition for a $100,000 grant for job-skills training

- Creation of a mural capturing residents' vision of what a healthy community should look like, painted by forty youths under the direction of a local artist
- Successful advocation for additional evening and weekend bus service, increased police patrols, and improved street lighting and trash pickup
- Successful obtaining of funding for youth sports programs
- Establishment of computer classes

As residents experienced success in achieving immediate community priorities, they also began to participate in larger health department initiatives that would improve their neighborhoods. Residents thus served on a regional Partnership for Health advisory board and an environmental health advisory board. Other residents worked with the health department to develop new community health indicators that better reflected the concerns of local residents. Resident advocates were key to both obtaining funds to build the Center for Health in North Richmond and implementing a bucket brigade in which residents in a community where oil refineries proliferate were, and continue to be, trained to trap air samples to identify and report toxic chemical releases. (See El-Askari et al. 1998 and Minkler 2000 for a more detailed discussion of these and other outcomes.)

On another level, an important accomplishment of this project has been its success in helping to change attitudes in the health department itself about the value of a cross-disciplinary, strengths-based project like this one. Support for the HNP in the health department is now widespread as members of the different HNP neighborhoods teams have become more visible in local government and planning bodies, expressing their personal and community visions for their neighborhoods. Experienced HNP participants also have been actively promoting their perspective in health department planning processes, such as development of the county's chronic disease prevention plan. Finally, current HNP director Roxanne Carrillo is actively drawing on the lessons of the HNP in her role as a trainer with a new CDC-funded after-school empowerment program, Youth Empowerment Strategies (YES!), in several local elementary and middle schools (Wilson et al. in press; also see chapter 12).

Although these accomplishments represent important and tangible outcomes of the HNP, a continuing challenge has involved evaluating the impact of the HNP on individual-level health and well-being. Health department epidemiologist Chuck McKetney has successfully used Barbara Israel et al.'s (1994) scale for measuring perceived control (see also appendix 9) to examine changes in perceived control on the individual, organizational, and community levels. His research revealed significant increases in participating residents' perceptions about their ability to influence their lives, their community's control over decisions affecting it, and so forth. At the same time, he noted that the plethora of health interventions operating in the county simultaneously (for example, close to a dozen different prenatal programs) made it impossible to detect with any certainty the actual impacts of the HNP in particular health domains. Finally, even in an area in which significant health behavior changes did appear to result from the project (such as a significantly higher participation rate in a new Healthy Families Program in areas where the NHAs were active), cuts in funding for the data base established to track these changes made further follow-up impossible (personal communication from Chuck McKetney, August 2002). Because a major goal of projects such as the HNP is to build individual and community capacity toward the ultimate end of helping to eliminate health disparities, difficulties presented in the area of project evaluation remain a major challenge.

## Adapting and Replicating the Model

In 1999, building on the lessons of the Healthy Neighborhoods Project in Contra Costa County, the public health division of neighboring Berkeley's Health and Human Services Department began to lay the groundwork for a similar project. Like Contra Costa, Berkeley is ethnically and culturally diverse, with great disparities in wealth and health status between the predominantly white population living in the hills and the disproportionately African American, Latino, and other racial-ethnic populations living in the flat lands of West and South Berkeley (Namkung and Ducos 1999). Like Contra Costa, the city has a wealth of assets, including its diversity; its role as home to one of the world's top universities; and a long tradition of social activism, high-level civic engagement, and its own city-run public health department. A receptive health officer and director of the Maternal Child and Adolescent Health Program (MCAH) helped create an environment in which a replication project could be mounted, as did the city's recent hiring of one of the founders of the HNP.

As Saul Alinsky (1972) and other organizers (see chapter 10) have pointed out, however, a key to successful organizing often rests with timing and the presence of a catalytic event that increases receptivity to change. In Berkeley, such an event took place with the release and wide publicizing of the 1999 *City of Berkeley Health Status Report* (Namkung and Ducos 1999), which uncovered and analyzed the city's racial-ethnic health disparities. The twenty-year gap in male life expectancy between the mostly white men living in the hills and the mostly African American men in the flat lands grabbed headlines, as did the finding that Berkeley had larger racial and ethnic health disparities than any of the surrounding Bay Area regions (Namkung and Ducos 1999).

Key local policymakers such as Congresswoman Barbara Lee and Alameda County Supervisor Keith Carson used the occasion of the report's release to call a town hall meeting on the topic of health disparities in the city. Approximately 220 South and West Berkeley residents, policymakers, health care providers, merchants, university students, and members of the faith community participated in this lively meeting. Residents representing many different racial and ethnic groups from the flat land neighborhoods and elsewhere voiced their strong conviction that they themselves needed to do something about the disparities problem, including organizing, collecting their own data, and working to address racism. Serving at the time as a consultant to the health department, one of the chapter authors (Walton) recognized the HNP model as an ideal fit and began by providing technical assistance to health department staff in areas such as principles of capacity building and expansion of diverse cultural and language services before working on the development of community teams. She worked closely, for example, with the public health division's MCAH program in its efforts to create a community-based public health approach to better address health disparities. In her subsequent role as director of the division's new Community Capacity Building Program, Walton was well positioned to help the HNP model become a reality.

The town hall meeting provided an excellent starting place for this process; and a cross-section of sixty participants, most of them residents, voluntarily chose to meet monthly, eventually forming the Community Action Team advisory group. Adapting the HNP model, Walton provided technical assistance to the South and West Berkeley communities with the support of the public health staff in the development of two resident-driven Community Action Teams (CATs) funded by the city and the federal government. The CATs went through intensive training and other steps (such as the creation of a community survey instrument) similar to those of the original HNP but modified to focus more heavily on social and economic determinants of health. As part of their work, the Berkeley CATs also organized a well-attended racial and ethnic community health summit, which provided residents, policymakers, and others with opportunities for education, small group work, and the encouragement to speak openly about racism, politics, and other root causes of the racial and ethnic health disparities in their community. Aware that racism is experienced by residents beyond their local borders (as when they shop for groceries or go to banks or health care facilities in neighboring cities), the CATs expanded their invitation list beyond the city limits. This regional approach helped them build networks with other collaboratives, such as the Alameda County Health Disparities Work Group.

As noted, among the results of this process were CAT member participation in the South and West Berkeley Health Disparities Forum, along with city, state, and federal policymakers; Berkeley city government representatives; local private and nonprofit health providers; businesses; and UC Berkeley's School of Public Health. With the ambitious goal of eliminating health disparities in South and West Berkeley through collaborative efforts and the implementation of policy and institutional change, the forum has convened for two years and joined forces with the Mayor's Task Force on the Uninsured and other local groups and organizations to strengthen efforts to eliminate disparities and improve health care access. The forum also has supported the city's MCAH program in its efforts to secure funding for prevention programs to eliminate racial and ethnic health disparities.

Members of the CATs also are making a difference, in part through their active involvement with the city's Neighborhood Services Initiative, which promotes dialogue with community residents and businesses to improve city services. CAT representatives also now participate on other coalitions and collaborations throughout the city, introducing their model and methods of educating about health disparities.

The CATs have conducted door-to-door surveys and used these interaction opportunities to offer immediate referrals and subsequent follow-up for residents who need health and other city services. CAT members are working with Berkeley youth programs to recruit and train hard-to-reach young people, involve them in action planning around health disparities, and foster their participation in an assortment of youth-guided leadership and capacity building activities. As one indication of the perceived value of the work of the CATs, the city of Berkeley health status reports now include the work and results of the CATs in their documentation (Namkung et al. 2003).

Like the original Healthy Neighborhoods Project, the Berkeley project has developed innovative ways of addressing some of the logistical and practical problems it has confronted. For example, a respected community-based health care provider, Lifelong Medical Care, now provides free health and dental coverage for the CAT organizers until they are full-time employees and covered by city benefits. This organization also serves as a fiscal agent for the CATs so that they can respond to funding opportunities on short notice and provide stipends for the intensive participation of some residents.

The Berkeley replication project has faced numerous challenges, among them the fact that if CAT members are hired as staff they must follow city policy and can no longer contact their local council members or lead a media advocacy campaign without permission from the City Manager's Office. As we will discuss, institutional culture and systems changes are needed on the municipal level if resident-staff organizers are to be able to implement effective community organizing campaigns without the limitations under which they currently operate.

Despite such obstacles, however, the project has been highly effective in meeting its goals and objectives. Among the factors that may be contributing to this level of success is the fact that, with many people of color occupying the highest leadership positions in the department as well as many key staff positions, the public health division mirrors the diversity of the city it serves. This diversity helps provide a safe environment in which staff members can discuss the difficulties and

challenges involved in confronting and strategizing around the complicated concept of racism. At monthly MCAH staff meetings and retreats, for example, literature is provided and regular discussions are held on topics such as different forms
of racism (Jones 2000), cultural humility (Tervalon and Murray-Garcia 1998),
unequal health and medical treatment by race-ethnicity (Institute of Medicine
2002), and the social determinants of health. Concepts such as institutionalized
racism, personally mediated racism, and internalized racism (Jones 2000) are discussed and used to help determine strategies. In this way, organizing for change
and grappling with the difficult issue of racism are not merely left for community
forums; the health department actively engages with them internally as well. In
the words of MCAH Director Vicki Alexander, "It takes incredible courage,
trust, faith, social consciousness and commitment from the leadership of all levels of the health department, as well as undying willpower to prevent this issue
from getting isolated and buried" (personal communication, May 2003).

As staff and CAT members speak publicly about these issues and their efforts
to implement their action plans, unexpected tears may run down their cheeks and
voices raise in passion. Yet this, too, indicates their depth of connection. For many
health department staff members and other project participants, the poor health
conditions of African Americans in South and West Berkeley are a deeply personal issue that directly affects their own families and communities.

## Lessons Learned and Implications for Public Health Practice

This chapter began by suggesting that three key areas are critical to the development
of effective community–health department partnerships and, over the long term,
to improved health outcomes in low-income communities: resident-driven community development; an increase in the community-based capacities of public health
staff, particularly with respect to cultural humility; and cultural and systems
change within public agencies. We now highlight several lessons from the original Healthy Neighborhood Project and its replication in a neighboring county to
underscore the importance of each of these areas. As already noted, the importance of an ongoing and steadfast commitment to high-level resident involvement
in leadership, decision making, and control has been widely documented in the
literature (see Israel et al. 1998, Lasker et al. 2001, Minkler et al. 2001) and similarly was illustrated throughout the HNP and its Berkeley replication. But commitment to the process of sharing power must be unwavering, consistent, and
authentic. Resident engagement relies on the strategic development of capacities
on the part of both community members and institutional players. Finally, successful partnerships are reliant on the full understanding and buy-in of agency chains
of command in order to avoid derailing the process when turning over control
becomes too risky.

## CULTURAL HUMILITY AS A
## CRITICAL PUBLIC HEALTH CAPACITY

*Our organizations will change only when we undergo personal and social change; when we recognize who we are, where we come from, and the baggage we carry with us; when we recognize that we are not culture neutral; when we find ways to confront the often uncomfortable subjects of race and racism in ways that lead to understanding and action; when we find new ways to communicate and listen effectively; and most importantly, when we find ways to increase our personal and professional power by sharing it with those we serve.*

—Calvin Freeman, 1996, 1

As noted in chapter 1, the Institute of Medicine (1988, Gebbie et al. 2002) has been a critical voice in both articulating the importance of involving local health department staff in community-based public health interventions and ensuring that the public health work force is well trained in cultural competence and participatory approaches to facilitate this work in today's increasingly diverse communities. Similarly, in their study of more than four hundred local health departments, Edith Parker and her colleagues (2003) identified communicating with minority populations, pointing out community strengths as well as weaknesses, enhancing community input into problem identification and planning, and creating partnerships with community groups and agencies as among twenty-seven core public health competencies.

Integral to the achievement of each of these is cultural humility, a quality that our experience with the HNP suggests is perhaps the single most important element for partnership synergy with low-income communities of color. Indeed, to paraphrase N. Peled-Elhanan (2002) the commitment to and increasing skillfulness of the HNP staff in "being willing to hold back your ideologies, or your truth, or your personal and national narrative, and make room in yourself for the truth and the narrative of the other," was vital to project success.

Our experience underscores the centrality of culture in any change process and the need to recognize that culture includes "the realms of feeling, spirit, and relationships" (National Community Development Institute 2002, 2). This may mean finding participatory and other processes that are rooted in the cultures of the various communities involved. And it points up the importance of helping staff understand and build culturally sensitive relationships before becoming immersed in collaborative planning and decision making.

### PUBLIC HEALTH LEADERSHIP AND SYSTEMS CHANGE

*Engaging in a genuine partnership with communities requires giving up a degree of control over outcomes.*

—Wendel Brunner, Ph.D., M.D.,
Contra Costa County public health director, 2001

A critical counterpart to the relationship building and cultural humility capacities of staff involved in resident partnership development is committed public health leadership, which in turn is vital to systems change. An important lesson of the HNP in both Contra Costa County and the city of Berkeley involves the need for high-level leadership in the department to commit to sharing power and making important internal systems changes so that projects like this one can succeed.

The highly visible role of the Contra Costa County public health director, for example, including his leveraging of funds from categorical programs for the HNP, was critical to the ability of the project to materialize in the first place. The director's role also laid the groundwork for long-term, sustainable changes in how the department's community wellness and prevention programs were structured and managed, and it set an important precedent for other departments throughout the state.

Facilitating synergistic partnerships between health departments and communities means supporting nontraditional work hours for some health department staff, carving out funds for refreshments and child care, and in other ways accommodating local community needs. But it also may mean finding ways to address a civil service system whose rigid job classifications and requirements often preclude the hiring of local residents who have received training and shown immense promise in their work with projects like the HNP. In Contra Costa and Berkeley, staff members did tackle the civil service system to open up job opportunities for residents. All of the community organizers, who are fully trained, are now employed in full-time benefited positions, maintaining the same flexibility in hours and encouraged and allowed to maintain their identity as residents.

Yet even when progress is made in hiring, significant job-related challenges remain. In Berkeley, as we have noted, institutional culture and systems changes are needed on the municipal level so that resident and staff organizers have the freedom to mount community organizing campaigns without being hamstrung by bureaucratic rules and regulations preventing or severely compromising such activity.

A final lesson from the HNP experience involves the critical need for planning for sustainability. As funds for health departments undergo dramatic redirection in the face of real or perceived bioterrorism and severe economic downturns, levels of support initially received for programs like this one may prove impossible to sustain. On the inside, it will be even more important to build strong relationships between health departments and other city and county offices so that the latter begin to view such projects as beneficial for their own work—for example, as sources of trained residents who can be resources across multiple domains. At the same time, however, creative and diversified fundraising plans must be developed to enable such programs to thrive even if government funding is reduced. Health department staff should pursue the growing number of foundations and other philanthropic organizations that now support comprehensive community-based health initiatives and that may be vital to the future of such programs.

## Conclusion

Local health departments committed to authentic, meaningful engagement with residents cannot be wary or hesitant about the commitment it takes to begin such partnerships. As this chapter suggests, there are many perils on such a journey. From the personal process of cultural humility and acknowledgment of institutionalized racism, to leadership commitment, to sweeping systems changes, to exposing painful truths about the racial and ethnic health disparities that affect our neighborhoods, following this path requires courage. Yet as this chapter also demonstrates, the payoffs for doing so may be substantial for both communities and health departments themselves.

The Healthy Neighborhoods Project and its replication in Berkeley illustrated how two health departments attempted to engage meaningfully with local communities through community-driven efforts to help address locally identified problems. By identifying and building on community assets and attending to issues of race, ethnicity, and racism both in the community and internally, and by recognizing and responding to the need for system change and responsive leadership as well as high-level community participation, both case studies show the challenges and the promise of partnership approaches to addressing complex health and social problems.

*Editor's note:* After this book went to press in late 2003, the Public Health Division of the Contra Costa County Health Services Department created a new unit entitled "Community Collaborations." Created and staffed by The California Endowment/Public Health Institute's ambitious Partnership for the Public's Health initiative, the new unit currently is expanding to include the Healthy Neighborhoods Project.

### References

Alinsky, S. D. 1972. *Rules for Radicals*. New York: Vintage.

Brunner, W. 2001. "Community-Based Public Health: A Model for Local Success." *Community-Based Public Health Policy and Practice* 1 (September): 2–3.

Chavez, V., B. Duran, Q. E. Baker, M. M. Avila, and N. Wallerstein. 2003. "The Dance of Race and Privilege in Community Based Participatory Research." In *Community Based Participatory Research for Health*, edited by M. Minkler and N. Wallerstein, 81–97. San Francisco: Jossey-Bass.

El-Askari, G. A., J. Freestone, C. Irizarry, K. L. Kraut, S. T. Mashiyama, M. A. Morgan, and S. Walton. 1998. "The Healthy Neighborhoods Project: A Local Health Department's Role in Catalyzing Community Development." *Health Education and Behavior* 25, no. 2: 146–59.

Ellis, G. A., R. L. Hobart, and D. F. Reed. 1996. "Overcoming a Powerful Tobacco Lobby in Enacting Local Smoking Ordinances: The Contra Costa County Experience." *Journal of Public Health Policy* 17, no. 1: 28–46.

Ellis G. A., D. F. Reed, and H. Scheider. 1995. "Mobilizing a Low-Income African American Community around Tobacco Control: A Force Field Analysis." *Health Education Quarterly* 22, no. 4: 443–57.

Eng, E., J. Briscoe, and A. Cunningham. 1990. "Participation Effect from Water Project on Immunization." *Social Science and Medicine* 30, no. 12: 1349–58.

Freeman, C. 1996. "Building Multicultural Organizations." *Public Health Watch* (summer).

Gebbie, K., L. Rosenstock, and L. M. Hernandez. 2002. *Who Will Keep the Public Healthy? Educating Public Health Professionals for the 21st Century.* Washington, D.C.: Institute of Medicine.

Horwitz, C. 2002. *The Spiritual Activist: Practices to Transform Your Life, Your Work, and Your World.* New York: Penguin.

Institute of Medicine. 1988. *The Future of Public Health.* Washington, D.C.: National Academy Press.

Israel, B. A., B. Checkoway, A. J. Schulz, and M. Zimmerman. 1994. "Health Evaluation and Community Empowerment: Conceptualizing and Measuring Perceptions of Individual, Organizational, and Community Control." *Health Education Quarterly* 21, no. 2: 149–70.

Israel, B. A., A. J. Schulz, E. A. Parker, and A. B. Becker. 1998. "Review of Community-Based Research: Assessing Partnership Approaches to Improve Public Health." *Annual Review of Public Health* 19: 173–202.

James, S. A., A. Schulz, and J. van Olphen. 2001. "Social Capital, Poverty, and Community Health: An Exploration of Linkages." In *Social Capital and Poor Communities,* edited by S. Saegert, J. P. Thompson, and M. R. Warren, 165–88. New York: Sage Foundation.

Jones, C. P. 2000. "Levels of Racism: A Theoretic Framework and a Gardener's Tale." *American Journal of Public Health* 90, no. 8: 1212–15.

Kawachi, I., B. P. Kennedy, K. Lochner, and D. Prothrow-Stith. 1997. "Social Capital, Income Inequality, and Mortality." *American Journal of Public Health* 87, no. 9: 1491–98.

Kreuter, M. W., N. A. Lezin, and L. A. Young. 2000. "Evaluating Community Based Collaborative Mechanisms: Implications for Practitioners." *Health Promotion Practice* 1, no. 1: 49–63.

Lasker, R. D., E. S. Weiss, and R. Miller. 2001. "Partnership Synergy: A Practical Framework for Studying and Strengthening the Collaborative Advantage." *Milbank Quarterly* 79, no. 2: 179–205.

McIntosh, P. 1989. "White Privilege: Unpacking the Invisible Knapsack." *Peace and Freedom* (July–August).

McKnight, J. 1995. "Do No Harm." In *The Careless Society: Community and Its Counterfeits,* 101–14. New York: Basic Books.

McKnight, J., and J. Kretzmann. 1990. *Mapping Community Capacity.* Evanston, Ill.: Northwestern University, Center for Urban Affairs and Policy Research.

Minkler, M. 2000. "Participatory Action Research and Healthy Communities." *Public Health Reports* 115, nos. 1 and 2: 191–97.

Minkler, M., M. Thompson, J. Bell, and K. Rose. 2001. "Contributions of Community Involvement to Organizational-Level Empowerment: The Federal Healthy Start Experience." *Health Education and Behavior* 28, no. 6: 783–807.

Namkung, P., and J. Ducos. 1999. *City of Berkeley Health Status Report, 1999.* Berkeley, Calif.: Health and Human Services, Public Health Division.

Namkung, P., J. Ducos, V. Alexander, and K. Tehrani. 2003. *City of Berkeley Health Status Report, 2002, Low Birth Weight.* Berkeley, Calif.: Health and Human Services, Public Health Division.

National Community Development Institute. 2002. *Culturally-Based Framework*. Oakland, Calif.: National Community Development Institute.

Parker, E., L. H. Margolis, E. Eng, and C. Henriquez-Roldán. 2003. "Assessing the Capacity of Health Departments to Engage in Participatory, Community-Based Public Health." *American Journal of Public Health* 93, no. 3: 472–76.

Peled-Elhanan, N. 2002. "Not Being Afraid of Another Person's Truth: We Have Betrayed Our Children." *Jerusalem Post*, November 28, p. 9.

Sanders-Phillips, K. 1996. "The Ecology of Urban Violence: Its Relationship to Health Promotion Behaviors in Black and Latino Communities." *American Journal of Health Promotion* 10, no. 4: 308–17.

Shortell, S. M., A. P. Zukoski, J. A. Alexander, G. J. Bazzoli, D. A. Conrad, R. Hasnain-Wynia, S. Sofaer, B. Y. Chan, E. Casey, and F. S. Margolin. 2002. "Evaluating Partnerships for Community Health Improvement: Tracking the Footprints." *Journal of Health Politics, Policy, and Law* 27, no. 1: 49–91.

Tervalon, M., and J. Murray-Garcia. 1998. "Cultural Humility vs. Cultural Competence: A Critical Distinction in Defining Physician Training Outcomes in Medical Education." *Journal of Health Care for the Poor and Underserved* 9, no. 2: 117–25.

Vanier, J. 1989. *Community and Growth*. New York: Paulist Press.

Wallerstein, N. 2002. "Empowerment to Reduce Health Disparities." *Scandinavian Journal of Public Health* 30, supp. 59: 49–91.

Wilson, N., M. Minkler, S. Dasho, R. Carillo, N. Wallerstein, and D. Garcia. In press. "Training Students As Participants in Community Based Participatory Research: The Youth Empowerment Strategies (YES!) Project." *Journal of Community Practice*.

# Community Organizing with the Elderly Poor in San Francisco's Tenderloin District

*Chapter 15*

IN INNER-CITY, single-room occupancy hotel (SRO) neighborhoods such as San Francisco's Tenderloin District, large numbers of low-income elders live at the bottom of the housing ladder. Often just a step removed from homelessness, many of these residents confront daily the interrelated problems of poor health, social isolation, and powerlessness as a result of poverty and social marginalization.

Yet the elderly residents of impoverished and high-crime "Tenderloin districts" around the nation also possess many strengths and competencies. This chapter presents a case study of the Tenderloin Senior Organizing Project (TSOP), a community organizing effort that for sixteen years served as a vehicle for individual and community empowerment in a population previously labeled *unorganizable*. After briefly describing the project's setting, the chapter examines TSOP's theoretical underpinnings and historical development. I devote particular attention to TSOP's evolution from a program that tried to empower the elderly to one in which elders and their neighbors could empower themselves. Project outcomes are described, as are a number of the problems and challenges that TSOP faced in the course of its history. The chapter closes with a look at issues of sustainability and replicability as well as lessons learned.

## Background

A culturally diverse, mixed-use, residential area, the forty-five-block district known as the Tenderloin is home to large numbers of elders on small fixed incomes, younger people with physical and mental disabilities, immigrants, and homeless people. Three hundred times more densely populated than the city as a whole, this neighborhood for years has had the highest crime rate in San Francisco. The city's failure to enforce housing codes or building ordinances, the absence of any major grocery store chain, and the highest density of alcohol outlets in the city (California Department of Alcohol Beverage Control 2003) contribute to the prevalence of inadequate and unsafe housing, undernutrition, and alcoholism.

Although Tenderloin residents suffer from a plethora of unmet needs, the neighborhood also has many strengths, including multiculturalism. For years the district has had its own multilanguage newspaper. Several large and well-respected churches, a comprehensive and progressive local health center, and an active neighborhood planning coalition and housing clinic were among the potential allies that early TSOP organizers identified as in their effort to create an environment in which residents could become empowered.

TSOP's overall goal was to facilitate such empowerment by assisting elderly residents and their neighbors as they worked to organize and improve their community. The project's objectives were to draw out residents' competence, self-confidence, and leadership skills (Ferrante 1991) and reduce social isolation by enhancing social support networks in Tenderloin SRO hotels and other low-income residences.

## Theoretical Base

Three major conceptual domains guided the project from its inception. The first, social support, is based on the large body of evidence demonstrating the critical role of social support and social interaction on health status (Bloomberg et al. 1994, Heaney and Israel 2002, Seeman 2000). Whether they buffer stress or contribute to an increased sense of control over destiny (Syme 1991), interventions that build supportive networks may be particularly important in neighborhoods like the Tenderloin, where social marginality and isolation are endemic.

Many social support theories tend to focus on the individual and his or her supportive network as the sole unit of analysis. Thus, empirical studies often overlook the macrolevel changes that may take place as individuals and communities, empowered by increased social support, work collectively to attack shared problems that have contributed to their oppression. By applying theories of social support to the Tenderloin, TSOP staff and volunteers attempted to look beyond individual-level outcomes of increased social support to focus as well on institutional- or community-level changes (Minkler 1992).

This perspective is aligned with TSOP's second theoretical underpinning—the approach to empowerment theory that Brazilian educator Paulo Freire (1968, 1973) calls "education for critical consciousness." As discussed in chapter 12, Freire's educational methodology centers on a relationship of equality and mutual respect between group participants and teacher-learners, with the latter using a process called problem posing to ask questions that challenge members of the group to look for root causes and other consequences of the problem under discussion and eventually develop a plan of action. Although TSOP was conceived of, in part, as a Freirian project, with the idea that student facilitators would use this approach when leading hotel-based support and discussion groups, regular applications of the methodology proved difficult. Ongoing discussions of the root causes of problems, for example, often proved impractical when residents were motivated to organize quickly around problems that demanded immediate action. Consequently, although Freire's education for critical consciousness continued to provide an important philosophical and ideological base for the project, the method per se was not employed regularly or rigorously (Minkler 1992).

Of greater day-to-day usefulness in TSOP's work was a third, more eclectic, approach to community organization best typified by the philosophy and methods of Saul Alinsky (1969, 1972) and supplemented by the work of John L. McKnight (1987, 1993; see also chapter 9) and Michael Miller (1993). As discussed in chapter 11, Alinsky viewed the low-income community as powerless and disfranchised in relation to the "haves" and to society as a whole. The goal of his approach was to facilitate a process whereby people who came together around a shared interest or concern could collectively identify a specific issue or target, garner resources, mobilize an action campaign, and through their collective action help realign power in the community.

Recently, TSOP has drawn on the work of several post-Alinsky theorists and organizers who go considerably farther than he did in identifying and stressing the strengths of the local community and developing creative methods for capacity building. Among TSOP's conceptual underpinnings are John L. McKnight and John P. Kretzmann's (chapter 9) asset-based community development and newer, more egalitarian approaches often called woman-centered organizing (see chapters 11 and 13). Similarly, TSOP has borrowed from community organizer and theorist Michael Miller (1993) the notion that "action rooted in deeply held values is more likely to be sustained than that which relies solely on addressing a specific injustice." Miller stresses the relationship between community organizing and democratic citizenship, arguing that discussions of values should form part of the community organizing process. Through such discussions, community members ideally begin to challenge values such as rugged individualism, consumerism, and a status system that exploits the poor and causes them to internalize their oppression. By helping residents see their work in relation to deeper values and ideologies, TSOP has attempted to apply Miller's approach and make it a fourth conceptual project base.

## Project Origins and Evolution

Originally known as the Tenderloin Senior Outreach Project, TSOP was established in 1979 with the dual goals of (1) improving physical and mental health by reducing social isolation and providing relevant health education and (2) facilitating, through dialogue and participation, a process whereby residents would work together to identify common problems and seek solutions (Wechsler and Minkler 1986). Specific methods included helping residents form discussion and support groups (and later tenants' associations and interhotel organizations and coalitions) that could increase community competence and problem-solving ability and bring about concrete changes (for example, reductions in the neighborhood crime rate) that in turn could promote individual and community well-being (Minkler 1992).

Architects of what was to become TSOP began by conducting a community assessment, which revealed that forty-three different helping agencies and organizations existed in the forty-five-block area. Of these agencies, residents seemed to universally respect one in particular—St. Boniface Church. Following Alinsky's (1972) admonition to organizers to establish their legitimacy by linking themselves with a preexisting organization, the first project volunteers (students in a graduate community organizing class at the University of California at Berkeley) became St. Boniface volunteers and as such approached hotel managers about the possibility of serving refreshments in the hotel lobby one morning a week as a means of encouraging resident interaction. With the help of these inducements, they formed an informal coffee hour and discussion group in one hotel; the group met weekly and included a core of eight to twelve residents and two outside facilitators. As levels of trust and rapport increased, members began to share personal concerns about issues such as fear of crime, loneliness, rent increases, and their sense of powerlessness.

Student facilitators used a combination of organizing and educational approaches to help foster group solidarity and eventually community organizing. A Freirian problem-posing process was used as appropriate, for example, to help residents engage in dialogue about shared problems and their causes and to generate potential action plans. Similarly, facilitators followed Alinsky's (1972) admonition to create dissatisfaction with the status quo, channel frustration into concrete action, and help people identify specific, winnable issues. Finally, drawing on social support theories that stress the importance of social interaction opportunities per se, the student facilitators attempted to create a group atmosphere conducive to meeting the social as well as the political and task-oriented concerns of group members.

As the first hotel discussion group became an established entity, more student volunteers were recruited, and seven more groups were organized in other Tenderloin hotels. To provide coordination and continuity for the project, staff secured a small foundation grant to fund a part-time director; and TSOP became incorporated as a nonprofit organization with a twelve-member board of directors. Recognizing the importance of building on community assets, TSOP invited representatives of a popular neighborhood church, the powerful local planning coalition, and the neighborhood health clinic to join the board, along with community residents and allies from the business and professional communities.

Among the early issues identified and confronted by several of the hotel groups was the problem of undernutrition, particularly lack of access to fresh fruit and vegetables. After much discussion of alternative approaches, the residents of three hotels contracted with a local food advisory service and began operating their own hotel-based minimarkets one morning per week. In a fourth hotel, residents organized and ran a modest cooperative weekly breakfast program, thereby qualifying their hotel for participation in a food bank where large quantities of food could be purchased in bulk at reduced prices. Still other residents worked with TSOP staff to produce a no-cook cookbook of inexpensive and nutritious recipes. Later published by the San Francisco Department of Public Health, the cookbook was distributed free of charge to hundreds of Tenderloin residents; and more than one thousand copies were sold outside the community to generate additional money for the project. Early activities like these were important in making tangible changes (such as improved food access) but, more significantly, by contributing to resident feelings of control, competence, and collective ability to bring about change. Moreover, these early accomplishments gave residents the self-confidence needed to confront more difficult challenges in the future.

Although each hotel group developed and retained over time its own unique character, several common trends among the groups were evident. In all but one hotel group, for example, decreased reliance on outside facilitators was observed over time, with broader resident participation in discussion and decision making. TSOP members witnessed hotel residents' increasing concern about their neighbors in the building, particularly during stressful times, as when several hotels were temporarily evacuated in the aftermath of San Francisco's October 1989 earthquake. Residents of TSOP hotels arranged to go in groups to homeless shelters rather than be separated from their supporters. In one such hotel, a resident who had described herself as a loner before joining TSOP, said she now knew all of her 102 fellow residents and could tell the hotel manager which ones needed special assistance.

Another trend observed in the groups, and one critical to TSOP's evolution, was residents' realization of the need to look beyond hotel boundaries and work on shared problems with residents of other hotels and community groups. TSOP residents of several hotels thus identified crime and safety as their key area of concern and formed an interhotel coalition to begin work on this problem. The coalition in turn started the Safehouse Project, recruiting forty-eight neighborhood businesses and agencies to serve as places of refuge, demarcated by colorful posters, where residents could go for help in times of emergency. Coalition members also convinced the mayor to increase the number of police patrol officers in the neighborhood and, through this and other measures, helped effect a dramatic reduction in crime, including an 18 percent reduction in the first twelve months after the coalition's inception ("Safehouses Now Easing the Fears of Elderly Residents" 1982).

Two other outcomes of TSOP's organizing around the crime issue are worthy of note. First, having experienced success in increasing personal safety and well-being, the TSOP elderly began turning their attention to the safety needs of other vulnerable groups. Elderly TSOP members, for example, had their Safehouse materials translated into Cambodian and Vietnamese, and they arranged for articles about the project to appear in the Asian-language pages of the community newspaper. They were also able to recruit several Asian merchants in the neighborhood to open safehouses, bringing the total to more than one hundred at the height of the project.

Second, even though the Safehouse Project received considerable local and national publicity, several of the project's resident founders began to question the narrowness of the crime prevention approach they had developed. Their discussions of the root causes of the high crime rates in poverty neighborhoods and their involvement, albeit sporadically, in areas such as advocacy for the homeless, job training for the unemployed, and voter registration reflected increasing appreciation of the need to work toward broader social change. As E. Richard Brown (1991) notes in critically analyzing the TSOP experience, "Successful actions that resulted in desired changes in the health related environment may reduce the needs to which community members originally responded, but they may also increase community members' organizational skills, experience, leadership, and feelings of empowerment. They thus may encourage further action for more far reaching goals of social change."

## Increasing Community Capacity: Progress and Challenges

TSOP's commitment to "starting where the people are" (Nyswander 1956) by helping residents organize around issues, such as crime and nutrition, that they themselves had identified was in keeping with the organization's commitment to empowerment. Yet even with resident-initiated goals and activities, TSOP staff needed to be aware of the danger of slipping into the inadvertent creation of dependency. By the mid-1980s, for example, the cooperative breakfast program and hotel-based minimarkets, as well as a health promotion resource center that TSOP residents planned and originally ran themselves, had begun to look more and more like direct service activities. Although residents remained interested in reaping the benefits of these programs, they lost interest in running them themselves; and project volunteers and staff were alternating their organizing roles with direct service functions.

TSOP staff discussed with residents the increasing tensions and contradictions between the organization's desired role in stimulating community organization and leadership development and its de facto service role. In the words of former project director Diana Miller, "We needed to clarify that what we do is build public power. [TSOP's role] was getting distorted because the organizers were spending a lot of time and energy on mutual aid programs" (Vanover 1991, 45).

After these discussions, and with the support of the board of directors, TSOP began gradually to terminate its direct service programs. The health promotion resource center, for example, was spun off to another community-based organization, while the minimarkets and cooperative breakfast program were gradually phased out. At the same time, and in a further effort to clarify the project's mission, TSOP formally changed the O in its name from *Outreach* to *Organizing* and adopted a new mission statement that stressed the organization's values and its commitment to drawing out and building on the skills of residents and creating community competence through organizing.

TSOP's new operational model, which remained in place until the project's closure in 1995, involved entering new hotels and residences only at the request of residents. Through personal conversations, the TSOP organizer clarified the organization's role: not advocacy on behalf of residents but helping residents advocate on their own behalf. He or she would begin conversations about some of the advantages of organizing over seeking help and challenge residents to take the next step—that is, speak to a few of their neighbors and help form a small committee made up of individuals identified as potential leaders. Working with committee members on ways to think organizationally (Miller 1993), or strategically and tactically, the organizer would help residents form a tenants' association, which in turn would identify issues, assess resources, and mobilize to achieve collectively set goals (Ferrante 1991). A total of fourteen tenants' associations were established with the help of TSOP and achieved a number of impressive victories.

Critical to TSOP's goal of fostering community empowerment and problem-solving ability was its emphasis on leadership training. Through one-on-one and small-group activities, residents were helped to improve interpersonal skills, learn to facilitate meetings, and discover ways of working through (or against) bureaucracies to bring about change.

Early approaches to leadership training included a day-long leadership training conference attended by eighty residents and three media workshops in which TSOP members met with journalists and reporters, who helped them practice articulating their concerns to the press. Of greatest importance, however, was the ongoing nurture of individual and small-group leadership, including the extensive use of role plays before confrontations with landlords, meetings with city officials, and so on. In these trial runs, TSOP members could practice creating and responding to alternative hypothetical scenarios and learn to function effectively as leadership teams. Such exercises, and the selection and preparation of backup leaders in the event that a designated leader was ill on the day of a planned action, were among the strategies that enabled TSOP to develop a strong leadership cadre from among its membership.

More advanced leadership training was undertaken during the later years of the project, with twenty TSOP members attending intensive national leadership training programs sponsored by the San Francisco–based Organize Training Center. Led by a prominent Alinsky-style organizer, the four-day training covered topics such as issue selection, values and critical reflection, and negotiation processes. Reporting back on the experience, one elderly participant said, "The workshop gave me an overall theoretical construct in which to place the things our tenants' association had learned from our TSOP organizer . . . so I could better grasp how one thing (such as values) ties into the next (such as action). I saw how our individual work can lead to building part of a community. Who would have thought an atheist in an apartment in a major city would be sharing concerns with a Lutheran pastor who ministers to farmers in rural Nebraska?" (Miller 1993).

Although TSOP has been concerned with individual and community empowerment since its inception, the model's change over time reflected the organization's more sophisticated understanding of what empowerment entails and the preconditions necessary for its achievement. By helping residents create their own tenants' organizations and cross-group organizations rather than playing a direct role in their creation, and by offering resources (such as leadership training) as requested, the newer TSOP model was more effective in fostering true community organizing and empowerment.

TSOP continued to experience its share of problems. Residents became tired of or burned out on some issues they had earlier decided to tackle; there were occasional power plays in groups; leadership turned over because of illness, transiency, and other problems. Ethical issues also arose, as when one very elderly and disabled resident strongly opposed closing down the cooperative breakfast program, which for him was a high point of the week. When TSOP shifted to a pure community organizing project, it also discovered that its goals (for example, community empowerment and leadership development) were less attractive to most traditional foundation and corporate sponsors than were tangible deliverables such as hotel-based minimarkets and health promotion resource centers. Moreover, even progressive foundations that understood and applauded TSOP's new directions tended to avoid refunding the same project, so new sources of income continually had to be located. With an overworked board and no staff or volunteers specifically devoted to raising money, TSOP's two full-time organizers found themselves unable to respond to many requests to help organize in new buildings because they were too busy raising funds.

## Project Accomplishments and the Problem of Evaluation

As with many efforts aimed primarily at community organization and empowerment, separating TSOP's methods from its process outcomes is difficult. Equally
difficult is determining project impact on health and social outcomes such as malnutrition, depression, and social isolation in a neighborhood where concurrent
adverse developments (such as cutbacks in supplemental security income checks
and escalating violence deriving, in part, from the drug epidemic) have often con-
spired to exacerbate these problems. Finally, many residents' strong objection to
being studied meant that project staff members were reluctant to engage in or allow
formal evaluations until very late in the organization's history. In spite of these
limitations, however, a number of project outcomes can be examined.

TSOP's greatest achievement was its formation of eight hotel-based support
groups and fourteen tenants' associations. The support groups met weekly over
periods ranging from six months to, more typically, several years and averaged
eight to twelve regular members. All but one of these groups moved from staff
or student volunteer facilitation to resident facilitation or cofacilitation and from
discussion of issues to taking concrete action to bring about change.

These groups achieved a number of tangible victories. Members of one support group organized a protest against a sudden (and illegal) 30 percent increase
in rent, which as a consequence of resident organizing was reduced to 10 percent.
In another hotel, residents demanded and got a change in the landlord's harsh eviction policy. In a third, they pressured successfully for architectural changes to make
their shared bathrooms wheelchair accessible. Support-group organizing also
focused on accommodating the purely social and spiritual needs of residents and
included the planning of elaborate holiday parties and memorial services for
some group members who had passed away.

Finally, resident organizing sometimes led to cross-group activities (for
example, with the formation of a Tenderloin chapter of the Nuclear Freeze and
of the interhotel coalition Tenderloin Tenants for Safer Streets) and to increased
involvement with and on behalf of younger groups. On an early visit to TSOP,
Gray Panthers' founder Maggie Kuhn called the project "the best example I've ever
seen of the Gray Panthers' motto—'age and youth in action.'" She made this comment in reference to the fact that elderly TSOP support-group members had increasingly broadened their focus to work with younger disabled people, persons who
were homeless or unemployed, and neighborhood children.

In several instances, TSOP support groups formed the basis of subsequent tenants' associations that were able to build upon the former groups' effective leadership base and prior collective organizing efforts. The early victories of one such
organization included abolishing a hated furniture rental policy, instituting substantial rent rebates, and reducing pet deposits from $300 to $100 (Goldoflas 1988).

Other tenants' associations were formed in buildings where no previous organizing had taken place.

Victories achieved by the fourteen tenants' associations that TSOP helped to create included the following (Ferrante 1991, Miller 1993):

- Appealing to the city's rent board and winning $10,000 in compensation for a hotel elevator that had been out of service for five months
- Getting management to install in a hotel lobby a vending machine with low-cost, nutritious foods
- Successfully protesting a provision in a new lease agreement that would have limited residents' rights to freedom of speech and expression
- Winning improved pest control and upgrading substandard plumbing and wiring
- Getting an agreement for lead-based paint removal
- Helping to win an out-of-court settlement against a prestigious local law school that owned four neighborhood buildings and had reneged on promised internal security
- Getting hot water turned on in a building that had gone without it for ten years

Like the earlier TSOP support groups, the tenants' associations went beyond their buildings' borders to work with other groups, organizations, and agencies on problems affecting the larger community. Through collaboration with several local businesses and the San Francisco Department of Public Health, for example, residents were able to secure the cleanup of a vacant lot that had become such a noxious and rat-infested dumping ground that its odor had prevented neighbors from opening their windows (Miller 1993). Similarly, after the death of a resident at a local intersection, tenants' association members successfully negotiated with the San Francisco Department of Parking and Traffic Safety for a senior crossing sign and an increase in pedestrian crossing time.

Unfortunately, it is difficult to measure actual changes in health and quality of life that may be attributed, at least in part, to TSOP organizing efforts. In a few instances, TSOP was able to collect hard data on project accomplishments. An early evaluation of the minimarkets, for example, included twenty-four-hour diet recalls that demonstrated a significant increase in participants' consumption of fresh fruit and vegetables (Wechsler and Minkler 1986). Similarly, the chief of police attributed the marked decline in the neighborhood crime rate during the first two years of TSOP organizing in large part to tenant organizing and the increased community solidarity that it inspired.

Qualitative data, albeit often anecdotal, has suggested potential impacts on health and well-being. Many residents, for example, reported that, as a consequence of group participation through TSOP, they no longer felt depressed and lonely. A formerly depressed woman in her early sixties commented, "I can't tell you what a difference the group had made in my life. When I moved to the Tenderloin three years ago, my husband had just left me. All I kept thinking was, 'Who's going to want me now?' I think I would still be alone in my room if it weren't for [TSOP]."

A number of residents attributed changes in health habits to their involvement with TSOP, including smoking cessation, decreased alcohol consumption, and improved adherence to medical regimens. A mentally disabled resident who had frequently failed to take her prescribed medication reported that she had become religious about taking it now that she was heavily involved in several TSOP activities that relied upon her leadership skills. And a younger TSOP member remarked, "TSOP is the only group I belong to not because I'm poor or disabled or HIV positive but because of my strengths." Although such stories are difficult to translate into hard outcome data, they provide important anecdotal evidence of the effectiveness that TSOP groups and activities may have had in improving health and particularly in reducing depression among participants.

TSOP's focus on developing leaders and on increasing the problem-solving capacity of individuals and groups resulted in some important outcomes in terms of community empowerment. Management recognized several tenants' associations, for example, as the organized voice of building residents. In some of these residences, landlords continued to meet regularly with the associations to discuss the latter's concerns well beyond the project's formal closure, whereas in other buildings tenants' associations continued to have a regular hand in decision making on any issues that might affect them.

Effective tenants' association outreach to and collaboration with other community groups, local businesses and agencies, and government bodies such as the Department of Public Health, the Department of Housing and Urban Development, and the Department of Public Safety indicated, in part, association members' growing sophistication in problem solving. The formation of interhotel groups and coalitions such as Tenderloin Tenants for Safer Streets and the TSOP Leaders' Council suggests a growing identity with the community beyond individual buildings; this, too, appears to have contributed to neighborhood empowerment. Joint mobilization to bring down the crime rate, arrange for vacant lot cleanup, and in other ways improve quality of life for members of the neighborhood are outcomes that may illustrate the increased problem-solving ability, on the community level, that TSOP helped to foster.

An extensive formal evaluation based on structured interviews with residents, unstructured interviews with key informants, and documents review was conducted during TSOP's final year of operation (Shaw 1995). The survey research component of the study compared 150 residents of TSOP-organized and nonorganized buildings and included a modified version of Barbara Israel et al.'s (1994) scale for measuring perceptions of control on the individual, organizational, and community levels (see also appendix 9). Significant differences between the two groups were found along fourteen dimensions, including social isolation, morale, feelings of safety, perceived ability to improve building living conditions, and overall quality of life. Unfortunately, however, the study failed to document statistically significant changes in health or sense of empowerment and also pointed to major organizational limitations, including lack of adequate strategic planning.

Although the evaluation produced important data on numerous aspects of TSOP's accomplishments and problems, the largely quantitative nature of the study may have limited its ability to capture some of the essence of the project. An alternative approach grounded in the philosophy and methods of empowerment or participatory evaluation (see chapter 20) might have overcome these difficulties. As Stephen Fawcett et al. (1996) note, empowerment evaluation works toward the competing ends of "maximizing community control" and "understanding . . . the process outcomes of a community initiative" or organizing effort (183). Like other forms of participatory evaluation, empowerment evaluation ideally involves community members in all phases of the evaluation process and values both qualitative and quantitative data so that the stories of community members and others become a critical part of the data base. In both these respects, empowerment evaluation would, in retrospect, have been more in keeping with TSOP's philosophy and methods than was a more tradition survey research approach.

## Project Closure and Replication Efforts

TSOP's closure after sixteen years resulted from increased difficulty in raising the project's annual budget (approximately $100,000), most of it from private foundations. As suggested in the project evaluation, improved long-term strategic planning and earlier, more concerted efforts to develop a diversified funding base might have helped prevent the project's demise. At the same time, the general absence of government support for efforts such as TSOP and increased competition among community groups for individual, foundation, and corporate dollars as a consequence of severe government cutbacks make the closure of projects like this one all too common.

Several years before closure, however, and in response to growing numbers of requests for technical assistance from other community groups, TSOP developed a detailed project replication manual (Ferrante 1991). Outlining steps and barriers to starting and maintaining a grassroots organizing project, the guide includes discussions of topics such as the role of the organizer, choice of strategies and tactics, and the role of values in organizing, with illustrative case studies and quotations from TSOP residents. The manual was distributed upon request to organizers in the United States and Canada, and several replications have been attempted. A disabled veteran in New York City, for example, used the early TSOP model to help organize chronically schizophrenic veterans who had recently entered a residential treatment center (Pounder 1988). And in Vancouver, British Columbia, the Ministry of Health enthusiastically supported a TSOP-modeled, government-funded project in nine SRO hotels (Jones and Sommers 1994). Unfortunately, limited project staffing, especially in the final years, precluded following up these and other replication efforts. Such follow up is important, however, if we are to create a critical evidence base for the impact of projects like TSOP as they continue to be refined and adapted for use in other settings.

Fortunately, however, new technologies, including the Internet, have spread the word about this model and its potential for replication. TSOP thus is included as one of six projects featured in the United Nations' "Compendium of Community Programmes for Older Persons in Newly Aging Countries" (http://un.org/esa/socdev/ageing/agecoms4.html) and has been widely publicized through the United Kingdom–based organization ConsultAge. It also is one of two examples of community organizing models featured in a recent Internet review of health education models and theories (http://www.msucares.com/health/health/appal/htm), and is one of two case studies of locality development included in Jack Rothman, John Erlich, and John E. Tropman's (2001) classic text *Strategies of Community Intervention*. Vehicles like these provide an important means of disseminating the TSOP model, albeit without providing a means of tracking and monitoring new replications that may be underway.

## Conclusion

The TSOP experience offers a number of lessons for those concerned with community organizing for health. Prominent are (1) the importance of community, rather than outside organizer, definition of need; (2) the need for a preliminary community assessment as well as ongoing efforts to uncover and build upon community strengths; (3) the need to implement theories and methodologies flexibly, adapting them as necessary to ensure their greatest possible relevance in real-world contexts; (4) the importance of building comprehensive, participatory, and empowering strategies into community organizing project evaluation; and (5) the need for attending early on to broad strategic planning, including the development of a diversified funding base. Additionally, efforts to track project sustainability once funding is withdrawn and to follow and monitor replication efforts are important and often overlooked ways to determine additional long-term project outcomes.

The TSOP experience also demonstrates that even the most committed community organizing effort will have limited success in improving health and quality of life in neighborhoods like the Tenderloin without a broad societal commitment to the reduction of social inequalities. A project like TSOP can make significant inroads in helping reduce feelings of social isolation and powerlessness endemic in low-income, inner-city communities, especially because these feelings are often intimately tied to poor health. By helping to identify and nurture indigenous leaders and build tenants' associations and other structures that acted as a unified voice for residents, TSOP was able to help the people increase their power in fighting for and getting small but important changes in their health and living conditions. Furthermore, changes such as a drop (albeit temporarily) in the neighborhood crime rate, increased social support, and improvements in access to inexpensive, nutritious foods can have a direct bearing on malnutrition, depression, and other health and social problems prevalent in low-income communities.

Yet conditions in the Tenderloin District, like those in many inner-city neighborhoods in the United States, have actually deteriorated over the past two decades as a result of broader economic and social conditions over which even the best-organized communities have little or no control. Economic problems, combined with the politics of retrenchment that continue to the present, have taken a particular toll on the poor. Severe cutbacks in supplemental social security, subsidized housing, Medicaid, and a plethora of health and social service programs, combined with the growing epidemics of drugs, violence, and HIV/AIDS, wreak havoc on communities such as the Tenderloin.

Against this backdrop, the victories of organizations like TSOP take on added significance. Yet they also are dwarfed by the magnitude of the problems confronted, which can be adequately addressed only through a more fundamental societal-level commitment to reducing the social inequities that lie at the base of such problems. When poverty remains perhaps the single greatest risk factor for disease and premature death, and when the links among poverty, alienation, and numerous health and social problems are documented in study after study (Adler et al. 1994, James et al. 2001), our failure to deal with these more fundamental problems becomes increasingly troubling. Projects like TSOP do not operate in a vacuum; and without a broader social commitment to reducing social inequalities, the problems plaguing inner-city communities like the Tenderloin will continue largely unabated into the twenty-first century.

At the same time, however, while health educators and other concerned professionals increase our commitment to working for broader social change at the societal level, we must not lose sight of the real impact a project like TSOP can have in the lives of both individuals and communities. In the words of one elderly TSOP leader who credited the project with keeping her from succumbing to severe clinical depression, "I thought when you're way down like this, way down below the poverty level, you're powerless. But I realized you can make the big shots stand up and listen. It was amazing to me to learn that if you work together you can do something" (Ferrante 1991, 8).

## Acknowledgments

Portions of this chapter are based on Meredith Minkler, 1992, "Community Organizing among the Elderly Poor in the United States: A Case Study," *International Journal of Health Services* 22, no. 2: 303–16. Copyright © 1992 by the Baywood Publishing Company, Inc., Amityville, N.Y. All rights reserved.

## References

Adler, N. E., T. Boyce, M. A. Chesney, S. Cohen, S. Folkman, R. L. Kahn, and S. L. Syme. 1994. "Socioeconomic Status and Health: The Challenge of the Gradient." *American Psychologist* 49, no. 1: 15–24.

Alinsky, S. D. 1969. *Reveille for Radicals*. Chicago: University of Chicago Press.

———. 1972. *Rules for Radicals*. New York: Random House.

Bloomberg, L., J. Meyers, and M. T. Braverman. 1994. "The Importance of Social Interaction: A New Perspective on Social Epidemiology, Social Risk Factors, and Health." *Health Education Quarterly* 21, no. 4: 447–63.

Brown, E. R. 1991. "Community Action for Health Promotion: A Strategy to Empower Individuals and Communities." *Journal of Health Services* 21, no. 3: 441–56.

California Department of Alcoholic Beverage Control. 2003. Alcoholic beverage control files, San Francisco district office. Sacramento, July.

Fawcett, S. B., A. Paine-Andrews, V. Francisco, J. Schultz, K. P. Richter, R. K. Lewis, K. J. Harris, E. L. Williams, J. Y. Berkeley, J. L. Fisher, and C. M. Lopez. 1996. "Empowering Community Health Initiatives through Evaluations." In *Empowerment Evaluation: Knowledge and Tools for Self-Assessment and Accountability*, edited by D. Fetterman, S. Kaftarian, and A. Wandersman, 161–87. Thousand Oaks, Calif.: Sage.

Ferrante, L. 1991. *The Tenderloin Senior Organizing Project's Replication Manual*. San Francisco: Tenderloin Senior Organizing Project.

Freire, P. 1968. *Pedagogy of the Oppressed*, translated by M. B. Ramos. New York: Seabury.

———. 1973. *Education for Critical Consciousness*. New York: Seabury.

Goldoflas, B. 1988. "Organizing in a Gray Ghetto: The Tenderloin Senior Organizing Project." *Dollars and Sense* (January–February): 1–19.

Heaney, C. A., and B. A. Israel. 2002. "Social Networks and Social Support." In *Health Behavior and Health Education*, edited by K. Glanz, B. K. Rimer, and F. M. Lewis, 185–209. 3d ed. San Francisco: Jossey-Bass.

Israel, B., B. Checkoway, A. Schulz, and M. Zimmerman. 1994. "Health Education and Community Empowerment: Conceptualizing and Measuring Perceptions of Individual, Organizational, and Community Control." *Health Education Quarterly* 21, no. 2: 149–70.

James, S. A., A. Schulz, and J. van Olphen. 2001. "Social Capital, Poverty and Community Health: An Exploration of Linkages." In *Social Capital and Poor Communities*, edited by S. Saegert, J. P. Thompson, and M. R. Warren, 165–88. New York: Sage Foundation.

Jones, J., and J. Sommers. 1994. Grant proposal. Vancouver, Canada: Vancouver Second Mile High Society. Unpublished paper.

McKnight, J. 1987. "Regenerating Community." *Social Policy* 17, no. 3: 54–58.

———. 1993. "Local Social Community Development and Economic Development Issues." Paper presented at the annual meeting of the American Public Health Association, San Francisco, October 27.

Miller, M. 1993. *The Tenderloin Senior Organizing Project*. Louisville, Ky.: Presbyterian Committee on the Self-Development of People.

Minkler, M. 1992. "Community Organizing among the Elderly Poor in the U.S.: A Case Study." *International Journal of Health Services* 22 , no. 2: 303–16.

Nyswander, D. 1956. "Education for Health: Some Principles and Their Applications." *Health Education Monographs* 14: 65–70.

Pounder, R. F. 1988. "Social Learning for Schizophrenic Adults: The Lanchester Model." Ph.D. diss. prospectus, Teachers College.

Rothman, J., J. L. Erlich, and J. E. Tropman, eds. 2001. *Strategies of Community Organization.* 6th ed. Itasca, Ill.: Peacock.

"Safehouses Now Easing the Fears of Elderly Residents." 1982. *Los Angeles Times*, November 21.

Seeman, T. E. 2000. "Health Promoting Effects of Friends and Family on Health Outcomes in Older Adults." *American Journal of Health Promotion* 14, no. 6: 362–70.

Shaw, F. 1995. "Tenderloin Senior Organizing Project Evaluation." Woodland, Calif.: Wellness Foundation. Unpublished report.

Syme, S. L. 1988. "Social Epidemiology and the Work Environment." *International Journal of Health Services* 18, no. 4: 635–45.

———. 1991. "Control and Health: A Personal Perspective." *Advances* 7, no. 2: 16–27.

Vanover, J. 1991. "Some Seniors in San Francisco: An Interview with Diana Miller." *Organizing* (spring–summer): 44–47.

Wechsler, R., and M. Minkler. 1986. "A Community-Oriented Approach to Health Promotion: The Tenderloin Senior Outreach Program." In *Wellness and Health Promotion for the Elderly*, edited by K. Dychtwald. Rockville, Md.: Aspen Systems.

# Part VI

# Building and Maintaining Effective Coalitions

$A$s community organizer Tom Wolff (1995) points out, much recent work in community health and human services has been dominated by two catch phrases: coalition building and empowerment. Loosely used, seldom defined, and frequently mandated by funding sources, this "mismatched pair of phrases," he notes, often fail to describe the reality of our community coalition building efforts (13).

Although Wolff's concerns are accurate, well stated, and widely shared, he and other social change professionals also note the power of coalitions in bringing about change. Particularly in times of diminished fiscal resources and support, we need coalitions that can create a powerful unifying structure for organizations that share a goal or concern. Yet coalition work is also inherently complex and therefore difficult to study and evaluate (Wallerstein et al. 2002).

In chapter 16, Abraham Wandersman, Robert M. Goodman, and Frances D. Butterfoss expand and revise their earlier work to examine coalitions' growing popularity as well as their unique ability to address complex public health issues. Drawing on organizational theory in their conceptual framework, they consider how coalitions as organizations develop and thrive, looking in particular at resource acquisition, maintenance, production, and attainment of external goals. Wandersman and his colleagues argue that a coalition's membership is its primary resource, although external resources such as concerned public officials and funders and a variety of external groups and organizations may be important as well. They further argue that coalitions, like other organizations, should give special attention to issues of leadership, decision making, and conflict resolution. Both target activities (such as setting and fulfilling a coalition mission) and maintenance activities (for example, recruiting and training new members, facilitating leadership development, and fundraising) are vital to the production functions of a coalition. Finally, for many observers, coalition accomplishments are the bottom line in terms of coalition effectiveness and worth. Both short-term successes and longer-term impacts should be considered and evaluated, the authors argue, because both are necessary to long-range coalition viability and impact. The benefits and the costs of coalitions are considered in this chapter, as is an expanded discussion of the challenges involved in evaluating coalition effectiveness. Finally, the authors pose a series of helpful questions for health educators and other social change professionals about these powerful yet often difficult vehicles for social change.

Many of the principles and challenges laid out in chapter 16 are illustrated in a real-world context in chapter 17. Susan Klitzman, Daniel Kass, and Nicholas Freudenberg present an updated case study of New York City's Coalition to End Lead Poisoning and describe how this umbrella organization has sought to educate diverse constituencies and influence public policy over the past two decades. After a brief overview of the problem and the elements of a meaningful lead poisoning prevention effort, the authors describe the genesis and evolution of the coalition. Although its activities span several domains, its primary work has involved legal strategies, which include bringing a lawsuit against the city and helping to draft both local and state legislation to mandate worker training and certification in lead abatement. Arguing that "adversarial strategies sometimes are necessary to achieve change," the authors describe how the original lawsuit against the city helped bring coalition members to the table, making possible regular meetings with city officials and encouraging progressive city council members to introduce pertinent legislation. The protracted lawsuit also garnered media attention and sustained the coalition over time. Yet the authors also discuss the drawbacks of a litigation-driven approach, which can disempower community members who do not play an active role in the proceedings and create tense relationships between advocates and government, thus hampering communication and joint problem solving.

Chapter 17 presents a useful critical analysis of the structure and functioning of the coalition in relation to dimensions laid out in chapter 16. The coalition's relative informality, reflected in its fluid, dues-free membership, for example, has had a number of positive benefits. Members are unlikely to threaten to drop out as a way to get their positions adopted, and coalition resources are conserved for production rather than expended on maintenance functions. Yet this same informality has drawbacks as well, including a slow pace of production and a heavy reliance on a few founding members, whose departure could jeopardize the coalition's existence.

The chapter closes with a thoughtful look at lessons that can be drawn for coalition building around other public health concerns. Defining issues broadly and helping diverse groups feel a personal connection to the issue are essential in a coalition that is concerned with influencing public policy. Similarly, coalitions may need to respond to policy shifts by changing strategies and, in some cases, projecting a different image to the public. At a time when coalitions are formed—and dissolved—with increasing frequency, the experiences of New York City's Coalition to End Lead Poisoning are useful reminders of the long-term impact that such vehicles can have.

### References

Wallerstein, N., M. Polascek, and K. Maltrud. 2002. "Participatory Evaluation Model for Coalitions: The Development of Systems Indicators." *Health Promotion Practice* 3, no. 3: 361–73.

Wolff, T. 1995. "Coalition Building: Is This Really Empowerment?" In *From the Ground Up: A Workbook on Community Building and Community Development*, edited by G. Kaye and T. Wolff, 13–28. Amherst, Mass.: AHEC/Community Partners.

ABRAHAM WANDERSMAN
ROBERT M. GOODMAN
FRANCES D. BUTTERFOSS

# Understanding Coalitions and How They Operate as Organizations

*Chapter 16*

ALTHOUGH COALITIONS, partnerships, and consortia are popular strategies for dealing with complex health and social problems, bringing together diverse partners and running a successful coalition are very hard work. A consortium or coalition may be viewed as a type of organization; and like any organization, it needs resources, structures, processes, activities, and accomplishments to survive. Many of these components are derived from the surrounding community; therefore, they are essential elements of an open systems framework (so named because it is open to and interacts with the environment [Katz and Kahn 1978]). This chapter begins with an overview of the popularity and unique capabilities of coalitions in public health practice and as vehicles for community action. It then links the available research on coalitions to the open systems framework to clarify how coalitions operate. The chapter ends with a brief look at some key controversies over coalitions as well as directions, methods, and tools for obtaining and documenting results.

## The Rise of Coalitions as a Vehicle for Addressing Complex Public Health Issues

Substance abuse, smoking, violence, HIV/AIDS, and unplanned adolescent pregnancy are among the many complex health problems whose multiple causes are deeply embedded in our social fabric. As previous chapters have suggested, effectively addressing such problems requires concerted state and national efforts and societal-level commitment to broader social change. Additionally, as a number of the case studies in this book suggest, local community action has an important role to play. Effective community efforts to address complex health and social problems are commonly understood to require partnerships among numerous sectors.

Such partnerships may include schools, businesses, the media, the health sector, academia, the criminal justice system, government, and grassroots community groups.

In recent years, both government and private-sector funding agencies have required coalition formation as a core component of the programs they support (Green and Frankish in press). For example, the Robert Wood Johnson Foundation's Allies against Asthma Initiative was designed to tackle the problem of asthma through coalitions that integrate clinical, environmental, and community-derived approaches. In 2001, coalitions of community, academic, and medical partners were funded in seven cities (including San Juan, Puerto Rico) for four years, with the goal of developing viable community plans to reduce emergency department visits and hospital admissions for children with asthma. The needs assessments and community plans focused on improving adherence to national asthma guidelines and promoting preventive education and self-management of asthma for families affected by the disease. The health promotion grant initiatives of the W. K. Kellogg Foundation (1994), the Henry J. Kaiser Family Foundation (Tarlov et al. 1987), and the Fighting Back substance abuse prevention programs funded by the Robert Wood Johnson Foundation are among the major private-sector grant initiatives that have mandated coalition building as a key dimension of the efforts they support. On the U.S. government level, the CDC's PATCH health promotion program, the Native American tribal health promotion programs sponsored by the Office of Minority Health, and the hundreds of community partnerships funded by the Center for Substance Abuse Prevention are among numerous initiatives that require coalition building as a condition of funding. These and other public health efforts assume that programs designed, implemented, and owned by community coalitions will be far more effective than those developed by either government alone or a single group. Yet research with voluntary organizations suggests that coalitions vary in their effectiveness and are vulnerable to decline (Green and Frankish in press). Empirical evidence is needed to document how they operate, how they maintain their viability, and whether they actually improve the impact of public health initiatives.

## Unique Capabilities of Coalitions

Let's consider two definitions of coalitions. The first views a coalition as "an organization of individuals representing diverse organizations, factions, or constituencies who agree to work together in order to achieve a common goal" (Feighery and Rogers 1989, 1). The second sees a coalition as "an organization of diverse interest groups that combine their human and material resources to effect a specific change the members are unable to bring about independently" (Brown 1984, 4).

As both definitions suggest, coalitions are interorganizational, cooperative, and synergistic alliances. The word *coalition* is derived from two Latin roots:

*coalescere* (to grow together) and *coalitio* (a union). Coalitions unite individuals and groups in a shared purpose. But unity and purpose are common ingredients in many types of groups and cannot serve alone as distinguishing characteristics of coalitions. Some definitions emphasize that coalitions are multipurpose alliances that accommodate more than one mission or set of goals (Black 1983, Perlman 1979, Stevenson et al. 1985); exchange mutually beneficial resources (Allensworth and Patton 1990, Hord 1986); and direct their interventions at multiple levels, including policy change, resource development, and ecological change (McLeroy et al. 1988).

As a growing body of literature suggests, coalitions serve several important purposes:

1. They enable organizations to become involved in new and broader issues without having the sole responsibility for managing or developing those issues (Black 1983).
2. They demonstrate and develop widespread public support for issues, actions, or unmet needs and thus help create the political will to make hard choices (Klitzner 1991).
3. They maximize the power of individuals and groups through joint action. Coalitions can increase the critical mass behind a community effort by helping individuals achieve objectives beyond the scope of any one individual or organization (Brown 1984).
4. They minimize duplication of effort and services. This economy of scale can be a positive side effect of improved trust and communication among groups that would normally compete with one another (Brown 1984, Feighery and Rogers 1989).
5. They mobilize more talent, resources, and approaches to influence an issue than any single organization could muster alone. Such strategic devices enhance group leverage (Roberts-DeGennaro 1986a).
6. They provide an avenue for recruiting participants from diverse constituencies, such as political, business, human service, social, and religious groups as well as less organized grassroots groups and individuals   (Black 1983, Feighery and Rogers 1989).
7. They exploit new resources in changing situations (Boissevain 1974).

## Coalitions: Recent Criticisms

While the literature indicates that some coalitions have produced public health outcomes (see Wandersman and Florin 2000, Butterfoss et al. 1998), reviews also suggest that coalitions produce modest results at best and often few outcomes (see Hallfors et al. 2002, Kreuter et al. 2000). Such critiques have generated considerable controversy that includes questions about the overall purposes of coalitions and the theories that support their use. At least two prominent purposes have been offered: (1) coalitions are service-delivery mechanisms that can generate and implement needed strategies in a community and therefore produce public health and other outcomes, and (2) coalitions are collaborative systems-change agents that influence the delivery of intervention strategies among existing community agencies and organizations.

We generally support the second purpose for coalitions and caution against using them as direct service providers. We feel that coalitions are best viewed and operated as mediating social structures. According to the classic work of Peter L. Berger and Richard John Neuhaus (1977), mediating social structures act as powerful agents that link local citizen concerns and the larger formal institutions that influence the quality of community life (such as criminal justice agencies and school systems). For instance, in a recent study of strategies to address the reconstruction of homes damaged by road construction in a large southern city, local community partnerships served as a bridge between the community residents, whose homes were damaged, and the city government that was responsible for home repair (Yoo et al. in press). Previously, city policy had set unrealistically stringent deadlines for reporting damaged homes, but the partnership was able to influence a change in the policy. At one time, city inspectors often took many months to respond to claims, but the partnership helped change the wait to a matter of weeks.

This example illustrates that local citizen groups may best use coalitions to leverage power and influence with larger institutions (such as city government) that set the policies and procedures that hold sway over community life. Because coalitions, by definition, are composed of organizations that combine to increase their influence and reach, direct service provision can involve members in undesirable daily operations that take time away from issue advocacy. Although coalitions are typically made up of service organizations, member organizations may be better suited for service provision, thus freeing the coalition itself to function as a mediator between people and policy.

To be effective mediators, coalitions require organizational infrastructure and operative processes to plan and implement their activities effectively. In this chapter, we use an open systems framework of organizational functioning to understand how coalitions operate.

## The Open Systems Framework as a Model of Coalition Viability

How can we conceptualize the core elements of these synergistic working alliances? As noted, we employ Daniel Katz and Robert Kahn's (1978) open systems perspective as a theoretical framework to explain how organizations function and maintain momentum as they interact with the surrounding environment. The framework views organizations as mechanisms for processing resources from the environment, making them into products that, in turn, can positively affect that environment.

Using Katz and Kahn's work as a departure point, John Prestby and Abraham Wandersman (1985) developed a framework of organizational viability that suggests four components of organizational functioning: (1) resource acquisition, (2) maintenance subsystem (organizational structure), (3) production subsystem (actions or activities), and (4) external goal attainment (accomplishments) operating in an open environment. This model indicates that any organization that fails to obtain adequate and appropriate resources, develop an organizational structure for obtaining resources and conducting work, mobilize resources efficiently and effectively, turn out appropriate products (for example, action or member benefits), or accomplish something will eventually cease to operate. The elements of the open systems framework are diagrammed in figure 16.1.

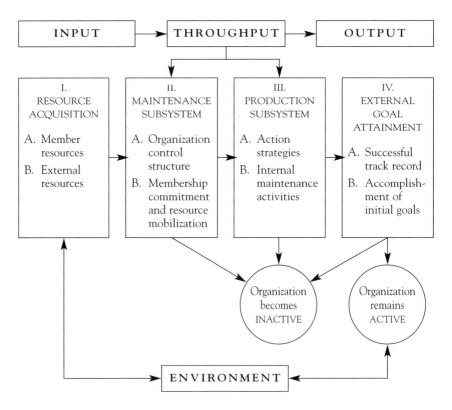

*Figure 16.1.* An open systems framework of organizational characteristics related to coalition funding.

## RESOURCE ACQUISITION

For a coalition to maintain itself, it must acquire the resources to keep going. For coalitions, resources consist primarily of those brought to the organization by its members and those recruited from external sources.

### MEMBER RESOURCES

A coalition's membership is its primary asset. Several variables related to members have been associated with organizational maintenance (Prestby and Wandersman 1985), including size of membership, depth of members' attachment to the mission, and members' personal and political efficacy.

Each member brings a different set of resources and skills to the coalition. For instance, one member may provide transportation to or space for meetings, another may contribute staff support, a third may assist in fundraising, and a fourth may provide access to and influence with relevant policymakers (Knoke and Wright-Isak 1982). Pooling member assets is especially significant when participation is voluntary and the coalition has few material resources of its own (Knoke and Wood 1981, Prestby and Wandersman 1985). Although member diversity enables the coalition to reach and represent a larger constituency, such diversity may also lead to diversity in assumptions and needs and eventually to conflict. Roz Lasker, Elisa Weiss, and Rebecca Miller (2001) propose that pooling diverse resources is one of the main determinants of synergy, a characteristic that enables coalition members to achieve together what they could not accomplish alone. Research has also shown that coalition staffing and structure are related to resource mobilization, which is related to effective implementation of coalition strategies (Kegler et al. 1998a, 1998b).

Effective implementation and maintenance of a coalition require not only motivated and involved members but also members with the skills or capacity to participate in a partnership and gain legitimacy (Gray 1985). For instance, a coalition that worked with problem youth demonstrated that the competence and performance of members were positively related to coordination among participating organizations and negatively related to conflict (Hall et al. 1977). Similarly, a skills training program conducted with members and chairpersons of an advocacy coalition resulted in members' increased reporting of issues, improvements in chairpersons' ability to conduct action-oriented meetings, and overall improved effectiveness of the consumer organization (Balcazar et al. 1990).

### EXTERNAL RESOURCES

Coalitions also benefit by linking with external resources, especially those concerned with policy, planning, and services (Butterfoss et al. 1993). Examples of external resources include elected officials and government agencies, religious and civic groups, neighborhood and community development associations, foundations, and national sources of technical assistance. These resources can provide expertise, facilities for meetings, mailing lists, referrals, additional personnel for special projects, grant funding, loans or donations, equipment and supplies, and co-sponsorship of events (Chavis et al. 1987, Prestby and Wandersman 1985, Braithwaite et al. 2000). Such external support may be reduced when granting sources undergo funding cutbacks or when the coalition has a small, overworked, inefficient staff; inadequate communication channels; or inflexible organizational policies (Whetten 1981).

A coalition's relationships with external resources may be classified along four dimensions: formalization (the degree of official recognition of the relationship), standardization (the degree to which procedures for links are specified), intensity (the frequency of interactions and flow of resources), and reciprocity (the degree of mutual exchange of resources). High levels of these dimensions are related to greater satisfaction with the collaborative relationship but may also produce more conflict (Marrett 1971). Collaboration with external resources may also be conceptualized along a continuum from mild to intense links: the stronger the link, the greater the trust and investment of time and resources among member agencies (Andrews 1990).

Access to local communities is an important link for many coalitions (Roberts-DeGennaro 1986b), particularly those concerned with health promotion. Such coalitions often benefit by linking with individuals and organizations active in community affairs. For instance, Prestby and Wandersman's (1985) study of block associations demonstrated that those that endured tended to have strong links with local community organizers and other neighborhood associations. Exchange of needed resources with other community organizations occurred more often in active associations (Chavis et al. 1987). Finally, Paul Florin, Roger Mitchell, and John Stevenson (1989) reported that improved links with several other community organizations was an important intermediate outcome of a substance abuse task force. Members of this group reported higher levels of participation, satisfaction, and positive expectations and had greater intent to participate in the future.

## MAINTENANCE SUBSYSTEM

Organizational structure is the aspect of a coalition that obtains resources and organizes members. If coalitions are to be viable, they must be able to set goals, administer rewards, and mediate between members' individual needs and the task requirements of the organization. Leadership; formalized rules, roles, and procedures; and processes for decision making and problem resolution are important mechanisms for accomplishing these tasks.

### LEADERSHIP

Strong central leadership is an important ingredient in the implementation and maintenance of coalition activities (Butterfoss et al. 1993). Regardless of size, coalitions tend to have a few core leaders who dominate activities (Roberts-DeGennaro 1986b). Ronald Braithwaite et al. (2000) note that the most successful rural substance abuse coalitions have strong leadership committed to a common goal. When leaders attend to and support individual member concerns and are competent in negotiation, garnering resources, problem solving, and conflict resolution, the coalition tends to be more cohesive in reaching peripheral members and maintaining coalition operations (Brown 1984). Other important qualities of leadership include the following (Butterfoss et al. 1993):

- Personal resources (such as self-efficacy), membership in other community organizations, and level of education
- A high degree of political knowledge, commitment, and competence
- Proven administrative skill in setting agendas, running efficient meetings, garnering resources, and delegating responsibilities
- Skill in communication and interpersonal relations
- The ability to promote equal status and encourage overall collaboration in the member organizations
- Flexibility
- Easy access to the media and decision-making centers of the community

Effective coalition leadership requires a collection of these qualities and skills, which usually exists not in one or two individuals but in a team of committed leaders. A steering committee of coalition work group leaders is one way to bring leaders and staff together to accomplish the work of the coalition.

FORMALIZED RULES, ROLES, AND PROCEDURES
Many authors assert that formalization is necessary for the successful implementation and maintenance of collaborative activities. Formalization is the degree to which rules, roles, and procedures are defined precisely. The higher the degree of formalization, the greater the investment of resources and exchanges among agencies, satisfaction with the effort itself, and willingness of member agencies to take responsibility and be committed. Examples of formalization include written memoranda of understanding, bylaws, and policy and procedures manuals; clearly defined roles; mission statements, goals, and objectives; and regular reorientation to the purposes, goals, roles, and procedures of collaboration (Butterfoss et al. 1993, Goodman and Steckler 1989). Formalization often results in routinization or persistent implementation of the coalition's operations. The more routine the operations, the more likely they are to be sustained (Goodman and Steckler 1989). In addition, structuring a coalition to be action-focused through work groups and task forces is associated with increased resource mobilization and implementation of strategies (Kegler et al. 1998a).

DECISION MAKING AND PROBLEM RESOLUTION PROCESSES

Participants' influence in making decisions is vital to a coalition. Wandersman (1981) describes a continuum of group decision-making power that moves from advice to control. Advisory power means that the coalition develops recommendations but that professionals and government officials have the final responsibility for decision making. Control means that the coalition itself has final decision-making power.

Cheri Brown (1984) suggests that small, single-issue coalitions may adopt a decision-by-consensus method, whereas larger, multi-issue coalitions may aim for a working consensus (two-thirds majority) when time is limited. She advises coalitions to encourage open discussions and urge members to share decision making. Otherwise, group members may not understand or be committed to the issues under discussion. They may sabotage a decision by withholding objections initially and then failing to support the decision later. She also urges coalitions to avoid overrepresentation in decision making by limiting the maximum number of votes allotted to each member organization.

Strong, effective coalitions depend on shared leadership and shared decision making. Influence in decision making is related to increased satisfaction and participation as well as more positive benefits (Butterfoss et al. 1996, Mayer et al. 1998). Shared decision making can be affected by a status differential in the group—that is, one professional or organization has more authority or greater resources than others do (Andrews 1990, 157). Howard Zuckerman and Arnold Kaluzny (1990) suggest that key stakeholders and leaders of an alliance be extensively involved in a joint decision-making process. Consensus and agreement require relationships among participants that are "collegial and egalitarian" and a manager who seeks to "balance constituencies rather than to control subordinates."

Prestby and Wandersman (1985) found that active block associations in the Neighborhood Participation Project in Los Angeles were more likely to use a democratic decision-making process, whereas inactive associations used an autocratic or mixed democratic-autocratic process. The Block Booster Project in Nashville, Tennessee, reported that active block association members felt they had a greater influence in deciding on group policies and actions than did inactive block association members (Chavis et al. 1987). Active block associations used consensus and formalized decision-making procedures more often and were more decentralized than inactive block associations were.

Decision making frequently involves conflict, negotiation, and compromise. Arlene Andrews (1990) warns that the group's problem-solving approach must be clearly defined so that solutions will not conflict with participants' individual responsibilities. In addition, conflict (usually interpersonal) is reduced when a consensus is reached by using group techniques, such as nominal group process. Brown (1984) provides extensive guidelines for managing conflict and maintains that "almost every decision by an existing coalition, or one in the process of forming, necessitates negotiation." She suggests that conflicts should not be suppressed because they can be energizing, forcing both sides to develop new options and new ways of working together (26, 27).

Richard Hall and colleagues (1977) report that conflict and coordination both appear to be consequences of frequent interorganizational interactions. Personnel competence, performance, quality of communications, and compatibility of philosophy were all positively related to coordination and negatively related to conflict among youth-oriented organizations.

Terry Mizrahi and Beth Rosenthal (1992) argue that conflict is an inherent characteristic of coalitions. It may arise between the coalition and its targets for social change or among coalition partners over issues such as leadership, goals, benefits, contributions, and representation. Conflict may lead to staff turnover, avoidance of certain activities, and difficulty in recruiting members (Kegler et al. 1998b). Mizrahi and Rosenthal (1992) identify four dynamic tensions that account for conflict in coalitions: (1) mixed loyalties of members to their own organizations and to the coalition, (2) the autonomy a coalition requires and its accountability to its member organizations, (3) lack of clarity about the coalition's purpose as either a means for specific change or a model for sustained interorganizational cooperation, and (4) members' diverse interests (see appendix 3).

Michael Edelstein (1992) suggests that several aspects of coalitions may be useful for understanding the context in which conflicts emerge:

1. Voluntary versus required formation: some coalitions are entered into voluntarily, whereas others are formed because they are required (for example, to obtain funding).
2. Reactive versus proactive formation: some coalitions form in reaction to a crisis, whereas others form to develop a new program or fill a gap.
3. Confrontation versus cooperation: some coalitions take an adversarial approach to the power structure, whereas others attempt to work with it.
4. Previous history of coalition partners: some coalition functioning will be influenced by the previous history of the coalition partners.
5. Consensus versus dissensus: some coalitions work with similar members (such as representatives of local community-based organizations that work on domestic violence), whereas some attempt to coalesce potentially opposing partners (such as public health educators who work in a substance abuse coalition with representatives from the beer and wine industry).

How the coalition manages these dynamics affects its cohesiveness and effectiveness. Conflict transformation is the process whereby resolution of conflict strengthens the coalition and builds capacity. Research shows that conflict transformation can be an effective part of coalition planning and contribute to goal attainment (Mayer et al. 1998).

VOLUNTEER-STAFF RELATIONSHIPS

Although not all coalitions have the resources to employ them, staff members can reduce the burdens of a coalition's membership. Staff members often support the coalition, encourage membership involvement, and build community capacity (Sanchez 2000). When a coalition employs staff, staff members and volunteers should be clear about their respective roles and decide if staff members are given latitude to carry out daily tasks (Brown 1984). Ellen Feighery and Todd Rogers (1989) suggest that staff roles should be clarified as soon as a coalition is formed. They believe that, in the early stages of the coalition, staff must help educate some volunteer members about issues that influence the coalition's mission and strategies and must guide them to assume new roles and responsibilities.

Staff effectiveness may be judged by how well staff members balance their provision of technical assistance with volunteers' ability to make informed decisions. A staff is more likely to improve the atmosphere of a coalition when it appreciates the voluntary nature of coalitions and has organizational and interpersonal skills to facilitate the complex collaborative process (Croan and Lees 1979). Some research suggests that coalitions with staff members who play a supportive rather than visible leadership role have higher levels of implementation (Kegler et al. 1998b). Studies have shown that staff competence is associated with increased perception of volunteer benefits (Rogers et al. 1993, Butterfoss et al. 1996, Kegler et al. 1998a).

There is sparse literature on different types of volunteer roles in coalitions. A volunteer can be an instrumental founding board member, a committee chair or dependable member, or an occasional participant who works on a single activity. We believe that each role has its own challenges, benefits, and costs and has a different relationship with staff. Additional research is needed to fill this gap in the literature.

COMMUNICATION PATTERNS

Smooth internal communication between membership and staff may be the essential ingredient in a well-functioning coalition. Open communication helps the group focus on a common purpose, increases trust and sharing of resources, provides information about programs, and allows members to express and resolve misgivings about planned activities (Andrews 1990, Feighery and Rogers 1989). Viable coalitions often have frequent meetings, which volunteer members are actively encouraged to attend (Benard 1989, Hord 1986), and a well-developed system of internal communication to keep staff and volunteers informed (Andrews

1990, Cohen et al. 1991, Croan and Lees 1979, Rogers et al. 1993; Kegler et al. 1998a).

Membership commitment and resource mobilization are key aspects of the operation of organizations, especially when they depend on voluntary effort. As Marilyn Gittell (1980) concludes, "We need to know more about why people join organizations and what encourages them to devote time and energy to those organizations' aims" (263). Political economy theory suggests that a social exchange takes place in organizations: participants will invest their energy in an organization only if they expect to receive some benefits. Following are some potential benefits and costs of participation:

### Benefits
- Increased networking, information sharing, and access to resources (Hord 1986, Kaplan 1986)
- Involvement in an important cause and attainment of desired outcomes from the coalition's efforts (Rich 1980, Zapka et al. 1992)
- Enjoyment of the coalition's work (Benard 1989)
- Receipt of personal recognition (Rich 1980, Roberts-DeGennaro 1986b, Wandersman and Alderman 1993)

### Costs
- Time given to coalition lost to other obligations (Bailey 1986, Rich 1980)
- Lost autonomy in decision making, expenditure of scarce resources, tensions involved in working to overcome any unfavorable image held by other partners (Schermerhorn 1975)
- Lack of direction from coalition leadership or staff, perception of lack of recognition or appreciation, burnout, lack of necessary skills, pressure for additional commitment (Wandersman and Alderman 1993)

Several studies have systematically studied the benefits and costs for individuals of participation in voluntary organizations. Prestby et al. (1990) found two main sources of motivation: personal gain (such as learning new skills and gaining personal recognition) and social-communal benefits (such as improving the neighborhood and helping others). In a related study, Wandersman et al. (1987) found that members and nonmembers agreed that the greatest benefits were making a contribution and helping others rather than satisfying self-interest or making personal gains. Active participants reported receiving significantly more social-communal benefits and personal benefits than less active participants did (Prestby et al. 1990). There are, however, costs involved in participation: personal costs (such as time, effort, and the things people give up in other parts of their lives to participate) and social-organizational costs (such as interpersonal conflict and lack of organizational progress) (Wandersman et al. 1987). Less active members report more social-organizational costs than more active members do (see Prestby et al. 1990). For those less active members, such costs may block more active participation.

Several studies have also looked at the ratio of benefits to costs. Prestby et al. (1990) found that the more actively a person participated, the higher the benefit-cost ratio was. Research also supports the fact that satisfied and committed members will participate more actively in the coalition (Butterfoss et al. 1993, 1996; Roberts-DeGennaro 1986a, 1986b; Rogers et al. 1993; Mayer et al. 1998).

In addition to understanding the costs and benefits of individual participation, it is useful to examine the costs and benefits for an organization that participates in a coalition. In other words, what does an individual organization get out of being in a coalition? Matthew Chinman and Abraham Wandersman (1999) provide a detailed review of the literature on costs and benefits in voluntary organizations.

## PRODUCTION SUBSYSTEM

A coalition must engage in two types of activities: (1) target activities, or those that work directly toward the consortium's intended goals and products; and (2) maintenance activities, or those that clarify processes and sustain and renew the infrastructure.

### TARGET ACTIVITIES

If a coalition is to survive, it must produce more than a sense of safety in numbers or camaraderie among members; it must engage in the tasks and produce the products for which it was created. Early in its existence, the coalition should create a mission statement, set up committees, perform a needs assessment, and develop a comprehensive plan. Marshall Kreuter, Nicole Lezin, and Laura Young (2000) note that many collaborative efforts fail to produce rigorous plans. Research has shown, however, that quality plans contribute to successful implementation (Kumpfer et al. 1993, Butterfoss et al. 1996, Kegler et al. 1998a).

In its implementation phase, the coalition carries out actual activities (training, advocacy, education programs). For example, a community partnership to prevent alcohol and other drug problems might develop after-school activities, parent training, media or red ribbon campaigns, and coping skills programs; or the partnership might advocate for policy change. Analyses show that coalitions tend to select activities that promote changes in awareness rather than more difficult policy-change strategies (Florin et al. 1993). Assuming that interventions are logically linked to planned outcomes, the likelihood of achieving those outcomes depends on the extent to which strategies are implemented and reach the intended populations. Adaptations of previously evaluated interventions (best practices) increase the likelihood that interventions will lead to community change and desired long-term outcomes (Green 2001, Cameron et al. 2001).

## MAINTENANCE ACTIVITIES

To sustain momentum and rebuild itself, a coalition has to recruit and orient new members, train leaders, prepare leaders-in-waiting to take over when necessary, address and resolve conflict, engage in public relations, celebrate accomplishments, and raise funds (Prestby and Wandersman 1985). Many voluntary organizations, including coalitions, are vulnerable in this area because maintenance activities do not always have the glitz, visibility, or priority of target activities.

Tension frequently arises between target and maintenance activities. For example, how much time should be spent on each type of activity when people have limited energy? Although we cannot say that a known best ratio exists, we believe that both target and maintenance activities are necessary for viability but insufficient for total coalition effectiveness. Perhaps understanding the importance of both types of activities can help members balance their time and energy. For example, staff might spend more time on maintenance activities, and volunteers might focus on target activities.

## EXTERNAL GOAL ATTAINMENT

What has the coalition accomplished? For many, including coalition members and funders, this is the bottom line. Has the coalition taken any actions that have achieved its initial goals and objectives? For example, has it reduced the incidence of substance abuse? Has it improved the training of public health professionals?

## SHORT- AND LONG-TERM CHANGES

Program evaluators often discuss the short- and long-term effects of an initiative. In program evaluation terms, *outcome evaluation* attempts to determine the short-term or direct effects of the program. In contrast, *impact evaluation* is concerned with the long-term, ultimate effects desired by a community organizing effort or program. In alcohol and other drug prevention programs, impacts can include reduction in overall drug use and a decrease in drunk driving–related fatalities. (In the public health field, the terms *outcomes* and *impacts* are used in the opposite way.)

Several analysts emphasize that coalitions need to accomplish quick wins and short-term successes to increase member motivation and pride and enhance credibility (Brown 1984, Croan and Lees 1979, Hord 1986). Once a coalition attains a quick win, it may direct its efforts toward more complex tasks (Cohen et al. 1991). Short-term successes should not, however, be mistaken for ultimate solutions to complex health problems and social concerns (Sink and Stowers 1989). A focus on quick wins and easy interventions may explain why some coalitions are not able to achieve systems or health outcomes change (Kreuter et al. 2000).

In addition to evaluating the outcomes produced by programs, some coalitions are concerned with system change, such as alterations in service delivery and system reform (Kagan 1991). Most researchers and practitioners agree that effective health promotion and disease prevention efforts require change at multiple levels, especially environmental and policy change (McLeroy et al. 1998). Different types of community changes have been described, such as changes in programs, policies, and practices (Fawcett et al. 1997). Further, as coalition interventions become more complex, assessment of such coalitions must focus on multiple levels and take community readiness into account (Goodman et al. 1996). Coalitions create change in communities by developing the skills of individuals, increasing the sense of community, and providing new ways to solve community problems. Coalitions also create changes in links among organizations and in the physical and social environment of a community (Kegler et al. 2000). Measurement of system change, such as new community links and cross-referrals among agencies, is difficult.

## CONTROVERSIES ABOUT COALITIONS
## AND SOME DIRECTIONS FOR OBTAINING RESULTS

The positive news is that coalitions can and do work, and some have demonstrated positive public health outcomes and impacts (Kegler et al. 2000, Butterfoss et al. 1998, Kreuter et al. 2000, Wandersman and Florin 2000). But many evaluations have shown disappointing results (see Hallfors et al. 2002, Saxe et al. 2002). Potential explanations have been cited in both this chapter and the general literature for the disappointing findings associated with coalitions and other collaborative partnerships (Roussos and Fawcett 2000, Mittelmark 1999, Kreuter et al. 2000, Berkowitz 2001). For example, design issues and secular trends make detection of community change difficult. Often coalitions do not focus on activities that will lead to sustained community change. Coalitions do not always employ staff who are versed in how to manage these organizations or know when to ask for technical assistance and training.

Coalitions may fail to show accomplishments in any of the following ways:

1. Theory failure: they use a coalition strategy when it is inappropriate for meeting a certain goal or have an incomplete conceptualization of the appropriate use of coalitions in addressing social and health concerns.

2. Implementation failure: they do not functioning well as organizations or implement strategies well.

3. Evaluation failure: their evaluations are poorly designed, use inappropriate comparison groups, or choose measures not sensitive to change.

4. System or resource failure: they design or implement good strategies, but those strategies are not supported by adequate resources or institutional backing.

## METHODS AND TOOLS FOR OBTAINING MORE RESULTS

For any intervention to succeed, whether at the individual level (such as therapy) or organizational level (such as violence prevention programs for a school), coalitions must choose both a good intervention and a good structure to deliver it. For example, achieving therapeutic outcomes requires using both evidence-based treatment strategies and a trained therapist to deliver the treatment. Similarly, good prevention programs catalyzed by any organization, including collaborations, require an intervention that is grounded in theory and best practice as well as a good organizational structure and a process to facilitate delivery of the intervention. Federal agencies have been promoting community agencies' and collaborations' use of evidence-based practices.

Coalitions need processes for planning and implementing effective interventions and evaluating and documenting results. Empowerment evaluation is a promising approach for helping coalitions accomplish this goal.

> The goal of empowerment evaluation is to improve program success.
> By providing program developers with tools for assessing the planning,
> implementation, and evaluation of programs, program practitioners
> have the opportunity to improve planning, implement with quality,
> evaluate outcomes, and develop a continuous quality improvement
> system, thereby increasing the probability of achieving results.
>
>                                                   (Wandersman 1999, 96)

Progress has been made in developing empowerment evaluation methods for building the capacity of community stakeholders to better plan, implement, and self-evaluate programs (Fetterman et al. 1996). Abraham Wandersman, Pamela Imm, Matthew Chinman, and Shakeh Kaftarian (2000) have developed a system called Getting to Outcomes, a results-based accountability approach that uses ten accountability questions and answers to help practitioners achieve results. Thomas Backer (2003) has edited a book about evaluating collaborations that includes methods for using data (Francisco et al. 2003) and working with evaluators (Guerra 2003). In sum, methods and tools for improving the planning, implementation, and evaluation of programs are being developed to help practitioners. In other words, researchers are refining the content of interventions.

What about structures that support (or undermine) the delivery of the program—the community collaboration? We need a set of empowerment and participatory evaluation methods and tools that help community collaborations become more effective and efficient organizationally. Concepts, methods, and tools that collaborations can use to build their capacity to become more organizationally effective and efficient are now available (see Backer 2003, Backer and Kunz 2003, Butterfoss in press, Maldrud et al. 1997, Norman 2003, Wolff 2003). Handbooks and manuals for developing and sustaining effective coalitions are also widely available (Dowling et al. 2000, Kaye and Wolffe 1995, Sofaer 2001, Winer and Ray 1994).

### CHALLENGE TO EVALUATORS

Ultimately, if coalitions are to contribute to the improved health status of the community, they must evaluate their impact on social and health systems and community outcomes. Thorough evaluation is one mechanism frequently cited for improving outcome effectiveness. Clearly, there is a great need for additional conceptualization and new methodological tools in the assessment of coalition functioning and outcomes. (See Backer 2003 and other chapters in this book for a discussion of promising developments in empowerment evaluation.)

### CHALLENGE TO COALITION LEADERS

The complex issues that many coalitions address take concerted and long-range efforts. Therefore, successful activities and programs probably need to be repeated. This requires institutionalization of the program or community organizing effort. The latter can be institutionalized either in the coalition or in one of its member agencies. In addition, institutionalization of the coalition itself (or its functions) should be a long-range consideration for most coalitions and a mark of coalition success. Robert Goodman and Allan Steckler (1989) have used an open systems framework to assess program institutionalization.

## Conclusion

Community coalitions and partnerships are exciting experiments in social change and powerful weapons in the battle to solve complex challenges in public health. We know they can work. They are at their best when they are accountable; are being used appropriately (good theory of change); and have thoughtful and energetic leaders who pay attention to coalition infrastructure, functioning, strategic planning, quality implementation, and self-evaluation of initiatives.

Coalitions form at the local level when grassroots groups seek safety or power in numbers. They may form when opportunities for new funding arise or cutbacks necessitate consolidation or cooperation. The basic idea is that working together can move us forward. But knowing how to make a coalition really work is paramount. The challenges to an effective coalition are enormous. Collaboration has been called an "unnatural act between unconsenting adults." While this remark is made in humor, it reflects a truism that collaboration is challenging because of turf issues, personalities, group dynamics, power, and status. Therefore, a coalition that attempts to achieve stability faces even more challenges.

Although the research literature on coalitions as organizations is still relatively thin, we believe that enough exists to suggest that, if a coalition is to be successful, its members and their roles need to be organized. The resources of a coalition (its greatest potential) must be organized in a structure that clarifies roles and relationships and produces activities that work toward the goals of the coalition to sustain and renew the organization. A successful coalition yields perceivable accomplishments and effects.

Health educators and other social change professionals engaged in coalition building and maintenance may benefit from reviewing how their consortia operate as organizations. What resources do members bring? What additional external resources are necessary? Are both target and maintenance activities occurring simultaneously? Do members feel that the benefits of participation outweigh the costs for themselves as individuals and for their organizations? Posing such questions, as well as others described in appendix 3, can help us be realistic about the costs and the many benefits of coalitions and make these social change vehicles realize their full potential.

## Acknowledgments

Portions of this chapter are based on "Understanding Coalitions" by Abraham Wandersman (April 1993), commissioned by the Community Based Public Health Evaluation Team at the University of Minnesota and funded by the W. K. Kellogg Foundation, adapted by permission of the author and Thomas M. Scott, director of the Center for Urban and Regional Affairs, Minneapolis.

## References

Allensworth, D., and W. Patton. 1990. "Promoting School Health through Coalition building." *Eta Sigma Gamma Monograph Series* 7, no. 2.

Andrews, A. 1990. "Interdisciplinary and Interorganizational Collaboration." In *Encyclopedia of Social Work*, edited by A. Minahan et al, 175–88. 18th ed. Silver Spring, Md.: National Association of Social Workers.

Backer, T. E., ed. 2003. *Evaluating Community Collaborations*. New York: Springer.

Backer, T. E., and C. Kunz. 2003. "The Human Side of Evaluating Collaborations." In *Evaluating community collaborations*, edited by T. Backer, 37–55. New York: Springer.

Bailey, A. 1986. "More Than Good Intentions: Building a Network of Collaboratives." *Education and Urban Society* 19, no. 1: 7–23.

Balcazar, R., T. Seekins, S. Fawcett, and B. Hopkins. 1990. "Empowering People with Physical Disabilities through Advocacy Skills Training." *American Journal of Community Psychology* 18, no. 2: 281–96.

Benard, B. 1989. "Working Together: Principles of Effective Collaboration." *Prevention Forum* (October): 4–9.

Berger, P., and R. Neuhaus. 1977. *To Empower People*. Washington, D.C.: American Enterprise Institute.

Berkowitz, B. 2001. "Studying the Outcomes of Community-Based Coalitions." *American Journal of Community Psychology* 29, no. 2: 213–27.

Black, T. 1983. "Coalition Building—Some Suggestions." *Child Welfare* 62, no. 3: 263–68.

Boissevain, J. 1974. *Friends of Friends*. Oxford: Blackwell.

Braithwaite, R., S. Taylor, and J. Austin. 2000. *Building Coalitions in the Black Community*. Thousand Oaks, Calif.: Sage.

Brown, C. 1984. *The Art of Coalition Building: A Guide for Community Leaders*. New York: American Jewish Committee.

Butterfoss, F. D. In press. "The Coalition Technical Assistance and Training Framework: Helping Community Coalitions Help Themselves." *Health Promotion Practice*.

Butterfoss, F. D., R. Goodman, and A. Wandersman. 1993. "Community Coalitions for Prevention and Health Promotion." *Health Education Research* 8, no. 3: 315–30.

————. 1996. "Community Coalitions for Prevention and Health Promotion: Factors Predicting Satisfaction, Participation and Planning." *Health Education Quarterly* 23, no. 1: 65–79.

Butterfoss, F. D., A. L. Morrow, J. Rosenthal, E. Dini, R. C. Crews, J. D. Webster, and P. A. Louis. 1998. "CINCH: An Urban Coalition for Empowerment and Action." *Health Education and Behavior* 25, no. 2: 213–25.

Cameron, R., M. Jolin, R. Walker, N. McDermott, and M. Gough. 2001. "Linking Science and Practice: Toward a System for Enabling Communities to Adopt Best Practices for Chronic Disease Prevention." *Health Promotion Practice* 2, no. 1: 35–42.

Chavis, D., P. Florin, R. Rich, and A. Wandersman. 1987. "The Role of Block Associations in Crime Control and Community Development: The Block Booster Project." Final report to the Ford Foundation, New York.

Chinman, M., and Wandersman, A. 1999. "The Benefits and Costs of Volunteering in Community Organizations: Review and Practical Implications." *Nonprofit and Voluntary Sector Quarterly* 28, no. 1: 46–64.

Cohen, L., N. Baer, and P. Satterwhite. 1991. "Developing Effective Coalitions: A How-to Guide for Injury Prevention Professionals." Paper presented at a meeting on maternal, child, and adolescent health, U.S. Department of Health, Washington, D.C., January.

Croan, G., and J. Lees. 1979. *Building Effective Coalitions: Some Planning Considerations*. Arlington, Va.: Westinghouse National Issues Center.

Dowling, J., H. J. O'Donnell, and Wellington Consulting Group. 2000. *A Development Manual for Asthma Coalitions*. Northbrook, Ill.: CHEST Foundation and the American College of Chest Physicians.

Edelstein, M. 1992. "Building Coalitions for Sustainability: An Examination of Emergent Partnerships Addressing Environmental and Community Issues." Paper presented at the annual meeting of the Environmental Design Research Association, Boulder, Colo., April.

Fawcett, S., R. Lewis, A. Paine-Andrews, V. Francisco, K. Richer, E. Williams, and B. Copple. 1997. "Evaluating Community Coalitions for Prevention of Substance Abuse: The Case of Project Freedom." *Health Education and Behavior* 24, no. 6: 812–28.

Feighery, E., and T. Rogers. 1989. "Building and Maintaining Effective Coalitions." *How-to Guides on Community Health Promotion*, no. 12. Palo Alto, Calif.: Stanford Health Promotion Resource Center.

Fetterman, D. M., S. J. Kaftarian, and A. Wandersman, eds. 1996. *Empowerment Evaluation: Knowledge and Tools for Self-Assessment and Accountability*. Thousand Oaks, Calif.: Sage.

Florin, P., R. Mitchell, and J. Stevenson. 1989. "Rhode Island Substance Abuse Prevention Act Questionnaire." Providence: University of Rhode Island, Department of Psychology.

Francisco, V., J. A. Schultz, and S. Fawcett. 2002. "How to Make Sense of Results from Collaboration Evaluations." In *Evaluating Community Collaborations for Serving Youth at Risk: A Handbook for Mental Health, School and Youth Violence Prevention Organizations*, edited by T. Backer, 163–78. Rockville, Md.: Center for Mental Health Services.

Gittell, M. 1980. *Limits of Citizen Participation: The Decline of Community Organizations*. Beverly Hills, Calif.: Sage.

Goodman, R. M., and A. Steckler. 1989. "A Framework for Assessing Program Institutionalization." *Knowledge in Society* 2, no. 1: 57–71.

Goodman, R. M., A. Wandersman, M. Chinman, P. Imm, and E. Morrisey. 1996. "An Ecological Assessment of Community-Based Interventions for Prevention and

Health Promotion: Approaches to Measuring Community Coalitions." *American Journal of Community Psychology* 24, no. 1: 33–61.

Gray, B. 1985. "Conditions Facilitating Interorganizational Collaboration." *Human Relations* 38, no. 10: 911–36.

Green, L. 2000. "Caveats on Coalitions: In Praise of Partnerships." *Health Promotion Practice* 1, no. 1: 64–65.

Green, L. W., and C. J. Frankish. In press. "Finding the Right Mix of Organizational, Decentralized, and Centralized Control in Planning for Health Promotion." In *Community Health Promotion*, edited by B. Beery, E. Wagner, and A. Cheadle. Seattle: University of Washington Press.

Guerra, N. G. 2003. "Evaluating Collaborations in Youth Violence Prevention." In *Evaluating Community Collaborations*, edited by T. Backer, 129–45. New York: Springer.

Hall, R., J. Clark, P. Giordano, P. Johnson, and M. Van Roekel. 1977. "Patterns of Interorganizational Relationships." *Administrative Science Quarterly* 22: 457–73.

Hallfors, D., H. Cho, D. Livert, and C. Kadushin. 2002. "Fighting Back against Substance Abuse: Are Community Coalitions Winning?" *American Journal of Preventive Medicine* 23, no. 4: 237–45.

Hord, S. 1986. "A Synthesis of Research on Organizational Collaboration." *Educational Leadership* 43 (February): 22–26.

Kagan, S. L. 1991. *United We Stand: Collaboration for Child Care and Early Education Services*. New York: Teachers College Press.

Kaplan, M. 1986. "Cooperation and Coalition Development among Neighborhood Organizations: A Case Study." *Journal of Voluntary Action Research* 15, no. 4: 23–34.

Katz, D., and R. L. Kahn. 1978. *The Social Psychology of Organizations*. 2d ed. New York: Wiley.

Kaye, G., and T. Wolffe. 1995. *From the Ground Up: A Workbook on Coalition Building and Community Development*. Amherst, Mass.: AHEC/Community Partners.

Kegler, M., A. Steckler, S. Malek, and K. McLeroy. 1998a. "Factors That Contribute to Effective Community Health Promotion Coalitions: A Study of Ten Project ASSIST Coalitions in North Carolina." *Health Education and Behavior* 25, no. 3: 338–53.

———. 1998b. "A Multiple Case Study of Implementation in 10 Local Project ASSIST Coalitions in North Carolina." *Health Education Research* 13, no. 2: 225–38.

Kegler, M., J. Twiss, and V. Look. 2000. "Assessing Community Change at Multiple Levels: The Genesis of an Evaluation Framework for the California Healthy Cities and Communities Project." *Health Education and Behavior* 27, no. 6: 760–79.

Klitzner, M. 1991. *National Evaluation Plan for Fighting Back*. Bethesda, Md.: Robert Wood Johnson Foundation.

Knoke, D., and J. R. Wood. 1981. *Organized for Action: Commitment in Voluntary Associations*. New Brunswick, N.J.: Rutgers University Press.

Knoke, D., and C. Wright-Isak. 1982. "Individual Motives and Organizational Incentive Systems." *Research in the Sociology of Organizations* 1: 209–54.

Kreuter, M., N. Lezin, and L. Young. 2000. "Evaluating Community-Based Collaborative Mechanisms: Implications for Practitioners." *Health Promotion Practice* 1, no. 1: 49–63.

Kumpfer, K., C. Turner, R. Hopkins, and J. Librett. 1993. "Leadership and Team Effectiveness in Community Coalitions for the Prevention of Alcohol and Other Drug Abuse." *Health Education Research* 8, no. 3: 359–74.

Lasker, R., E. Weiss, and R. Miller. 2001. "Partnership Synergy: A Practical Framework for Studying and Strengthening the Collaborative Advantage." *Milbank Quarterly* 79, no. 2: 179–205.

Maldrud, K., M. Polacsek, and N. Wallerstein. 1997. *A Workbook for Participatory Evaluation of Coalitions*. Albuquerque: University of New Mexico and New Mexico Partnership for Healthier Communities.

Marrett, C. 1971. "On the Specification of Interorganizational Dimensions." *Sociology and Social Research* 56: 83–99.

Mayer, J., R. Soweid, S. Dabney, C. Brownson, R. Goodman, and R. Brownson. 1998. "Practices of Successful Community Coalitions: A Multiple Case Study. *American Journal of Health Behavior* 22, no. 5: 368–77.

McLeroy, K. R., D. Bibeau, A. Steckler, and K. Glanz. 1988. "An Ecological Perspective on Health Promotion Programs." *Health Education Quarterly* 15, no. 4: 351–77.

Mittelmark, M. 1999. "Health Promotion at the Communitywide Level: Lessons from Diverse Perspectives." In *Health Promotion at the Community Level*, edited by N. Bracht, 3–26. 2d ed. Thousand Oaks, Calif.: Sage.

Mizrahi, T., and B. Rosenthal. 1992. "Managing Dynamic Tension in Social Change Coalitions." In *Community Organization and Social Administration: Advances, Trends, and Emerging Principles*, edited by T. Mizrahi and J. D. Morrison. New York: Haworth.

Norman, A. J. 2003. "Multicultural Issues in Collaboration: Some Implications for Multirater Evaluation." In *Evaluating Community Collaborations*, edited by T. Backer. New York: Springer.

Perlman, J. 1979. "Grassroots Empowerment and Government Response." *Social Policy* 10: 16–21.

Prestby, J. E., and A. Wandersman. 1985. "An Empirical Exploration of a Framework of Organizational Viability: Maintaining Block Organizations." *Journal of Applied Behavioral Science* 21, no. 3: 287–305.

Prestby, J., A. Wandersman, P. Florin, R. Rich, and D. Chavis. 1990. "Benefits, Costs, Incentive Management, and Participation in Voluntary Organizations: A Means to Understanding and Promoting Empowerment." *American Journal of Community Psychology* 18, no. 1: 117–49.

Rich, R. 1980. "The Dynamics of Leadership in Neighborhood Organizations." *Social Science Quarterly* 60, no. 4: 570–87.

Roberts-DeGennaro, M. 1986a. "Building Coalitions for Political Advocacy." *Social Work* 31 (July–August): 308–11.

———. 1986b. "Factors Contributing to Coalition Maintenance." *Journal of Sociology and Social Welfare* 13, no. 2: 248–64.

Rogers, T., B. Howard-Pitney, E. Feighery, D. Altman, J. Endres, and A. Roeseler. 1993. "Characteristics and Participant Perceptions of Tobacco Control Coalitions in California." *Health Education Research* 8, no. 3: 345–57.

Roussos, S., and S. Fawcett. 2000. "A Review of Collaborative Partnerships as a Strategy for Improving Community Health." *Annual Review of Public Health* 21: 369–402.

Sanchez, V. 2000. "Reflections on Community Coalition Staff: Research Directions from Practice." *Health Promotion Practice* 1, no. 4: 320–22.

Saxe, L., C. Kadushin, E. Tighe, A. Beveridge, A. Brodsky, D. Livert, and D. M. Rindskopf. 2002. *The Front Lines of the War against Drugs: Can Research Help Direct Policy?* Waltham, Mass.: Heller School for Social Policy and Management.

Schermerhorn, J., Jr. 1975. "Determinants of Interorganizational Cooperation." *Academy of Management Review* 18, no. 4: 846–56.

Sink, D., and G. Stowers. 1989. "Coalitions and Their Effect on the Urban Policy Agenda." *Administration in Social Work* 13, no. 2: 83–98.

Sofaer, S. 2001. *Working Together, Moving Ahead: A Manual to Support Effective Community Health Coalitions.* New York: Baruch College, School of Public Affairs.

Stevenson, W., J. Pearce, and L. Porter. 1985. "The Concept of Coalition in Organization Theory and Research." *Academy of Management Review* 10, no. 2: 256–68.

Tarlov, A., B. Kehrer, D. Hall, S. Samuels, G. Brown, M. Felix, and J. Ross. 1987. "Foundation Work: The Health Promotion Program of the Henry Kaiser Family Foundation." *American Journal of Health Promotion* 2, no. 2: 74–78.

Wandersman, A. 1981. "A Framework of Participation in Community Organizations." *Journal of Applied Behavioral Science* 17, no. 1: 27–58.

Wandersman, A., and J. Alderman. 1993. "Incentives, Costs, and Barriers for Volunteers: A Staff Perspective for Volunteers in One State." *Review of Public Personnel Administration* 13, no. 1: 67–76.

Wandersman, A., P. Florin, R. Friedmann, and R. Meier. 1987. "Who Participates, Who Does Not, and Why? An Analysis of Voluntary Neighborhood Associations in the United States and Israel." *Sociological Forum* 2, no. 3: 534–55.

Wandersman, A., and P. Florin. 2000. "Citizen Participation and Community Organizations." In *Handbook of Community Psychology*, edited by J. Rappaport and E. Seidman, 247–72. New York: Plenum.

Wandersman, A., P. Imm, M. J. Chinman, and S. J. Kaftarian. 1999. *Getting to Outcomes: Methods and Tools for Planning, Evaluation, and Accountability*. Rockville, Md.: Center for Substance Abuse Prevention.

Whetten, D. 1981. "Interorganizational Relations: A Review of the Field." *Journal of Higher Education* 52, no. 1: 1–27.

Winer, M., and K. Ray. 1994. *Collaboration Handbook: Creating, Sustaining and Enjoying the Journey*. St. Paul, Minn.: Wilder Foundation.

W. K. Kellogg Foundation. 1994. "Working Together toward Healthy Communities." Brochure for the Community-based Public Health Initiative. Battle Creek, Mich.: W. K. Kellogg Foundation.

Wolff, T. 2003. "A Practical Approach to Evaluation of Collaborations." In *Evaluating community collaborations*, edited by T. Backer. New York: Springer.

Yoo, S. Y., N. E. Weed, M. L. Lempa, M. Mbondo, R. Shada, and R. M. Goodman. In press. "Collaborative Community Empowerment: An Illustration of a Six-Step Process." *Health Promotion Practice*.

Zapka, J. G., G. R. Marrocco, B. Lewis, J. McCusker, J. Sullivan, J. McCarthy, and F. X. Birch. 1992. "Inter-Organizational Response to AIDS: A Case Study of the Worcester AIDS Consortium." *Health Education Research* 7: 31–46.

Zuckerman, H., and A. Kaluzny. 1990. "Managing beyond Vertical and Horizontal Integration: Strategic Alliances As an Emerging Organizational Form. Ann Arbor: University of Michigan. Unpublished paper.

SUSAN KLITZMAN
DANIEL KASS
NICHOLAS FREUDENBERG

*Chapter 17*

# Coalition Building to Prevent Childhood Lead Poisoning

## A Case Study from New York City

How CAN public health professionals working in advocacy organizations influence public policy in order to promote health and prevent disease? What methods are effective when the targets for behavior change are institutions and policymakers as well as patients, clients, and consumers? What are some of the opportunities and constraints involved in advocacy work? How should advocacy organizations respond over time to changing public health priorities and needs? In this chapter, we address these questions using a case study of the New York City Coalition to End Childhood Lead Poisoning (NYCCELP). In the 1980s, several public health advocates and other advocates from around New York City formed the NYCCELP to respond to the problem of childhood lead poisoning. The coalition has managed to sustain itself for two decades. This chapter describes the thinking and efforts that drove the coalition's formation as well its intended and actual direct and indirect achievements.

### The Public Health Scope of Childhood Lead Poisoning

Lead poisoning continues to be a significant environmental disease among young children, despite dramatic declines in its magnitude and severity in both the United States as a whole (CDC 1997, 2000) and New York City in particular (Klitzman and Leighton 1999). Still, according to the CDC (2003), in 1999–2000, an estimated 2.2 percent of U.S. children between the ages of one and five (approximately 500,000) had elevated blood lead levels (BLLs)—greater than or equal to ten micrograms per deciliter (µg/dL). Similar prevalence rates have been reported for New

York City children (New York City Department of Health and Mental Hygiene 2002); and although they are continuing to decline, almost five thousand young children in the city had elevated BLLs in 2002 (Frieden 2003).

Since the reduction of lead in gasoline and the banning of lead-containing solder in food storage cans, the single greatest remaining source of childhood lead exposure is lead-based paint—in particular, dust and paint chips from old and deteriorating paint. Other sources, such as exposures in their country of origin among immigrant children (Geltman et al. 2001) and soil and exterior paint, may also be important for specific population subgroups. Through normal hand-to-mouth activity, toddlers can ingest lead dust that has contaminated easily reachable surfaces. An estimated 38 million U.S. housing units contain lead-based paint; 24 million have significant lead-based paint hazards. Of those with hazards, 1.2 million house low-income families with children under six years old (Jacobs et al. 2002).

Although lead is toxic to all humans, its effects are particularly dangerous to children younger than six. Their still-developing nervous systems are damaged by very small amounts of lead exposure. Children also absorb lead from their digestive systems six times more efficiently than adults do and, because of their small size, receive far greater effective doses. Recent studies have demonstrated that even children with BLLs lower than 10 µg/dl suffer persistent intellectual impairment (Canfield et al. 2003, Lanphear et al. 2000). At higher levels, they show a variety of development delays and learning disorders, including delayed speech development and verbal processing, poor attention span, and decreased IQ scores. Behavioral disorders, including juvenile delinquency, have similarly been linked to childhood exposures to lead (Goyer 1993, Needleman et al. 2002). Inside the body, lead can be stored in the bones for long periods of time and released when calcium is liberated, as during pregnancy and lactation.

Childhood lead poisoning continues to be disproportionately concentrated among very young, poor, urban children of color living in older, distressed housing (CDC 1997). In 2000, of the 817 newly identified New York City children with BLLs at or above the environmental action level (one test greater than or equal to 19 µg/dL or two persistent tests between 15 and 19 µg/dL), almost two-thirds (519 cases) were between the ages of six months and six years. Of these, about 90 percent were African American, Hispanic, or Asian; 94 percent lived in zip codes where the percentage of pre-1950 housing was at least 28 percent above the national average; and 74 percent lived in areas where the proportion of poor children was at or above the citywide average of 17 percent (New York City Department of Health and Mental Hygiene 2002)

The societal cost of childhood lead poisoning includes medical costs for affected children and exposed mothers, costs of special education, lost lifetime occupational productivity, victims' personal injury claims, and a host of related expenses (Schwartz 1994) estimated at $43.4 billion annually (Landrigan et al. 2002). An increase of 10 μg/dl in a child's BLL reduces the value of his or her future earnings by approximately $37,000 (Grosse et al. 2002).

## Elements of a Meaningful
## Lead Poisoning Prevention Program

Childhood lead poisoning is a fully preventable public health problem; its causes and control methods are well understood. This notion is implicit in the U.S. Department of Health and Human Services' (2000) "Healthy People 2010" goal of reducing to zero the number of children between the ages of one and six with BLLs greater than or equal to 10 μg/dl by the year 2010. Achieving this goal requires a multifaceted approach that combines public health, medical, and housing interventions and incorporates both primary prevention strategies (controlling lead hazards before a child is poisoned) and secondary prevention strategies (acting after a child has an elevated BLL). At the secondary prevention level, identifying cases depends on screening children for BLLs as early as possible and at regular intervals. Successful screening programs depend on regulatory requirements, such as those in place in New York State since 1993 (Official Compilation 1993); access to medical care; and knowledgeable medical care providers and informed parents. When cases are identified, further exposure to lead dust must be minimized by care-fully evaluating and controlling lead hazards in dwellings and other places frequented by affected children. Where the potential for lead paint exposure is found, corrective action is required to ensure that peeling or chipping paint is removed and lead-containing dust is safely remediated. Where lead paint remains, leaking roofs and pipes, unstable plaster, and damaged ceilings, all of which cause paint to deteriorate, must be repaired. So successful remediation requires a regulatory and enforcement infrastructure, as has emerged in New York City since 1970 (RCNY 1960, 1993).

In terms of primary prevention, New York City was one of the first jurisdictions in the United States to ban the use of lead-based paint for interior residences, a step it took in 1960 (RCNY 1960). But agreement among the various local stakeholders on how best to assure the appropriate and safe remediation of existing lead-based paint hazards has remained elusive. Among the many reasons is the fact that 55 percent of the city's housing units (about 1.6 million) were built before 1950 (when lead-based paint was widely used). Since 1980, little new, lead-free, low-income housing has been built. Many older units are situated in poor neighborhoods and are in deteriorating condition. Owners of many high-risk properties may lack the resources for ongoing maintenance and repair. In addition, court decisions in the 1980s (NYCCELP v. Koch 1989) and 1990s (*Juarez v. Wavecrest Management Team, Ltd.* 1996) increased the potential liability faced by property owners and many municipalities (including New York City) for damages suffered by lead poisoned children. As a result, property owners, government agencies, and elected officials can be reticent to embrace new regulatory mandates without adequate resources or legal protections.

Although a general consensus exists on what needs to be done, little agreement has emerged on how to go about doing it, who should bear the cost, and how to appropriately make interim progress on the problem while waiting for permanent solutions. It is clear, however, that prevention efforts must involve the coordination of public health agencies, medical practitioners, landlords, housing inspectors, health educators, and social workers and that these efforts must be driven by enforceable local policies that are designed to protect those children at greatest risk. In answer to a call for improved local policy to prevent childhood lead poisoning, a coalition in New York City was born.

## The Formation of a Citywide Coalition

NYCCELP was created at a time of widespread lead poisoning, growing medical evidence that exposure to very low levels of lead causes serious health problems, and lack of confidence in the city government's willingness to confront the problem. Some fourteen years before the coalition's creation, scientists, housing activists, social workers, and parents of lead-poisoned children formed Citizens to End Lead Poisoning. This group, in concert with a militant Puerto Rican organization, successfully mounted pressure to force the city to develop an agency infrastructure to screen and medically treat poisoned children and educate health care providers about lead poisoning. Although the group did not last, the problem of lead poisoning did, and the city's response to the problem waned (Freudenberg and Golub 1987)

In the early 1980s, several organizations emerged to address neighborhood environmental quality concerns. The Washington Heights Health Action Project organized a local coalition against lead poisoning that met for two years and helped to improve screening and educational services in northern Manhattan. The Lead Poisoning Prevention Project began in 1981 at Montefiore Medical Center in the Bronx with the aims of educating the community about lead, inspecting apartments, offering blood lead screening, and providing follow-up medical care.

These two organizations' successes in mobilizing people on this issue, as well as their failures in making substantive changes in city policies on lead poisoning, created the impetus for a citywide coalition against lead poisoning. In 1983, leaders of these two community-based efforts called together a group of housing activists, health professionals, and staff members from advocacy groups to form a new organization dedicated to making lead poisoning once again a citywide political issue. The group called itself the New York City Coalition to End Lead

Poisoning. Its members initially included social workers, community organizers, health educators, physicians, and housing activists. It later expanded its membership to include legal advocates, construction trade unions, and private consulting firms.

## The Coalition's Activity

The coalition's first task was to review the city government's entire lead poisoning control program. After nine months of meetings with officials at the Department of Health and the Department of Housing Preservation and Development, reviewing data on program performance, and consulting with medical experts about lead poisoning, NYCCELP wrote a report titled "The Problem That Hasn't Gone Away: Childhood Lead Poisoning in New York City." One week before its scheduled release, a newly formed interagency task force on lead poisoning, convened by the mayor's office, urgently asked the coalition not to release its report. The task force also outlined several new initiatives on lead poisoning, including more community education, more screening, and better interagency coordination. After much discussion, NYCCELP decided to release the report, hoping it would generate additional political support for stronger city action. The report recommended actions that addressed each of the essential elements of a preventive program.

In the months following the release of the report, NYCCELP members worked with another consortium of public health and advocacy groups to craft a budget proposal that would offer initial funding for implementing its recommendations. Although the city council ultimately increased the budget for lead poisoning control by $300,000, the funds were allocated to study control measures that would, in the opinion of the coalition, serve only to delay needed apartment repair. Little money was allocated to crucial screening, education, and lead paint abatement.

In early 1985, the coalition decided to initiate a lawsuit against the city. This decision was based on the coalition's perception that city government had failed to act decisively to prevent lead poisoning and refused to meet with coalition members after release of the report. With representation by Bronx Legal Services, a class-action lawsuit was filed on behalf of five lead-poisoned children and their parents against the mayor and the commissioners of health and housing preservation and development. Although monetary awards were requested, the broader hope was that the lawsuit would force the development of improved policy and enforcement of city regulations. Filed in a mayoral election year, the lawsuit, so the coalition hoped, would politicize the issue of lead poisoning and force candidates to define their position on this and other related public health and housing issues.

Eighteen years have passed since the lawsuit was filed. The courts have ruled in favor of the coalition and the plaintiffs multiple times. The city has been held in contempt of court for failing to comply with orders to enforce city housing and health codes in ways the courts have interpreted were necessary to comply with the city's mandate to protect the health of children. For example, in 1989, the courts interpreted the law, Local Law 1 of 1982, as requiring complete removal of all lead-based paint, even intact paint (NYCCELP v. Koch 1989). In 1998, after losing its final appeal, the city published rules to implement Local Law 1 in response to court orders. Many public health and housing representatives, including some coalition members, expressed grave concerns about this policy. These included the risk that new hazards could be created by disturbing intact paint, the cost of abating an estimated 1.6 million dwellings, and fear that many landlords might abandon their properties because rents would be insufficient to cover abatement costs. To address these concerns, the city council speaker and the mayor proposed legislation employing a lead-safe approach (addressing current hazards, such as peeling paint) rather than a lead-free approach (removing all lead-based paint). The bill received support from several real estate organizations but drew heavy criticism from many public health professionals and advocates. Although many elements of the bill were viewed as protective (including the focus on inspecting for and addressing peeling lead-based paint in multiple dwellings where young children reside), the bill failed to address other important issues, including lead-dust hazards, worker training, and clearance dust testing. Nonetheless, the city council passed the measure. The legislation, Local Law 38 of 1999, became effective in November 1999; and shortly thereafter NYCCELP filed another lawsuit, charging that the city council had failed to comply with environmental review requirements. After a lengthy court battle, the Court of Appeals ruled in NYCCELP's favor (New York State Court of Appeals 2003).

The lawsuit has had several anticipated and unanticipated benefits in the ongoing struggle to prevent child lead poisoning. Perhaps most important, according to Andrew Goldberg, an attorney who represented plaintiffs from the mid-1980s until the mid-1990s, "the litigation always kept us at the table. It's important in a fight where there's such unequal bargaining power (i.e., poor families versus a powerful real estate industry)" (personal communication, July 2, 2003). For example, in 1992, the mayor convened a task force, which included coalition members, to review city policy on lead poisoning. Although many suspected that the effort was intended to appease the city's critics, coalition members participated and helped to prevent a consensus on what they believed were ineffective approaches to the problem. The coalition also gained members from the ranks of this task force who had become frustrated at the disproportionate power of the real estate industry and profit-oriented environmental consultants.

Although the lawsuit has dragged on, it has helped to sustain the coalition. Success in the courts has helped legitimize the coalition in the media and among politicians and candidates. Status reports are discussed at meetings. Media coverage and legal affiliations have linked coalition members to organizations and efforts outside of New York City and strengthened the coalition's role in national alliances to address lead poisoning.

While the lawsuit has been the most sustained and visible part of NYCCELP's work, the coalition's activity has included other outward-reaching and inward-strengthening efforts. NYCCELP has, for example, developed community education curricula, conducted trainings, and cosponsored conferences. On the political front, members engage in state and local advocacy for improved enforcement and expanded budgets. They have also drafted legislation to mandate lead-abatement worker training and certification (because improper abatement can lead to serious lead exposure among already poisoned children) and set minimum standards for abatement procedures. NYCCELP has for years served as a referral service for families, helping them to navigate the Byzantine structures of city government and referring them to legal representation to redress hazardous conditions.

## A Critical Analysis of the Coalition

Despite its successes in court, NYCCELP members themselves are quick to point out the limitations of a litigation-driven approach. According to Goldberg, "Litigation . . . can suck the life blood out of an organization trying to do grassroots organizing. Meetings became dominated by discussions related to litigation strategies and alternatives" (personal communication, July 2, 2003). Current lead attorney Matthew Chachere concurs: "[It] can disempower constituents (i.e., parents) because they can't follow it or play a role; they can't go and lobby a judge. [There's] a danger when professionals (lawyers) handle everything, and there's nothing for them to do." He also notes that successful litigation does not automatically lead to desired changes: "[The original lawsuit] achieved a lot. But when push came to shove, it was scuttled by the actions of the city. . . . They revoked the laws. There were lots of great court orders, but they could not be enforced without organized community support" (personal communication, July 2, 2003). So litigation has created a hostile environment between advocates and government plaintiffs that has stifled communication, information exchange, and problem solving. It has made it impossible for various stakeholders to use their collective expertise in amicably crafting workable solutions, programs, and policies. It is not clear, however, whether such dialogue would have taken place without the lawsuit. In addition, the litigation has imposed significant demands on lead poisoning prevention efforts in government agencies, which, one could argue, has diverted resources away from direct public health activities. Countless hours have been spent in meetings, document review, and other preparation for litigation.

On the legislative front, while NYCCELP members have been active in help-ing to draft and lobby for state and local legislation, their efforts have met with varying success. As noted, New York State passed comprehensive lead legislation in 1993. Yet as of this writing, with the recent court decision nullifying Local Law 38, the city still does not have a workable law in place to protect those chil-dren at greatest risk from exposure to lead-based paint hazards. Most recently, NYCCELP was successful in lobbying for the passage of a new childhood lead poisoning prevention law, which passed the city council, overriding a mayoral veto.

Since its inception, NYCCELP has remained singularly focused on lead. While this clarity of purpose may have contributed to its legal successes, it may have simultaneously limited opportunities for expansion. We now recognize that multiple hazards, in addition to lead-based paint, exist in the home environment: pest-infestation, pathogenic mold, safety hazards, and poor indoor air quality. Many of these conditions share common underlying causes, such as inadequate main-tenance and water damage (Matte and Jacobs 2000, Krieger and Higgins 2002). Federal agencies such as the U.S. Department of Housing and Urban Develop-ment and the CDC have provided seed funding to demonstrate these connections and seek common solutions. Many localities are now experimenting with more comprehensive "healthy homes" approaches to inspection, education, and build-ing maintenance. A broader housing mission within NYCCELP may have allowed it to expand its reach and funding base in this and other areas.

Furthermore, in light of the continuing decline in overall BLLs, inflexible and costly approaches that are applicable to all dwelling units regardless of risk are being called into question. According to Health Commissioner Thomas Frieden, "Efforts that divert the focus away from . . . high need communities, however well-intentioned, carry the serious risk of slowing progress in the communities where most progress is needed" (Frieden 2003).

The structure of the coalition also bears critical scrutiny. Throughout its exis-tence, NYCCELP has depended principally on member resources. Because many of the organizations that its participants represent have stable staff and financial resources (for example, hospital- and university-based programs and legal offices), NYCCELP has received only minimal funding to hire staff. Membership is fluid. Members are not charged dues. Leaders are democratically selected, but there is little concentration of power in their positions. Attendance at meetings is spo-radic, and there is no mechanism for expulsion. The voluntary and flexible nature of the coalition's structure has contributed positively to its work and survival in two important ways: (1) members do not threaten to drop out, which has added to the coalition's stability; and (2) scarce human resources are not expended on operations but are directed instead toward the primary objective of influencing city-wide lead poisoning prevention policy.

The coalition's informality also has its drawbacks. Flexible membership increases a coalition's risk of collapse or co-optation. NYCCELP has survived these threats because several original founding members have maintained strong, central roles throughout its existence and because key departing members were able to pass the torch to new attorneys, community and parent members, and organizations. Recently, a conscious effort was made to broaden NYCCELP's base of support to include labor organizations (such as the Central Labor Council of New York City and the New York Committee for Occupational Safety and Health), racial justice organizations (such as the NAACP), and child advocacy organizations (such as the Children's Defense Fund and the Citizen's Committee for Children).

For much of its history, NYCCELP's office was physically located in a lead-safe house, ensuring its connection to families suffering the effects of lead poisoning. For a time, however, its offices moved out of the house; and the organization, according to Megan Charlop, a NYCCELP board member, lost a critical connection to people suffering problems that reflected gaps and failings in the public health and housing systems. During this time, she says, the organization "lost steam, lost volunteers, and had fewer community-based activities." Since NYCCELP's board of directors voted to move its offices back to a lead-safe house, "NYCCELP has been reinvigorated, has more volunteers, and is thriving. Our parents' education program is doing well, and we have pieced together funds to maintain a part-time staff position" (personal communication, July 14, 2003).

As Abraham Wandersman and his colleagues argue in chapter 16, "a coalition's membership is its primary asset." NYCCELP depends almost entirely on the financial and material resources of its organizational members. Individuals and organizations contribute time for mobilization, advocacy, legal representation, report writing, education, and other work products as well as postage and transportation expenses. This has ultimately helped to sustain the coalition in several ways:

- Members have had to work in their own base organizations to convince their boards or supervisors of the importance of the issues and the relevance of the proposed activities. The net effect has been that member organizations have expanded their own missions to better incorporate child lead poisoning prevention.
- The coalition generally has not opted to engage in activities its members are not capable of sustaining, thereby leading to more successes, fewer failures, and less frustration.
- Each member organization pledges its support fully aware of its own resource limitations and is less likely not to deliver on its promises. This has helped to solidify the partnerships and minimize internal divisiveness.

- Contributions of resources have been balanced among organizational members; whereas some member organizations are able to offer financial support, others can mobilize volunteer labor.

## Lessons for Coalitions
## Addressing Public Health Concerns

Several lessons can be drawn from the history of the NYCCELP that are relevant to broader public health efforts. As noted in chapter 16, those seeking to change policy must define issues broadly so as to invite participation by constituencies diverse enough to have a political impact. If broad support for policy changes is lacking, policymakers tend to dismiss the problem as insignificant. Because NYCCELP organized around an understanding that lead poisoning is a symptom of poor housing, it was able to attract the participation of community development groups, tenant organizations, housing organizers, and legal advocates. By recognizing the connection between lead poisoning and the broader vulnerability of low-income children to other negative health outcomes, NYCCELP has been able to draw the membership and support of child welfare and racial and environmental justice organizations and advocates. By recognizing the connection between safe lead remediation and worker training and protections, NYCCELP has been able to attract powerful labor organizations and advocates. And by recognizing that the solutions to lead poisoning must include community education and mobilization, NYCCELP has invited the participation of talented educators and organizers. Thus, the range of skills and capacity to participate, which chapter 16 identified as crucial to the effective implementation and survival of coalitions, has been ensured. Table 17.1 illustrates the dimensions of lead poisoning and the potential constituencies affected and therefore involved in a coalition effort. This conceptualization of the problem helped the coalition to engage a wide variety of groups not previously involved in lead poisoning prevention. If public health advocates are to reach beyond those groups already concerned about an identified problem, they must learn how to describe the issue in terms that appeal to new constituencies' self-interests (see chapters 10 and 11).

Public health advocates must also understand how different groups influence the policy process. City council members, for example, respond to pressure that emanates from their own districts. City agency personnel may be responsive to data and persuasion but are just as influenced by their agency heads, who in turn must respond to the mayor's office. The mayor's attention is captured by the media. The coalition has worked to effect policy change through each of these avenues, mindful of their interconnections (Freudenberg and Golub 1987).

Coalitions must also be able to respond to changes in the policy arena with appropriate internal redirection of resources, modifications of strategies, and,

*Table 17.1*
Framework for Coalition Building on Lead Poisoning

| Dimension of Lead Poisoning Problem | Constituencies Involved |
| --- | --- |
| Poor housing | Housing and tenant groups |
| Neighborhood deterioration | Neighborhood associations and community development groups |
| Child health | Child health advocacy groups, parents, providers |
| Public education | Parents, school officials |
| Public health and primary prevention issues | Public health professionals and advocacy groups |
| Political issues | Elected officials, political parties, political aspirants |
| Environmental issues | Environmental organizations |
| Legal problems and liabilities | Law organizations, public service law groups, private attorneys |
| Employment issues | Trade unions, community development agencies, private environmental consulting firms |
| Minority issues | Civil rights groups, environmental justice groups |

*Source:* Reprinted from "Health Education, Public Policy, and Disease Prevention: A Case History of the New York City Coalition to End Lead Poisoning," by N. Freudenberg and M. Golub, *Health Education Quarterly* 14 (4) (1987):387–401, by permission of Sage Publications, Inc. Copyright © 1987 by Sage Publications, Inc.

when necessary, modification of the public perception of the coalition and its members. NYCCELP has attempted to balance its role as plaintiff in advocacy lawsuits against New York City with its more unifying role as an educational body. The coalition has also been able to shift its attention from local organizing to city and state policy issues and back as opportunities and constraints at these levels have changed.

Another lesson is that adversarial strategies sometimes are necessary to achieve meaningful change in public health policy. Although most public health workers are more practiced in consensus building methods, refusal to consider confrontational approaches can limit the effectiveness of the best-intentioned interventions. While we are familiar with the efforts of powerful organizations to influence or silence national dialogue on major health issues (for example, the tobacco industry on smoking, the chemical industry on environmental risks), it is important for public health advocates to evaluate whether similar interests are aligned against public health efforts more locally. In New York City, efforts to improve policy and increase public resources to prevent lead poisoning have been opposed by powerful real estate interests. NYCCELP's adversarial legal strategies strove to minimize the influence of these interests by moving the debate to the courts, which were presumably less susceptible to real estate lobbying than the legislative bodies were.

In the twenty years of NYCCELP's existence, a great deal of progress has been made in the city, and indeed nationally, in addressing the risks of childhood lead poisoning. As noted, both the magnitude and severity of the disease have continued to decline at a rapid pace, even though the action level for environmental intervention has been lowered three times since 1985 (RCNY 1960, Klitzman and Leighton 1999). Between 1995 and 2002 alone, there was a nearly 80 percent decline in the number of New York City children aged six months to six years with elevated BLLs (Frieden 2003). Very few diseases have experienced such a rapid or sustained reduction. These improvements are due in part to the promulgation of numerous regulations and policies and to concerted efforts by the public health community in the government, medical, academic, and nonprofit sectors. For example, New York State now requires that blood lead testing be performed on all children at ages one and two, during routine medical visits, and that all test results be reported to state and local health agencies for surveillance purposes (Official Compilation of Codes, Rules, and Regulations of the State of New York 1993). Similarly, New York City's Department of Health and Department of Housing Preservation and Development have made significant programmatic improvements, including professionalization and training of lead-inspection staff, implementation of improved computerized surveillance and tracking systems, improved interagency coordination, more systematized inspection protocols and procedures, and enhanced supervision and program monitoring and reporting. Recently, the Department of Housing Preservation and Development announced targeted enforcement of regulations with regard to property owners who had buildings with two or more apartments with lead-poisoned children and violations (Wasserman 2003). Neighborhood institutions have emerged that educate and organize around lead paint hazards. The New York City school system has begun to assess and correct peeling paint hazards in kindergarten classrooms. National regulations require that building owners divulge knowledge of the presence of lead paint before property transfers (U.S. Department of Housing and Urban Development 1999). Public awareness in New York City of the problem of lead poisoning has never been greater. The extent to which these advances are directly attributable to the work of NYCCELP cannot be demonstrated empirically. More likely, a confluence of forces at the local, state, and national levels converged to bring about these changes. Perhaps, then, the most important lesson from the experience of NYCCELP is that without forceful, sustainable, broad-based coalition efforts that help to frame the content and tenor of the dialogue on this and other public health issues, such progress would have been slower in coming and less effective on arrival.

## Acknowledgments

We wish to acknowledge the assistance of several people who contributed to our understanding of the role of NYCCELP in addressing lead poisoning in New York City: Maxine Golub, Institute for Urban Family Health; Lucy Billings, formerly with Bronx Legal Services and currently a New York civil court judge; Matthew Chachere, Northern Manhattan Improvement Corporation; Megan Charlop, Montefiore Medical Center; Andrew Goldberg, MFY Legal Services; and Diana Silver, New York University.

The opinions expressed in this chapter are solely those of the authors and are not necessarily shared by the people just listed, nor do they reflect the positions of any of their current or former affiliations or employers.

An earlier version of this article appeared as N. Freudenberg and M. Golub, 1987, "Health Education, Public Policy, and Disease Prevention: A Case History of the New York City Coalition to End Lead Poisoning," *Health Education Quarterly* 14, no. 4: 387–401. Copyright © 1987 by S.O.P.H.E. Reprinted by permission of Sage Publications, Inc.

## References

Canfield, R. L., C. R. Henderson, Jr., D. A. Cory-Slechta, C. Cox, T. A. Jusko, and B. P. Lanphear. 2003. "Intellectual Impairment in Children with Blood Lead Concentrations below 10 Microg. per Deciliter." *New England Journal of Medicine* 348, no. 16: 1517–26.

Centers for Disease Control (CDC). 1997. "Update: Blood Lead Levels—United States, 1991–1994." *Morbidity and Mortality Weekly Report* 46, no. 7: 141–46.

———. 2000. "Blood Lead Levels in Young Children—United States and Selected States, 1996–1999." *Morbidity and Mortality Weekly Report* 49, no. 50: 1133–37.

———. 2003. *Second National Report on Human Exposure to Environmental Chemicals*. National Center for Environmental Health publication no. 02-0716. Atlanta.

Freudenberg, N., and M. Golub. 1987. "Health Education, Public Policy, and Disease Prevention: A Case History of the New York City Coalition to End Lead Poisoning." *Health Education Quarterly* 14, no. 4: 387–401.

Frieden, T. 2003. Testimony before the New York City Council. June 23.

Geltman, P. L., M. J. Brown, and J. Cochran. 2001. "Lead Poisoning among Refugee Children Resettled in Massachusetts, 1995 to 1999." *Pediatrics* 108, no. 1: 158–62.

Goyer, R. A. 1993. "Lead Toxicity: Current Concerns." *Environmental Health Perspectives* 100: 177–87.

Grosse, S. D., T. D. Matte, J. Schwartz, and R. J. Jackson. 2002. "Economic Gains Resulting from the Reduction in Children's Exposure to Lead in the United States." *Environmental Health Perspectives* 110, no. 1: 563–69.

Jacobs, D. E., R. P. Clickner, J. Y. Zhou, S. M. Viet, D. A. Marker, J. W. Rogers, D. C. Zeldin, P. Broene, and W. Friedman 2002. "The Prevalence of Lead-Based Paint Hazards in U.S. Housing." *Environmental Health Perspectives* 110, no. 10: A599–A606.

*Juarez v. Wavecrest Management Team, Ltd.* 1996. 88 N.Y. 2d 628, 640–41.

Klitzman, S., and J. Leighton. 1999. "Decreasing Childhood Lead Poisoning in New York City: 1970–1998." *Journal of Urban Health* 76, no. 4: 542–45.

Krieger, J., and D. L. Higgins. 2002. "Housing and Health: Time again for Public Health Action." *American Journal of Public Health* 92, no. 5: 758–68.

Landrigan, P. J., C. B. Schechter, J. M. Lipton, M. C. Fahs, and J. Schwartz. 2002. "Environmental Pollutants and Disease in American Children: Estimates of Morbidity, Mortality, and Costs for Lead Poisoning, Asthma, Cancer, and Developmental Disabilities." *Environmental Health Perspectives* 110, no. 7: 721–28.

Lanphear, B. P., K. Dietrich, P. Auinger, and C. Cox. 2000. "Cognitive Deficits Associated with Blood Lead Concentrations < 10 Microg/dL in U.S. Children and Adolescents." *Public Health Reports* 115, no. 6: 521–29.

Matte, T. D., and D. E. Jacobs. 2000. "Housing and Health—Current Issues and Implications for Research and Programs." *Journal of Urban Health* 77, no. 1: 7–25.

Needleman, H. L., C. McFarland, R. B. Ness, S. E. Fienberg, and M. J. Tobin. 2002. "Bone Lead Levels in Adjudicated Delinquents: A Case Control Study." *Neurotoxicology and Teratology* 24, no. 6: 711–17.

New York City Department of Health and Mental Hygiene, Lead Poisoning Prevention Program. 2002. "Surveillance of Childhood Blood Lead Levels in New York City." Retrieved July 2002. http://www.ci.nyc.ny.us/html/doh/pdf/lead/toc-es.pdf.

*In the matter of New York City Coalition to End Lead Poisoning, Inc., et al. v. Peter Vallone et al.* 2003. 100 N.Y. 2d 337, 794 N.E. 2d 672, 763 N.Y.S. 2d 530.

*NYCCELP v. Koch.* 1989. No. 42780/85. Sup. Ct. N.Y. County.

Official Compilation of Codes, Rules and Regulations of the State of New York. 1993. *Lead Poisoning Prevention and Control*, title 10, chap. 2, subchap. G, part 67.

Rules of the City of New York (RCNY). 1960. *Lead Paint*, title 24, sec. 173.13.

———. 1993. *Safety Standards for Lead Based Paint Abatement*, title 24, sec. 173.14.

Schwartz, J. 1994. "Societal Benefits of Reducing Lead Exposure." *Environmental Research* 66, no. 1: 105–24.

U.S. Department of Health and Human Services. 2000. *Healthy People 2010: Understanding and Improving Health*. 2d ed. Washington, D.C.: U.S. Government Printing Office.

U.S. Department of Housing and Urban Development. 1999. "Requirements for Notification, Evaluation and Reduction of Lead-Based Paint Hazards in Federally Owned Residential Property and Housing Receiving Federal Assistance; Final Rule." *Federal Register* 64, no. 178: 50139.

Wasserman, J. 2003. "18 Landlords Duck City on Lead Poison." *New York Daily News*, June 12.

# The Arts and the Internet as Tools for Community Building

## *Part VII*    and Organizing

DURING THE PAST two decades, many innovative tools and approaches have enriched community building and organizing; some were discussed in previous chapters, while others appear in the appendix (for example, user-friendly geographic information systems and community indicator development). In part 7, we focus on two approaches with particular potency for community building and organizing, especially as ways to reach new populations with our work.

The Internet has profoundly transformed many aspects of our lives. It is also transforming the ways in which we define and build communities and engage in grassroots organizing for health and social change (Hick and McNutt 2002). In chapter 18, Sonja Herbert takes a lively look at Internet support for advocacy and community organizing. Using web sites such as Environmental Scorecard, the Community Toolbox, Advocates for Youth, moveon.org, and compaspoint, she discusses Internet access to information, showing that the web provides tools for organizing and political action, helps disenfranchised groups grow new communities, and offers important resources for sustainability. But Herbert is also careful to provide "hazard signs" throughout the chapter, reminding us of the Internet's limitations in various organizing contexts and stages and raising concerns about the digital divide that continues to limit web access in many communities.

If the Internet is one of our newest tools for advocacy and community building and organizing, the arts are among the oldest. Yet texts on community organizing tend to overlook their impressive track record in building community and promoting social change. In chapter 19, Marian McDonald, Jennifer Sarché, and Caroline C. Wang consider the arts as a vehicle for social change, their import in social movements nationally and internationally, and theoretical bases for using the arts to stimulate community organizing and community building. The arts can promote organizing for health in a wide and interrelated variety of ways—

getting people involved, facilitating assessment, promoting healing and community building, and offering culturally competent approaches to addressing health disparities. Using case studies such as the NAMES Project AIDS memorial quilt, a Latino youth arts project in greater New Orleans (McDonald et al. 1998–99), and the Clothesline Project to promote awareness of violence against women, McDonald and her colleagues vividly illustrate the power of art in community health organizing. The chapter then turns to photovoice, a process in which groups are given inexpensive cameras and trained to use them to capture and reflect on strengths and concerns in their lives and communities. Subsequently, the photos become a basis for critical dialogue and action (Wang 1999). Of particular interest is the use of photovoice to reach policymakers. Although many diverse photovoice projects have illustrated the potential of this approach with groups of youth, rural Chinese women, and the homeless (http://www.photovoice.org, Wang 1999), the chapter highlights one in particular—the Flint Photovoice Project in Michigan—to demonstrate the potential of this technique from a policy advocacy perspective. The chapter concludes by arguing that the particular strengths of the arts should not be overlooked in today's challenging climate for organizing.

### References

Hick, S. F., and J. G. McNutt. 2002. *Advocacy, Activism, and the Internet: Community Organization and Social Policy.* Chicago: Lyceum.

McDonald, M., G. Antunez, and M. Gottemoeller. 1998–99. "Using the Arts and Literature in Health Education." *International Quarterly of Community Health Education* 18, no. 3: 269–82.

Wang, C. C. 1999. "Photovoice: A Participatory Action Research Strategy Applied to Women's Health." *Journal of Women's Health* 8, no. 2: 185–92.

# Chapter 18

# Harnessing the Power of the Internet for Advocacy and Organizing

I FIRST GLIMPSED how the Internet could advance community organizing in 1994, when I participated in planning sessions for the United Nations' International Conference on Population and Development. Using e-mail, advocates around the world could draft a common agenda (or at least complementary national agendas) before the international conference began. Many arrived in Cairo as trusted colleagues dedicated to solving remaining differences and lobbying governments to adopt the agreement. Women's rights advocates felt that a new international solidarity movement had begun. We quickly put the e-mail network into action again for the United Nations' Fourth World Conference on Women. These conferences convinced me that the Internet could strengthen advocacy efforts by allowing collaboration across geographic and time-zone barriers.

This chapter explores how social change movements continue to harness the advocacy potential of the Internet. Particularly, the international peace movement shows how our methods have matured beyond circulating clunky petitions, which may never reach their target or have the desired effect. My scope includes both advocacy efforts taking place entirely on line in virtual communities as well as organizing efforts that occur primarily off line. Following theories of community organizing, I address how the Internet improves access to key assessment information, supports community building, and an provides innovative means for political action and community organizing (Hick and McNutt 2002, McCaughey and Ayers 2003). Web site addresses accompany my points, for it is worth the risk of outdated links to provide concrete examples. Finally, despite my belief in the potency of the Internet for social change, I post a few caution signs. As advocates, we need to remember that access to a powerful new tool doesn't make it the right tool for every community, every target, or every stage of our organizing efforts.

## Increasing Access to Assessment Information

In my workshops for public health students, I stress that the Internet has affected community organizing primarily by expanding access to information. Their eyes roll. As experienced web users, they tend to assume that they will have open access to more information than they can deal with; thus, the Internet doesn't seem strategically or politically crucial to community organizing. They are won over, however, after we discuss cases in which the struggle for information *is* the political action. These include the electoral fight on whether California can collect data by race and ethnicity and the Bush administration's decision to strip comprehensive sexuality education information from federal health web sites. Even if information doesn't seem political, getting the right piece at the right time to the right people can be politically crucial.

Our advocacy goals determine what information is strategically important at the moment, but finding that information on the Internet can feel like bargain basement shopping: we slog through piles of junk, hoping to uncover a diamond in the rough. The key is to apply the rules of grocery shopping: never go in without a list, resist buying what you already have, and avoid flashy products with little value. My mother would add that it helps to shop at the same trusted stores regularly because knowing what they carry and how they organize it can save a great deal of time. Each section in this chapter highlights one type of information that advocates often shop for, including research on public health issues, our communities, the political environment, and media coverage.

### ASSESSING PUBLIC HEALTH ISSUES

The Internet provides unprecedented access to published research, such as medical studies and public health data. By conducting literature searches through Medline (http://medline.cos.com) or subscribing to online journal reviews, public health advocates can quickly get the latest information on scientific controversies. We can also find health and demographic data on line from local, state, and federal public health departments. The federal government's new web site on federal statistics (http://www.fedstats.gov), for example, allows advocates to determine which federal agency can best answer each type of data question. We can use the site to search the Department of Interior's web site for census data on Alabama (population breakdowns by age, ethnicity, income, educational levels, and so on) and then link to the Department of Health and Human Services' site to get corresponding public health data by issue or population. Easier access to public health information allows advocates to build stronger arguments for the need to address a particular problem or for tailoring an intervention to different populations. Further, by using online geographic mapping programs, advocates can turn raw data into a graphically vivid community overview, which can be influential at public meetings (see appendix 6). Box 18.1 illustrates one effective way of setting up a web site.

---

Box 18.1

## Environmental Defense Network
(http://www.scorecard.org)

Many activists use their web sites as issue education tools, but few take full advantage of web design and data base technology. The Environmental Defense Network's scorecard web site is an exception. By providing searchable access to many federal and state data sets, the site allows advocates to quickly research the environmental dangers in their area. In particular, advocates can search for information in the following ways:

- By geographic location
- By environmental issue (air pollutants, animal waste, toxic releases from industrial facilities, and so on)
- By health effect—for instance, by substances widely recognized or suspected to cause cancer
- By pollution source, providing information about industrial facilities such as what chemicals they use, what levels of emissions they are allowed, and their history of regulatory compliance
- By chemicals regulated under major environmental laws, including information on how and why the chemical is used in manufacturing and a list of product brand names including that hazardous chemical
- By regulatory control, indicating not only which government agency has authority over each issue or substance but by which law or regulation

Advocates can easily combine data to construct a complex environmental picture. For instance, after reviewing what chemicals the nearby polluters are emitting, advocates can link to the health effects of these substances and find the regulatory controls, which should limit exposure. Such content-rich and technologically advanced web sites make "community right to know" laws more powerful because the community has an accessible way to find out. Now advocates can spend limited resources building strong campaigns for change. Scorecard.org supports this goal by providing opportunities for advocates in the same geographic region or working on the same issue to find each other, linking to resources such as the web sites of environmental justice groups, and allowing advocates to send faxes to the most serious polluters in their area.

---

## ASSESSING OUR COMMUNITIES

Collecting official data is only one part of a full community assessment, which may include techniques reviewed elsewhere in this book such as asset mapping (chapter 9) and photovoice (chapter 19). The Internet can support these primarily off-line assessment methods by directing advocates to web sites such as http://www. photovoice.com/ for compelling case studies. The Internet also allows advocates to disseminate assessment results widely, including community photos whose duplication would otherwise be extremely expensive.

Certain assessment techniques, such as key informant interviews, can be conducted by e-mail. Internet-specific assessment methods, such as chat room discussions, topical bulletin boards, and straw polls to prioritize issues, are also useful but do not necessarily gather the same information as traditional community meetings or door-knocking surveys do. Online conversations often miss the subtleties of tone or body language that indicate when a community assessment or agenda setting process is missing the mark. Finally, as a result of the digital divide discussed later in this chapter, online conversations may be closed to key members of our communities. Therefore, unless our advocacy community and actions are entirely on line, we need to make sure that the Internet isn't the only source of information we use to set our advocacy agendas.

## ASSESSING THE POLITICAL CONTEXT

Once we identify the most pressing issues in the community, we craft ideal solutions and strategic advocacy approaches. Other chapters and appendixes discuss the wide range of processes to reach these ends, so I will simply highlight how the Internet can help us take four steps common to many community organizing campaigns: movement research, opposition research, policy research, and media research. I titled this section "Assessing the Political Context" because even when our solutions seem to be straightforward public health interventions, we present them in a political context and thus must be ready to advocate on their behalf. Working on reproductive health and sexuality education taught me there are very few uncontested public health programs, even if the battles are simply about securing funds to implement a shared idea.

## ASSESSING OUR ALLIES

Each year the National Women's Health Network (2003) establishes programmatic and policy priorities, reviewing what is most important to our constituency and discussing how each advocacy project may match our mission. As a small nonprofit, we ask ourselves whether we can make a unique contribution to advancing policy on a particular public health issue. Answering that question depends on assessing, for instance, what issues other breast cancer or reproductive rights advocacy groups are taking on this year. What activities would be redundant? With whom could we build a partnership to create a stronger, more unified political force? On whose toes might we step if we take a particular advocacy approach or position? We can answer some of these questions through our existing advocacy networks, but organizational web pages can also be extremely useful. We may find, for instance, that a state-based advocacy group has a solution for a women's health policy problem that could be applied nationally. Or we may not have to write talking points about a new contraceptive device if a trusted partner has posted those points earlier in the week.

### ASSESSING OUR OPPOSITION

Organizing legend Saul Alinksy (1972) frequently spoke of the need to "do your homework," which meant, among other things, learning as much as possible about your adversaries. While serving on the policy staff of the Sexuality Information and Education Council of the United States (SIECUS), I quickly learned the benefit of tracking our opponents' web sites (Daley and Herbert 1997). Before meeting them in legislative debates or on national news shows, we needed to know their current priorities, arguments, tactics, and core supporters. Our best offense frequently had to be a strong defense because they often highlighted our efforts for comprehensive sexuality education as a way of mobilizing their base or raising funds for their projects. Tracking the opposition's projects allowed us to prepare for future attacks. The Internet allows us to monitor our opposition undetected, which beats attending anti-choice or abstinence-only education events.

### ASSESSING THE NEWS COVERAGE

The news can be a powerful tool for influencing public health policy debates at the local, state, and federal levels (Themba 1999, Wallack et al. 1993). In chapter 23, Lawrence Wallack details the strategies of a media advocacy approach; so here I will simply touch on how the Internet can help advocates gain access to the news, including traditional and alternative news outlets.

Most advocates know a few news outlets in their community. Before the Internet, if we wanted to branch out to additional media or locate an appropriate reporter, we undertook a labor-intensive research process. This was particularly true if we were working on a national campaign or an issue in which policymakers outside our community held decision-making power. Although we could buy guides to the major news outlets, those guides are outdated quickly, and their cost makes them too expensive for most community groups or local libraries.

On the Internet, we can quickly find news outlets in our area by searching sites such as http://capitoladvantage.com. The major news outlets also have their own web sites that often allow advocates to search for current and past news stories by topic, reporter, and date. By reviewing this coverage, we can easily research whether our issue is on the public agenda, what perspectives have been overlooked, and which reporters might have an interest in a story.

Through e-mail, we can easily share the news coverage we find with other advocates. As part of my media advocacy work, I electronically search for news stories about child care and e-mail relevant links to hundreds of advocates each week. This gives them a heads-up on what issues policymakers or reporters might want to discuss. In contrast, before the Internet, I spent four hours every day clipping, photocopying, and faxing advocates the hard copies of articles related to reproductive rights. The Internet makes tracking the news more practical and timely. Not only can we more easily listen in on the public conversation surrounding our issues, but the Internet also makes it easier to join the debate. Many newspapers, for example, prefer readers to submit op-eds and letters to the editor electronically, which many advocates find easier than mailing a traditional letter. When submitting a letter, use a personal e-mail address because news editors are getting suspicious of letters e-mailed en masse from single web sites (Lee 2003).

In addition to making it easier to access the mainstream media, the Internet now makes it easier to find alternative news sources. During the war on Iraq, peace advocates used the Internet to follow international news coverage, which offered a dramatically different perspective. In fact, web sites such as http://www.alternet.org and http://www.indymedia.org are dedicated to collecting alternative perspectives on national and international events. The Internet even makes some alternative news venues possible, such as http://www.salon.com, or available to a much wider audience, such as http://www.youthradio.com. While the public affairs shows produced by youth are carried on some radio stations, the Internet allows their unique perspectives to be read or heard on line, dramatically broadening their potential audience and impact. Finally, many advocates expect that camera cell phones will allow advocates to report directly on protests and other organizing events as they happen. (For more information, see chapter 23 and the web site of Berkeley Media Studies Group, http://www.bmsg.org).

## CONDUCTING POLICY RESEARCH

Solving many public health problems requires policy change, often in legislative bodies (Milio 1998, Themba 1999). The Internet has made it much easier to track the status of legislation and regulations on both the state and federal levels. While making policy change still requires a great deal of community organizing and strategic pressure, organizations no longer need a lobbyist or a legislative tracking service just to find out which committee has taken what action on their bill. Instead, the U.S. Congress (http://thomas.loc.gov) and most state legislatures have official web sites that allow you to find your elected officials by typing in your zip code, research the legislative process, track legislation by topic or bill number, read the full text of each bill, and identify which subcommittees (and therefore elected officials) have jurisdiction over your issue. Activists can quickly discover which of several related bills best support their issues and, with a few keystrokes, urge key committee members to support a particular bill. A few innovative state legislative sites also provide advocates with e-mail updates if action is taken on particular legislation. Advocates can then track many more bills with fewer resources.

In addition to official legislative sites, many independent web sites monitor our legislative bodies. One such resource is Project Vote Smart (http://www.votesmart.org), which provides a comprehensive data base of elected officials, lists of key legislative votes by topic, and links to independently created voting records of elected officials by issue area. Finally, many community organizers will be targeting governmental bodies smaller than their legislature, such as their school board, public health department, or city council. In many communities, the Internet also provides access to the official calendars, meeting minutes, member positions, and actions of these policymaking bodies.

### APPLYING ASSESSMENTS TO OUR ADVOCACY AGENDA

We conduct public health, community, political, and media research to craft a well-informed advocacy agenda (Wallack et al. 1999). As discussed, the Internet provides valuable information on which to build our advocacy agendas. That said, I urge caution for four reasons. First, the Internet may not provide a full picture of our communities because all members of a community and all types of information are not on line. Second, people pass on information without determining its legitimacy. We should always check back with the supposed source or with web sites such as http://www.urbanlegends.com before forwarding e-mails. Third, the information may be accurate but shared before we have sufficiently considered a community-appropriate strategy. For instance, I received many e-mails requesting that I speak up on behalf of Amina Lawal, a Nigerian woman facing death by stoning for having sex outside of marriage. The facts were true, but the strategy was confusing. Some e-mails said that mass outside pressure was making the campaign more difficult for in-country organizers, while others said the pressure was turning the tide on her sentence. From thousands of miles away, I can't know if I was being an effective advocate. (For more information, see http://www.oprah.com/tows/pastshows/tows _2002/tows_past_20021004_b.jhtml.)

Finally, while circulating information is much easier via the Internet, circulation alone may not translate into community action. We still must combine our assessment information with sufficient community building and advocacy strategies to bring about successful public health changes.

## Community Building on the Internet

As noted in previous chapters, community building is a process of creating connections between people based on factors such as a shared neighborhood, membership in a group, demographic characteristics, common interests, and shared political concerns. The Internet clearly allows online communities to form and often strengthens offline communities.

My favorite virtual communities are the web sites where people play cribbage and the teen sections of the Advocates for Youth site (http://www.advocatesforyouth.org/). The cribbage sites stand out because a friend, who rarely left her house due to a serious disability, found a needed community there and in the process showed me how the Internet could bridge physical barriers. The Advocates for Youth site allows youth who share a common identity (ethnicity, sexuality, HIV status, advocacy interests, and so on) to support each other across boundaries of geography and anonymity. For instance, after incidents of high-profile violence on queer people, this web site receives thousands of hits, many from queer youth isolated in rural or conservative areas. For these youth, participating in a community that supports them is a political act.

The Internet also supports offline communities. Municipal web sites help residents navigate their neighborhood to find city services, religious communities, or social activities. Many social and political communities have replaced phone trees and newsletters with e-mail to announce activities, whether potlucks or protests. But making announcements and decisions off line remains crucial because not all community members can or choose to participate on line. Advocates who are on line can find and then share wonderful resources for their community building and community organizing efforts, such as the Community Tool Box. Developed by the Work Group for Community Health and Development at the University of Kansas, the Community Tool Box (CTB) (http://ctb.ku.edu/wg/) is one of the most comprehensive community building tools on the Internet. Established in 1995 and currently more than 6,000 pages long, it "promote[s] community health and development by connecting people, ideas and resources" (Fawcett et al. 2003, 167; see box 18.2).

As discussed in chapter 22, community building is typically an important precursor to effective community organizing efforts (see also Walsh 1997). When the Internet is discussed as an organizing vehicle, many advocates express concern that the community ties built on line are not sensitive or strong enough to motivate sustained political action. They may use the Internet for quick announcements but prefer to hold spaghetti dinners or kitchen table discussions to decide political strategy. Online advocates argue that some individuals may not require a deep sense of unity to take action and prefer to invest their advocacy time when their personal schedule permits. Personally, the time

*Box 18.2*
**Community Tool Box**
(http://ctb.ku.edu/)

This web site is a valuable stop for anyone interested in building community capacity or developing community organizing campaigns. Advocates no longer need bookshelves full of how-to manuals. Instead, on this site we can quickly find the tools that match our current needs. The designers' philosophy is to support advocates in developing sixteen core competencies, which provide the skeletal structure for the site:

Creating and maintaining coalitions
Assessing community needs and resources
Analyzing community-identified problems and goals
Developing a framework or model for change
Developing strategic and action plans
Building leadership
Developing an intervention
Increasing participation and membership
Enhancing cultural competency
Advocating for change
Influencing policy development
Evaluating the initiative
Implementing a social marketing effort
Writing a grant application for funding
Improving organizational management and development
Sustaining the work or initiative

In each section, advocates are offered how-to advice, case examples, and practical tools. The web site is easy to navigate, with searchable categories such as the following: learn a skill, plan the work (tool kits), solve a problem (a troubleshooting guide), and connect with others. This last option allows advocates to connect with others facing similar issues in community forums or to ask an advisor for guidance by e-mail. This site receives high marks because it is clearly designed and staffed by seasoned, community-focused professionals.

For more on the philosophy behind the Community Tool Box, see S. J. Fawcett et al., 2003, "Using Internet-Based Tools to Build Capacity for Community-Based Participatory Research and Other Efforts to Promote Health and Development," in *Community-Based Participatory Research for Health*, edited by M. Minkler and N. Wallerstein (San Francisco: Jossey-Bass), 155–78.

I am willing to put into an action on line is increased when I build a connection with other advocates, usually in person. For example, during annual meetings of the American Public Health Association, I attend the sessions of the progressive 1848 caucus to feel part of an activist community within the larger public health profession. This sense of connection makes me more likely to respond when called to action on the community list serve (Spirit of 1848 @yahoogroups.com). When deciding whether to invest in community building as part of our advocacy efforts, we must ask ourselves what combination of methods will work best for our community of advocates, our issue, our goals, and our political targets.

## The Internet and Political Action

*Internet activism methods work very well, until they don't work at all.*

An advocate I admire put succinctly what I feel as an activist on line. Our methods will remain effective only if used judiciously and strategically. Highlighted in this section are core Internet methods, with tips on employing them carefully. Moveon.org is discussed because it effectively and innovatively uses the Internet to support online and offline advocacy. In addition, the site http://www.netaction.org offers an extremely helpful virtual activist training tool, which covers every step, from setting up a Bcc (list-suppressed) list serve to establishing sufficient cybersecurity. Not covered here is hacktivism, the process of shutting down your opponents' web sites as a political strategy. (See Vegh 2003 for a case study of how Seattle protestors used hacktivism.)

### ONLINE COLLABORATIONS

E-mail remains the most popular online tool because advocates collaborate in smaller or more confidential groups to develop advocacy materials or campaign strategies. Threatened human rights activists, for instance, use e-mail to send urgent action requests to Amnesty International under the radar of government censors (Albert 2003).

### ACTIVIST LIST SERVES

On e-mail list serves, timely information can be cheaply and easily sent to a targeted audience. Overwhelmed advocates are unlikely to act, however, so send succinct alerts only when the update or action is of clear strategic importance. If your list is unmoderated and allows everyone to post messages, offer a digest version so members can scan daily summaries. Use subject lines carefully, date and sign everything, and link to your web site as a place to learn more or take direct action.

## CAMPAIGN WEB SITES

Organizational web sites become action centers with careful planning. Establish a take-action section, which briefly describes campaign goals, provides links to background information, and offers concrete steps for or direct links to taking action. Write and design materials specifically for a web format. Invest in searchable navigation systems. Collect e-mail addresses of supporters and allow them to donate on line to build the strength of your movement. Finally, alert advocates when a campaign goal, strategy, or target has changed. The Internet allows us to be quicker at launching, changing, and ending our campaigns. For instance, before the Internet it could take years before advocates learned that a particular boycott was over. Now we can just check CO-OP America's Boycott Action News (http://boycotts.org/).

---

*Box 18.3*

### Moveon.org

Established in 1998, Moveon.org has grown to include more than 1 million advocates worldwide, largely due to the organization's vigorous stand for peace (Packer 2003). With only four staff members, the web site defines the cutting edge of online advocacy, constantly inventing new ways to leverage the power of the Internet and its broad membership.

The backbone of the work is asking members to contact political targets by e-mail, phone, or fax or in person. More creatively, staff members have launched a virtual march to send antiwar messages to the U.S. Congress, an online democratic primary, and a process for advocates to suggest and prioritize possible future issues (Boyd 2003, Tierney 2003). They strategically offer advocates many levels on which to take action, from sending a simple e-mail or attending a speak-out to coordinating a candlelight peace vigil or signing up for in-person legislative visits. Moveon.org was perhaps most visible at the peace protests against the wars in Afghanistan and Iraq, when hundreds of thousands of activists downloaded protest placards.

The core strength of Moveon.org is that its staff members carefully assess each political goal and context to develop the appropriate strategy, whether an online campaign or an offline protest. Organizer Eli Pariser told the *New York Times* that "we've changed the way we do organizing—to move past emailing and phone calls and get people back out on the streets—and [we] use the Internet as a backbone for catalyzing that" (Packer 2003). Moveon.org has clearly heard the call from political theorists that sometimes social change requires us to put our bodies on the line, whether sitting in at lunch counters or escorting women into abortion clinics; and it is not possible to put our bodies on the line, online (McCaughey and Ayers 2003).

### DIRECT LINKS TO POLICYMAKERS

Many activist web sites are now offering direct links to policymakers, providing an online template letter that can be altered to fit your perspective. Gone are the letter writing tables outside our supermarkets or community meetings. Advocates wonder if e-mailed letters are as effective as postal mail or faxes. This depends on our targets. Some legislators, for example, log e-mail into the same computer system used to track other issue mail. Other policymakers see mass e-mail campaigns as spam. Learn what each target responds to and design your strategies accordingly. To get the attention of elected officials, you must identify yourself as a voting constituent. Examples of targeted letter writing campaigns can be seen at http://www.workingforchange.com/activism/index. One benefit of online submissions is that the sponsoring organization can track how many e-mails or faxes were sent to policymakers and which activists participated. Moveon.org provides an excellent example, regularly tracking the work of its million-plus members.

## Expanding and Sustaining Advocacy Efforts: Closing the Digital Divide

Successful advocacy efforts always keep an eye on the future. What battles will we face? Who must we involve? And how can we secure the resources to win? Two resources are always key: the participation of core community members and the financial resources to support our advocacy strategies. The more difficult challenge for social justice advocates today, however, is ensuring that all members of our communities participate in agenda setting and advocacy goals. Chapters 16 and 17 discuss building community coalitions as one important means of bringing diverse parts of the community together around shared issues or concerns. As I've already discussed, the Internet makes it easier for many advocates to participate politically; but if digital divides exist, work conducted primarily on line can block the participation of other community members (see chapter 6). As L. A. Kauffman, an organizer with United for Peace and Justice, says, "when we're online . . . a whole lot of people are not in the room" (Boyd 2003).

The term *digital divide* highlights the fact that many, primarily low-income, communities do not have access to computer technology or training. Digital divides are also created by generational gaps, educational gaps, English-language abilities, geographic location, mental and physical disabilities, and traditional socioeconomic barriers that keep some communities under-resourced. As social justice advocates, we must address digital divides to ensure equal participation in our movements. Such divides are issues in their own right, for they create new power differentials in our society. Until digital divides are erased, we must make sure the Internet is not our only method of conducting research, building community, sending alerts, setting our agenda, receiving feedback, or taking political action. Each of these core elements of community organizing and advocacy is too important to be left to a single modus operandi—even one as powerful as the Internet—if we are to ensure the broadest possible base of participants.

*Digital Divide Network* (http://www.digitaldividenetwork.org)
> This site provides an overview of digital divide issues and the movement to build bridges across them. You can also search for programs by zip code.

*Community Technology Centers Network* (http://www.ctcnet.org)
> This site lists community technology centers (CTCs) by region. CTCs stress that computer hardware or free Internet access at your local library alone don't erase digital divides. The CTCs focus on skills-building programs and community infrastructure development.

*Tech Soup* (http://www.techsoup.org)
> This site provides tips for technology planning, lists of where to donate or acquire computers, and links to web sites that can test your organizational site to see if it is accessible to disabled users.

## Sustainability Resources

Solving most public health problems will take years, and fortunately the Internet offers resources to sustain our efforts and organizations. My favorite organizational development web site is the Nonprofit Genie (http://www.genie.org), which offers tips on board development, interviewing consultants, choosing data base or financial software, volunteer management, and technology planning. Innovative ideas, of course, only go so far without financial resources. The Internet also offers avenues for increasing your organization's financial health:

- *Direct web site contributions.* Web sites can offer your organization increased visibility to attract donors while also serving as portals for donations, receiving them either directly or by linking to, for example, http://www.giveforchange.com.

- *Soliciting your supporters.* Many advocates now use their e-mail lists to request donations. As with house parties, direct mail, and telemarketing, successful pitches stress how donations will directly support advocacy goals. Moveon.org raised $200,000 in just two hours for Walter Mondale's last-minute bid to replace deceased Senator Paul Wellstone on the Minnesota ballot (Packer 2003).

- *Foundation prospecting.* Advocates now have access to the Foundation Center's library at http://www.fdncenter.org. This site includes many recent requests for proposals and subscription data bases of grant opportunities. Additionally, many foundations, private companies, and government agencies have web sites specifying their areas of interest and application guidelines.

## Conclusion

The Internet offers advocates a powerful tool for conducting agenda-setting research, building and supporting communities, and taking direct political action. Online resources can support both online and offline advocacy efforts. Online advocacy methods themselves can be combined with traditional assessment and organizing methods to ensure that all community members can participate. Finally, while online advocacy methods are innovative, we do well to respect four tenets of traditional community organizing. First, discussing the problem is not the same as working toward a solution. Politically minded people fill electronic bulletin boards with their frustrations but would do better to apply the motto of the Washington, D.C., Rape Crisis Center: "Turn your anger into change" (http://www.dcrcc.org/).

Second, urging people to take action isn't the same as supporting or empowering them to do this successfully. For instance, e-mailing advocates media talking points can't take the place of training them to discuss the issue confidently.

Third, it is always worth the time to develop a strategic advocacy plan. The Internet makes it quick, easy, and cheap to take action. But being effective isn't about volume; rather, it is about strategy. Finally, most social justice campaigns are long, so we must invest in building a movement of advocates, not just a large number of people who take action once. My favorite neighborhood diner has a sign posted, which applies here: "It is better to serve 1 customer 1,000 times, than 1,000 customers once." That said, the biggest strength of the Internet for social change is that we can enlist supporters who may never have participated in more time-consuming advocacy efforts. Our challenge is to leverage this broader membership and our new online methods successfully while not losing the strengths of offline community participation and traditional community organizing methods.

### References

Alinsky, S. D. 1972. *Rules for Radicals*. New York: Vintage.
Boyd, A. 2003. "The Web Wires the Movement." *Nation*, July 25.
Daley, D., and S. Herbert. 1997. "On-Line Activism: From Easy Education to Political Potency." *SIECUS Report* 25, no. 6: 27–33.
Fawcett, S., J. Schultz, V. Carson, V. Renault, and V. Francisco. 2003. "Using Internet Based Tools to Build Capacity for Community Based Participatory Research and Other Efforts to Promote Health and Development." In *Community Based Participatory Research for Health*, edited by M. Minkler and N. Wallerstein, 155–78. San Francisco: Jossey-Bass.

Hick, S. F., and J. G. McNutt. 2002. *Advocacy, Activism and the Internet: Community Organization and Social Policy.* Chicago: Lyceum.

Lebert, J. 2003. "Wiring Human Rights Activism: Amnesty International and the Challenges of Information and Communications Technologies." In *Cyberactivism: Online Activism in Theory and Practice,* edited by M. McCaughey, and M. Ayers, 209–231. New York: Routledge.

Lee, J. 2003. "Editors and Lobbyists Wage High-Tech War over Letters." *New York Times,* January 27, p. C10.

McCaughey, M., and M. Ayers, eds. 2003. Introduction. *Cyberactivism: Online Activism in Theory and Practice,* 1–24. New York: Routledge.

Milio, N. 1998. "Priorities and Strategies for Promoting Community-Based Prevention Policies." *Journal of Public Health Management Practice* 4, no. 3: 14–28.

National Women's Health Network. 2003. http://www.womenshealthnetwork.org.

Packer, G. 2003. "Smart-Mobbing the War." *New York Times,* March 9, sec. 6, p. 46.

Themba, M. N. 1999. *Making Policy, Making Change: How Communities Are Taking Law into Their Own Hands.* San Francisco: Jossey-Bass.

Tierney, J. 2003. "An Antiwar Demonstration That Does Not Take to the Streets." *New York Times,* February 26.

Vegh, S. 2003. "Classifying Forms of Online Activism: The Case of Cyberprotests against the World Bank." In *Cyberactivism: Online Activism in Theory and Practice,* edited by M. McCaughey and M. Ayers, 71–95. New York: Routledge.

Wallack, L., L. Dorfman, D. Jernigan, and M. Themba. 1993. *Media Advocacy and Public Health: Power for Prevention.* Newbury Park, Calif.: Sage.

Wallack, L., K. Woodruff, L. Dorfman, and I. Diaz. 1999. *News for a Change: An Advocate's Guide to Working with the Media.* Thousand Oaks, Calif.: Sage.

Walsh, J. 1997. *Stories of Renewal: Community Building and the Future of Urban America.* New York: Rockefeller Foundation.

MARIAN McDONALD
JENNIFER SARCHÉ
CAROLINE C. WANG

# Chapter 19

# Using the Arts in Community Organizing and Community Building

COMMUNITY ORGANIZING allows people who share a particular geographic space or identity to find shared issues and goals as well as resources they can use collectively to achieve those goals (see chapter 1). Literature, music, video, painting, photography, and other forms of artistic expression are powerful tools for community organizing in health and related areas (McDonald et al. 1998, Chavez et al. in press). They can draw attention to an issue, offer catharsis for a community after a crisis, pull communities together to create art, and communicate across cultural and language barriers. As Vivian Chavez and her colleagues (in press) note, "The cultural diversity, personal sensitivity, and passion that characterize some of the arts resonate with some key principles and commitments of health promotion." They also foster a high level of community participation (Freudenberg et al. 1995, Wallerstein 1999) and emphasize humor and fun as important components of our practice (Minkler 1994).

In this chapter, we consider diverse case studies involving the arts, including the AIDS memorial quilt and a Latino community's exploration of how the arts can foster community organizing for health. We also examine photovoice (Wang and Burris 1994; Wang 1999, 2003), which helps people "identify, represent, and enhance their community through a specific photographic technique" (Wang and Burris 1997, 369), and illustrate how communities can reach policymakers using this participatory approach to action research.

The arts and literature are also essential to various forms of education and have had great value in clinical practice and healing (Smith 1995). Although a review of such applications is beyond the scope of this chapter, a number of researchers discuss these topics in other publications (see McDonald et al. 1998, Winkler 1993, Kaplan 2000).

## Community Organizing for Change and the Arts as a Vehicle

Any group of people that identifies itself as a community and sets out to create collective change is engaged in community organizing. The variety of communities and goals requires diverse tools and methodologies, ranging from door-to-door canvassing and attending city council meetings to staging public protests or conducting mass-media campaigns. Groups decide on organizing strategies by looking critically at their target: they decide who is in a position to make the desired change, identify available resources, and decide how best to effect the changes they seek (see chapters 10 and 11). In each case study in this chapter, community groups chose the arts as their approach to accomplishing their goals.

Artistic expression has been universal to human culture throughout history (Clardy 2000). Artistic imagery taps into our visceral forms of knowing and reacting to the world and so carries a great deal of meaning (Riley 2001). The act of creating increases feelings of well-being and can facilitate feelings of belonging. Furthermore, the creation of art does not depend on language or education level but can be accomplished by anyone with will and desire (Kaplan 2000). The power of art for community organizing, then, lies in the power of the arts to communicate a message and elicit an emotional response as well as in the creation of art itself. As Lucy Lippard (2000) notes, the arts can "be redemptive and restorative, critical and empowering."

The arts have always played a role in community organizing and social change, although they are often seen as incidental or secondary, with little intrinsic social value. Poet and activist Audre Lorde (1984) challenged this view in her essay on the importance of poetry in people's lives, especially the lives of women: "For women . . . poetry is not a luxury. It is a vital necessity of our existence. It forms the quality of the light within which we predicate our hopes and dreams toward survival and change, first made into language, then into idea, then into more tangible action" (37). Lorde sees poetry and other forms of creativity and expression as necessary precursors to action. She shares this view with many artists, educators, and advocates throughout history and across the globe. They include African American jazz singer Billie Holiday, whose insistence on singing a song about southern lynchings shocked audiences; Chilean songwriter Victor Jara, who sang against the murderers in Chile's 1973 coup d'état; and Maya Ying Lin, Chinese American architect whose design for the Vietnam War Memorial helped to create the conditions for national healing.

## Legacy of the Arts in Social Movements

In the United States, the arts have played an important role in social movements. Woody Guthrie's melodic tributes to the working people ("This Land Is Your Land")

and biting criticisms of injustice ("Deportees") won him audiences in the strife-torn forties and a permanent place in U.S. culture (Guthrie 1958). Legendary African American actor and singer Paul Robeson resisted bigotry and repression with his masterful performances in the fifties, helping set the stage for the civil rights movement. The forceful refrain of the gospel–turned–civil rights song "We Shall Overcome" became an anthem of the fight against segregation and for civil rights and later was embraced by the labor, peace, and women's movements. "We Shall Overcome" was sung at rallies and in churches, on marches and in vigils. The song's power and longevity comes from its collective affirmation of determination, hope, and courage.

Although this book focuses on the United States, the nation's increasing diversity, combined with organizing successes in other countries, makes it important to look beyond our borders for lessons. In countries where democratic forces have challenged domination and foreign interference, the battle for control over cultural expression has been key. In Nicaragua, victory over dictator Anastasio Somoza helped put in place new and popular forms of expression, from a grassroots literacy campaign to a new song movement and the flourishing of murals and poetry workshops (Kunzle 1995, Black 1981, Cardenal 1982, Randall 1984). With the change of government in 1990 and a determined rollback of Sandinista influence, one of the first tactics of Managua's conservative mayor Arnoldo Aleman was to paint over some of the city's most impressive pro-Sandinista murals.

## Using the Arts and Literature in Organizing for Community Health

The arts have historically been deeply rooted in change processes, providing a rich tradition for those involved in health-related change. It is against this backdrop that the use of the arts in organizing around health can be understood. Health education theory and methodology offer invaluable insight into involving community members in organizing and advocating for better health in their communities. The constantly changing field of health education is seeking new and more effective ways to address the increasingly complex challenges of promoting and organizing for health (Clark and McLeroy 1995). Thus, it is necessary to consider the potential of the arts for advancing health education and therefore organizing for health.

## Theoretical Bases

To be effective, community organizing for health needs to begin with people's reality. Central to that reality is culture, which embodies people's history and aspirations (Ordones and Vanolli 1995). As Amilcar Cabral (1979), an African leader who fought for the independence of Guinea-Bissau, has noted:

Culture is the dynamic synthesis, at the level of individual or community consciousness, of the material and spiritual historical reality of a society or a human group, of the relations existing between [people] and nature as well as among social classes or sectors. Cultural manifestations are the various forms in which this synthesis is expressed, individually, or collectively, at each stage in the evolution of the society or group. (210)

More recently, the international women's movement has demonstrated, through a wide array of art and literature, the indispensable role of culture in the development of consciousness and identity (Randall 1991, Cheney et al. 1976, Rich 1993, Chicago 1985, hooks 1994, Whitehead 1996). Specifically, the development of voice has been advanced as a key element of the process of transforming women's lives (Randall 1991, Olsen 1978, Mairs 1994, Rukeyser 1996).

The creation of a voice to break the silence is central in the work of the late Brazilian adult educator Paulo Freire, whose writings have transformed our view of education and popular culture (Freire 1970, 1990a, 1990b; Boal 1972, 1979; see also chapters 2 and 12). Freire's philosophy and practice stem from the belief that change in human communities involves an interactive process between individuals and society: awareness begins in a person's own thinking and develops from that person's reflected-upon experience in a collective context. Of particular concern to Freire was education for critical consciousness, through which people who have been alienated from their culture are encouraged to identify, examine, and act on the root causes of their oppression. The Freirian notion of conscientization always involves group rather than individual transformation or consciousness raising. Initially developed as a literacy method for Brazilian peasants, his approach involved "teaching people to read, while at the same time teaching them to read the political and social situation in which they lived" so that they could then help transform it (Carroll and Minkler 2000). The use of pictures and other visual symbols to capture the themes generated in this process is central to the methodology (see chapter 12 and appendix 7).

A valuable guide for health education and community organizing, Freire's concept of empowerment rooted in critical consciousness and developed through practice has been applied in health education and community organizing projects around the globe (Minkler and Cox 1980; Wallerstein and Bernstein 1988; Wallerstein and Weinger 1992; Horton and Freire 1990; Werner and Bower 1982; Wang and Burris 1994; Laver et al. 1996–97, 1998; see also chapters 2 and 12).

The theoretical and practical legacy of feminism also provides numerous conceptual bases for using the arts in community health organizing. Feminism's tenets of the personal as political, the importance of relationships and process, and the embracing of diversity encourage creative and collective expression (Richardson and Taylor 1993, Rosen 2000, Ruiz and DuBois 1994).

Other theoretical and conceptual frameworks and approaches in health promotion draw on the use of arts and literature as well. The Health Belief Model, for example, posits that the individual's perceptions of a health issue is key to whether and how that person will act (Rosenstock 1990). One of the ways in which the arts affect society is related to its ability to open eyes anew, to change perceptions. Social learning theory offers another theoretical framework that underscores the utility of the arts and literature as educational and organizing tools. Social learning theory links an individual's likelihood of change to the person's belief in her or his ability to change (Perry et al. 1990). The arts affect self-efficacy in two ways. First, a positive identity of self and community expressed and reinforced through culture can give communities and individuals strength. For example, the sixties slogan "black is beautiful" reflected and reinforced pride and emerging power in the African American community. Second, the individual and personal process of creation can be empowering, opening up new vistas of self-confidence (Mairs 1994, Rukeyser 1996, Wang and Burris 1994).

The arts also promote health by developing and expanding social support. While the arts are often solitary activities in the creation stage, the act of sharing them is social and collective. By creating common reference points through culture, communities begin to break down isolation, share their common experience, and build collective vision. This community building process often is a critical precursor to community organizing (see chapters 4 and 6).

## The Arts in Urban Life

The arts play a particularly important role in urban health organizing. The physical environment of cities provides unique public places where people can express themselves—sidewalks, buildings, subways, and parks. Additionally, the population density of cities brings people into contact constantly, creating endless opportunities for common experiences and communication. For many people living in the city, popular culture is their only exposure to art forms.

A number of forms of art and literature have been used in cities to give voice to communities. They include community murals, guerilla theater, poetry slams, dance brigades, participatory video, and even graffiti (Boal 1979, Barnett 1984, Chavez et al. in press). The forms used are as diverse as communities themselves.

Today, diversity of culture, language, and ethnicity is common in most major urban areas. The arts can give voice to the heterogeneity of urban populations, breaking down barriers in the process. Ethnic, racial, and linguistic diversity exists in urban areas, alongside diversity of age, gender, economic status, and sexual orientation and identity. When organizing for urban community health, health professionals and activists need to address diversity directly rather than ignore or downplay it (Airhihenbuwa 1994). The arts can be effectively used to express and respect diversity in a process that can weave unity among the community's different threads.

## The Arts in the Practice of Community Organizing for Health

Health education leader Dorothy Nyswander's (1956) admonition to "start where the people are" suggests that organizers need to familiarize themselves with a people's cultural expressions as part of working with the community. As Freire asks, "How is it possible for us to work in a community without feeling the spirit of the culture that has been there for many years, without trying to understand the soul of the culture?" (Horton and Freire 1990, 131).

In the community, the arts can promote organizing for health in the following ways, often simultaneously:

1. *Get people involved.* Art forms and activities involve people who might otherwise be disinterested or intimidated by more explicitly health-oriented or community organizing activities. Simply put, the arts make getting involved fun. For example, rap contests have been conducted in the San Francisco Bay Area AIDS movement to involve youth in building AIDS awareness. Similarly, the New Orleans Children's Advocacy Program sponsored a poster contest for school-aged youth focused on violence prevention, adding children's poignant voices to the city's fight against crime ("Children Put Peace to Paper in Contest" 1996).

2. *Find out about a community.* The arts can be a valuable strategy for conducting community needs assessments and mapping community assets (Kretzmann and McKnight, 1993; see also chapter 9). Poetry and art workshops, offered to the community at low or no cost, can provide valuable insights into the community, its leaders, and its history.

3. *Change awareness and relay health education messages.* The arts are powerful messengers. Because they tap into people's feelings, they have the potential to shape consciousness. Furthermore, visual and oral representations are easy to grasp, regardless of educational background and training (Tolley and Bentley 1996). Positive messages can be developed and promoted in popular culture. An example is a 1990s song that gained air time in Spanish-speaking communities throughout the Americas, "Ponte El Sombrero" (put on your hat), which encourages condom use in a playful, nonthreatening way. This approach is sometimes referred to as *edu-tainment* or *enter-education* (Steckler et al. 1995). It relays the message through an already-established medium of popular and commercial culture, such as a television show, a film, or a song. Examples are the HIV-positive member of the cast on MTV's *Real World* or films such as *Erin Brockovich,* which

was based on the true story of a community with abnormally high cancer rates and its successful fight against toxic polluters.

While potentially very effective, the approach can be challenging for a number of reasons. First, communities typically don't have access to screenwriters, songwriters, and producers and hence have little control over the messages portrayed or solutions proposed. Although new approaches such as media advocacy (see chapter 23) are helping communities become far more savvy in using the media to highlight their concerns and issues, access remains a significant barrier. Second, edu-tainment overwhelmingly relies on commercial culture in which the recipient of the message is by design a detached listener or observer as opposed to an active agent. And because these vehicles are external to community, they can sometimes encourage a passive, consumer approach rather than empowerment.

4. *Attract attention to an issue.* A cultural manifestation of an issue will often catch people's attention, changing their perceptions, as in the AIDS quilt and the Clothesline Project. Begun by women in Massachusetts in 1990 to promote awareness of violence against women, the Clothesline Project urges victims and survivors of violence against women to create T-shirts that express feelings about the experience. A white T-shirt is used in memory of a murdered woman, a blue T-shirt for survivors of childhood sexual abuse, yellow for a battered woman, and so on. A series of these T-shirts is displayed on a clothesline in a public place, a graphic and moving statement about the issue (Clothesline Project 2003, "Ms.: The Many Faces of Feminism" 1994). Project steering committee chair Carol Chichetto explains, "The concept was simple—let each woman tell her own story in her own unique way, and hang it out for all to see. It was and is a way of airing society's dirty laundry" (Clothesline Project 2003, n.p.). Begun locally in Massachusetts with just thirty-one shirts, the project is now international, with some 35,000 to 50,000 shirts. Organizers took a simple, accessible medium and transformed it into a powerful voice against the pervasive problems of child sexual abuse, intimate partner violence, and violence against women.

5. *Promote community building.* The community building perspective (see chapter 4 and appendix 2) complements some of the most basic tenets of health education, such as the importance of starting where the people are and actively involving them in the development and implementation of new programs and initiatives (Freudenberg et al. 1995). To emphasize health education as a process of establishing and strengthening relationships, the framework allows for unfettered forms of community expression, a task to which the arts are particularly well suited. Cultural forms of expression rooted in the community help not only to give voice to concerns but to establish the collective life, whether through celebration, ritual, or grief (Ellis et al. 1995). Such community expressions can be powerful tools in achieving organizing goals.

They can be especially powerful in communities of color, where oppression has often belittled or suppressed traditional forms of expression (Duran and Duran 1995). Culture itself can become a battleground, and cultural norms can be arenas for asserting identify and defying imposed norms (Cabral 1979, Duran and Duran 1995, Aguirre-Molina et al. 2001, Torres and Cernada 2003).

6. *Promote healing.* The restorative powers of the arts have long been acknowledged. The creative process is both restorative and transformative, healing the one who undertakes it (Longman 1994). At the same time, the fruits of the creative process offer insights to others with similar experiences and help promote their healing though an interactive process.

The Vietnam War Memorial in Washington, D.C., provides a powerful example. The simple, stark wall etched with the names of the dead has become a mecca for millions who need to reflect on, cry about, or exorcise the war. It has promoted the healing, understanding, and forgiveness so elusive to the country in the years following the war (Randall 1991).

In working with war-traumatized Guatemalan children, M. Brinton Lykes (1997) found that drama, body movements, and play elicited opinions from children who had been silenced and terrorized by the violence of war. The opportunity to voice their fear, sadness, and anger through characters allowed them to express themselves and respond openly to the researcher's questions. Lykes hypothesized that, without the drama, the children would have been too afraid to express their experiences and true feelings; and their need for psychological and social support would have been harder to ascertain.

7. *Promote culturally competent health organizing efforts and address health disparities.* One of the major challenges facing community organizing for health is effectively addressing widespread health disparities based on race, ethnicity, gender, language, age, disabilities, geography, and sexual orientation. As documented extensively in the Institute of Medicine's 2003 report, racial and ethnic health disparities are widespread and require a number of urgent responses (Smedley et al. 2003, Betancourt et al. 2003). Health disparities can be addressed by promoting cultural and linguistic competence in health promotion and delivery, both important arenas for community health organizing (Betancourt et al. 2003).

*Cultural competence* is defined broadly as a set of skills that allows individuals or institutions to increase their appreciation of cultural differences and act sensitively, appropriately, and respectfully toward different cultures (Denboba et al. 1998, DHHS 1998). Increasingly, cultural competence is seen as an indispensable characteristic of health care professionals and the programs they deliver to communities (Mokuau 1998;, Office of Minority Health 2000; NAHH 2000, 2001a, 2001b; Betancourt et al. 2003).

The arts are a natural and effective vehicle for promoting cultural competence because people create in the forms and language that are most deeply rooted in their culture, experience, values, and history. The arts provide an intimate and immediate expression of what is culturally appropriate and meaningful for communities. Using the arts can greatly assist the development of culturally competent community health organizing.

8. *Empower*. This may be the most important aspect of using the arts in community organizing for health. When a person or a community becomes involved in a creative process, the result can be exhilarating. When one becomes the video maker, the poet, or the muralist and is transformed through that process, both the messenger and the audience can change (Boal 1979, Chavez et al. in press). An example is Teatro Campesino, the popular theater that arose alongside the United Farm Workers during the long strike in the grape fields in the seventies. When farmworkers took on the role of the boss in skits, the task was initially difficult for them. Once they assumed that role of power and strength, however, it carried over to their work to win the strike (NLCC 1996).

One argument for the effectiveness of the Health Empowerment though Arts and Literature (HEAL) framework is that it establishes a basis for incorporation and ownership of ideas, feelings, and processes (McDonald 2000). An old Chinese saying is often applied to the learning process: "If I hear it, I forget it. If I see it, I remember it. If I do it, I know it" (Werner and Bower 1982, chap. 11, p. 1). The HEAL framework adds the notion "If I create it, it is mine." Being able to communicate effectively through an art form, whether a play or graffiti, and whether the work is highly skilled or rudimentary, gives a person and a community a sense that they can do something valuable that is meaningful to others and establishes the voice that Freire and others have spoken of. This transformative nature of participation in the creative process can be invaluable for organizing around health issues.

We turn now to three case studies that illustrate in greater detail how the arts can be used to achieve these eight objectives in the context of community organizing and community building for health.

## Hand-Made Health Education:
## The NAMES Project AIDS Memorial Quilt

Among the best-known examples of the use of the arts in health promotion and community building and organizing is the NAMES Project's AIDS memorial quilt, which has successfully achieved all of the listed objectives. The AIDS quilt is the largest ongoing community arts project in the world (NAMES Project Foundation 1996). Its October 1996 display in Washington, D.C., covering the entire

National Mall, constituted both the largest AIDS event and the largest community art event in history. That was the last time the quilt was displayed in its entirety.

The AIDS quilt began in 1987, when gay activist and NAMES Project founder Cleve Jones organized a community meeting in San Francisco to come up with a way to commemorate those who had died in the AIDS epidemic. He began by making a quilt for a friend. He was quickly joined by thousands of others who were relieved to have the opportunity to express their grief constructively (Howe 1997). The quilt project grew quickly; and on October 11, 1987, it was displayed for the first time as part of the national march for lesbian and gay rights. At that time, the quilt covered a space larger than a football field.

The quilt soon elicited financial and volunteer support and grew from a memorial into a method for activism. The mission statement of the NAMES Project is "to use the AIDS memorial quilt to bring an end to AIDS." The project's stated goals are to "Provide a creative means for remembrance and healing. Illustrate the enormity of the AIDS epidemic. Increase public awareness of AIDS. Assist with HIV prevention education. Raise funds for community-based AIDS service organizations" (AIDS quilt web site 2003, n.p.).

The project's community organization method reflects feminist influences: the movement takes the personal experience of those whose loved ones have died of AIDS and converts it into a powerful political campaign to raise awareness about and money for AIDS victims (see chapter 11). The project is multicultural because it implicitly critiques how the marginalized status of most AIDS victims, initially gay men and increasingly poor people and people of color, slowed governmental reaction to the epidemic. The quilt is also a grassroots organizing effort in the sense that "People excluded from the mainstream of organized power . . . come together . . . to assert their needs" (see chapter 6). It provided a way for the marginalized victims, their families, and their friends to band together and form a community effort across the United States and eventually around the world.

Each quilt panel, created to remember the life of a person lost to AIDS, is the size of a human grave. Panels are made of a wide array of materials, from photographs, to love letters, to condoms, to stuffed animals, to wedding rings. As the AIDS epidemic grows, so does the quilt; new memorial panels are added each month (AIDS quilt web site 2003). The quilt has effectively addressed the challenge of organizing in diverse communities. Because there are no guidelines for panels other than size, participants are free to express themselves in ways that are appropriate to their cultures. A quick glance at the panels shows that they feature more than twenty languages, many different artistic styles, and a wide variety of materials. In this sense, the quilt is utterly inclusive. The money raised, which comes largely from private donations and foundations and to date is more than $3 million, goes to direct services for AIDS victims (AIDS quilt web site 2003).

In 2001, the quilt included 44,000 panels and covered an area the size of twenty-six football fields (AIDS quilt web site 2003). At its 1988 display in Washington, D.C., participants began the ritual of reading the names of the dead. At the historic October 1996 display, over 70,000 names were read—more names than appear on the Vietnam War Memorial.

The NAMES Project conducts a number of community-based, academic, high school, interfaith, and corporate programs as well as World AIDS Day and international displays. More than forty countries have participated, including Australia, Poland, Zambia, Thailand, Russia, France, Guatemala, and Puerto Rico (NAMES Project Foundation 1996). Nominated for a Nobel Peace Prize in 1989, the quilt project may be the world's most effective AIDS educator and organizer. As suggested, it also has been a potent community builder, helping both quilt creators and viewers feel an increased sense of community, which in turn has stimulated collective action.

> Perhaps the most powerful symbol for telling the story of the AIDS epidemic has been the "quilt." Separately, each patch, through word, picture or symbol, signified the very personal and intimate costs of the epidemic. Woven together, they conveyed a powerful collective story of loss and grief. Critical to this discussion, the ritualized story telling of the quilt preserved the memory of those who had died, while promoting connections to survivors. It is in the nexus between ritual and shared meaning that some part of communal experience is built. Ritual repeated over time creates a basis for historic memory.
>
> (Fabricant and Fisher 2002, 16)

## Community Building and Health Organizing in Greater New Orleans

The belief that the arts can play a role in community building and health organizing was the basis for the 1996 Summer Arts Discovery Program/Discubriendo El Arte in greater New Orleans. The program was the first stage of a community health organizing plan developed by the Latino Health Outreach Project/Proyecto Pro-Salud Latina (LHOP/PPSL), a collaboration of students and faculty at Tulane's School of Public Health and Tropical Medicine in New Orleans. Previously, there had been no community health organizing in the area's Latino community, whose population had been growing quickly for several years. Very few programs and services were available to this predominantly monolingual, Spanish-speaking group, and organized Latino political power was extremely limited.

At the invitation of local Latino community activists, LHOP/PPSL members (a multiracial, bilingual group) began their work at the Redwoods subsidized housing development in the summer, volunteering time and scrounging for art supplies. The predominantly Latino (87 percent) development, made up of some five hundred families, is located in Kenner, a city in the greater New Orleans metropolitan area. A local community organizer assisted with initial contacts and gave LHOP/PPSL rent-free space in the after-school tutoring center he had started in the complex.

The objectives of the Summer Arts Discovery Program/Discubriendo El Arte were threefold: gain entree into the community, begin community assessment, and offer something of value to the community. By visiting door to door in each housing unit, distributing bilingual fliers to announce the free workshops, and preregistering children, LHOP/PPSL members established recognition and familiarity in the community.

Community assessment and asset mapping included gathering as much information as possible about the organization, family life, community dynamics, and health education concerns of the Redwoods community. By implementing the Summer Arts Discovery Program/Discubriendo El Arte, the LHOP/PPSL team hoped to learn from the outreach process, the children's artwork and interactions, and contact with the parents. Art activities were designed around the themes of community, family, and school to elicit children's perceptions of their community.

The response to the arts workshops was positive. An average of twenty-five children participated in each session, with eighteen to twenty return participants. The group was able to establish rapport with the children as well as the mothers, who dropped the children off and picked them up. Interaction with mothers led to input about topics for future health education activities, such as cancer prevention and nutrition, and resulted in a series of *charlas* (talks) conducted in the following months.

Carrying out the program allowed the LHOP/PPSL team to make a number of useful observations about language preferences (the children preferred to use English in the workshops), family unity, gender roles, and recurrent themes. These insights helped team members plan future activities and gave them a realistic understanding of important community dynamics. As the initial stage of a community health organizing effort that went on for several years, the Summer Arts Discovery Program/Discubriendo El Arte accomplished the objectives of introducing LHOP/PPSL to the community and providing valuable data and insights for future efforts. Several women in the community became involved in community health activities as a direct result of the summer art workshops.

The program was carried out with donated labor and supplies, accomplishing a great deal on a shoestring. It is an example of how, with modest resources, effective health organizing using the arts can be conducted in underserved communities in great need of opportunities to develop and raise their voices.

## Photovoice for Community Organizing and to Reach Policymakers

As noted, photovoice is a process through which people can "identify, represent and enhance their community through a specific photographic technique" (Wang 1999, 185). Rooted in health education principles, critical education, feminist theory, and documentary photography (Wang and Burris 1994), photovoice is an increasingly popular approach in health promotion, community organizing, and community-based participatory research (Wang 1999, 2003). In photovoice, people are given cameras and asked to photograph their everyday health and work realities. They then engage in critical reflective dialogue about the pictures and their contexts, often using the mnemonic SHOWED as an aid (Shaffer 1983):

- What do you *see* here?
- What's really *happening* here?
- How does this relate to *our* lives?
- *Why* does this problem, concern, or strength *exist*?
- What can we *do* about it?

The goals of photovoice are to enable participants to (1) record and reflect on their personal and community strengths and concerns, (2) promote critical dialogue and knowledge about personal and community issues through group discussion of photographs, and (3) reach policymakers (Wang 1999, 185). First used in Yunnan, China, by sixty-two rural women, photovoice links photography with community assessment and empowerment to communicate needs determined at the grassroots level; the aim is to reach policymakers. In Yunnan, the photographs allowed the women to express themselves and became powerful advocacy tools (Wang et al. 1996). The methodology has since been applied in rural and urban settings around the world. In the United States, it has been used with youth in Baltimore (Strack and Magill 2004) and in neighborhoods surrounding Richmond, California (Wilson et al. in press); homeless people in Ann Arbor, Michigan (Wang et al. 2000, Wang 2003); neighborhood residents in Flint, Michigan (Wang 2000, Wang et al. in press), and Contra Costa County, California (Spears 1999); and people with mental illnesses in New Haven, Connecticut (Bowers 1999; see also *http://www.photovoice.com*).

Photovoice is designed to reach—and touch—policymakers. The Flint Photovoice Project in Michigan (Wang et al. in press) is an example. Catalyzed by leaders of a neighborhood violence prevention coalition, project organizers began by recruiting eight local facilitators and eleven professional photographers, who participated in a train-the-trainers session. These participants were introduced to the photovoice concept and method; discussed cameras, ethics, and power; and took part in a guided photo shoot. The facilitators and professional photographers then worked with four groups: ten youth involved in a study of adolescent resiliency, ten youth active as local community leaders, eleven adult neighborhood activists, and ten policymakers. We should note that organizers recruited policymakers at the project's outset to provide the political will to implement participants' policy and program recommendations in accordance with established photovoice methodology (Wang et al. in press). Flint Photovoice deviated from standard photovoice protocol by also involving a second group of policymakers to take photographs.

Organizers found that policymakers' experiential participation as photographers offered several advantages. To begin with, policymakers took it upon themselves to provide venues for display, such as legislative breakfasts, city hall, government agencies, and news programs. In addition, their "firsthand experience with photovoice gave them an innovative tool with which to explore and improve programs over which they had the most influence" (Wang et al. in press). For example, because the local health department director was involved in the project, he introduced the photovoice method as part of an ongoing gonorrhea control initiative whose goal was to tap the insights of consumers and providers. Finally, policymakers' participation set the stage for interactions in which participants representing widely disparate age, socioeconomic status, neighborhoods, and social power were able to communicate and collaborate. The long-term relationships established among diverse participants were some of the project's most powerful outcomes (Wang et al. in press).

Assessing the impact of the approach on programs or policies can be challenging because many interacting factors are at play. Yet effective use of photovoice has been credited in part with acquisition of funding for violence prevention and the renewal of funding for Flint area programs overall (Wang et al. in press). Additionally, as noted in chapter 12, including photovoice as a centerpiece of a proposed new youth empowerment project in northern California was an important factor in the project's successful competition for a $1.5 million CDC community-based prevention research grant (Wilson et al. in press).

Not all photovoice participants may be interested in policy-level outcomes, as illustrated by the Ann Arbor, Michigan, Language of Light Photovoice Project, which was conducted among homeless persons. Although they were excited by the well-attended public forums where they shared their photographs and perspectives with local community leaders, the general public, and journalists, participants (contrary to project organizers' initial expectations) elected not to focus on a core policy issue affecting homeless people—namely, a controversial plan to move the shelter to a remote area near the dump. Instead, the men and women living at the shelter chose to describe and vivify what gave them hope and what enabled them to survive emotionally and practically on the streets (Wang et al. 2000, Wang 2003). Both the shelter's sixty-day limit and the strong support that participants offered one another throughout the photovoice project appear to have contributed to the fact that ten of the eleven participants were able to leave the shelter and find their own housing. Project leaders respected the group's need to focus on individual, permanent housing solutions rather than public policy advocacy about transitional housing. Yet as projects in Yunnan, Flint, and the San Francisco Bay area have demonstrated, photovoice offers a potent tool for community organizing aimed at reaching policymakers when participating community members have an interest in working at this level.

## Conclusion

The arts can be a catalyst for change and growth in wide-ranging circumstances, providing a rich legacy for health organizers and promoters to draw on in their community organizing and community building efforts. As Vivian Chavez and her colleagues (in press) suggest about video, such an approach "has the potential to open communication and promote dialogue. Its images, sounds and music can motivate and inspire." It can also bring in new partners to share additional skills, which in turn may help attract the interest of funders, government agencies, health workers, youth, community coalitions, and others. Given the many challenges that continue to confront community health organizing, we need new ways to awaken and empower ourselves and our communities. The arts are some of our most effective tools.

### Acknowledgments

Portions of this chapter were adapted from M. McDonald, G. Antunez, and M. Gottemoeller, 1998–99, "Using the Arts and Literature in Health Education," *International Quarterly of Community Health Education* 18, no. 3: 269–82. The chapter authors gratefully acknowledge Giovanni Antunez and Megan Gottemoeller. They also thank Peter Solomon and Alyssa Lafosse for helpful suggestions and assistance with final editing.

### References

Aguirre-Molina, M., C. Molina, and R. Zambrana. 2002. *Health Issues in the Latino Community*. San Francisco: Jossey-Bass.
AIDS quilt web site. 2003. http://www.aidsquilt.org/Newsite/index.htm. Accessed June 28, 2003.
Airhihenbuwa, C. O. 1994. "Health Promotion and the Discourse on Culture: Implications for Empowerment." *Health Education Quarterly* 21, no. 3: 345–53.
Barnett, A. W. 1984. *Community Murals: The People's Art*. Cornwall, England: Art Alliance Press.
Betancourt, J., A. Green, and E. Carrillo. 2003. "Defining Cultural Competence: A Practical Framework for Addressing Racial/Ethnic Disparities in Health or Health Care." *Public Health Reports* 118 (July–August): 293–302.
Black, G. 1981. *Triumph of the People: The Sandinista Revolution in Nicaragua*. London: Zed.
Boal, A. 1972. *Categories de teatro popular*. Buenos Aires: Ediciones Cepe.
———. 1979. *Theater of the Oppressed*, translated by C. McBride. New York: Urizen.

Bowers, A. A. 1999. "People with Serious Mental Illnesses Using Photovoice: Implications for Participatory Research and Community Education." Paper presented at the annual meeting of the American Public Health Association, Chicago, November.

Cabral, A. 1979. "The Role of Culture in the Liberation Struggle." In *Communication and Class Struggle*, edited by A. Matterlart and S. Siegelaub. New York: International General.

Cardenal, E. 1982. "Defendiendo la cultura, el hombre, y el planeta." *Nicarauac*, 3: 149–52.

Carroll, J., and M. Minkler. 2000. "Freire's Message for Social Workers: Looking Back, Looking Ahead." *Journal of Community Practice* 8, no. 1: 21–36.

Chavez, V., B. A. Israel, A. Allen, R. Lichtenstein, M. DeCarlo, A. Schulz, et al. In press. "A Bridge between Communities: Video-Making Using Principles of Community-Based Participatory Research." *Journal of Health Promotion Practice*.

Cheney, J., M. Deihl, and D. Silverstein. 1976. *All Our Lives: A Women's Songbook*. Baltimore: Diana Press.

Chicago, J. 1985. *The Birth Project*. New York: Doubleday.

"Children Put Peace to Paper in Contest." 1996. *Times Picayune*, May 16, p. B1.

Clardy, B. 2000. *Prehistoric Art*. http://www.jlc.net/~brian/art/prehistoric.html. Accessed December 2000.

Clark, N. M., and K. McLeroy. 1995. "Creating Capacity through Health Education: What We Know and What We Don't." *Health Education Quarterly* 22, no. 3: 273–89.

Clothesline Project. n.d. *Bearing Witness to Violence against Women*. East Dennis, Mass: Clothesline Project.

———. 2003. http://www.clotheselineproject.org.

Denboba D. L., J. L. Bragdon, L. G. Epstein, K. Garthright, and T. M. Goldman. 1998. "Reducing Health Disparities through Cultural Competence." *Journal of Health Education* 29, supp.: 47–53.

Duran, E., and B. Duran. 1995. *Native American Postcolonial Psychology*. Albany: State University of New York Press.

Ellis, G., D. Reed, and H. Scheider. 1995. "Mobilizing a Low-Income African American Community around Tobacco Control: A Force Field Analysis." *Health Education Quarterly* 22, no. 4: 443–57.

Fabricant, M., and R. Fisher. 2002. "Agency Based Community Building in Low Income Neighborhoods: A Praxis Framework." *Journal of Community Practice* 10, no. 2: 1–22.

Freire, P. 1970. "Cultural Action and Conscientization." *Harvard Educational Review* 40, no. 3.

———. 1990a. *Education for Critical Consciousness*. New York: Continuum.

———. 1990b. *Pedagogy of the Oppressed*, translated by M. B. Ramos. New York: Continuum.

Freudenberg, N., E. Eng, B. Flay, G. Parcel, T. Rogers, and N. Wallerstein. 1995. "Strengthening Individual and Community Capacity to Prevent Disease and Promote Health: In Search of Relevant Theories and Principles." *Health Education Quarterly* 22, no. 3: 290–306.

Guthrie, W. 1958. *California to the New York Islands*. New York: Guthrie Children's Trust Fund.

hooks, b. 1994. *Outlaw Culture: Resisting Representations*. New York: Routledge.

Horton, M., and P. Freire. 1990. *We Make the Road by Walking: Conversations on Education and Social Change*. Philadelphia: Temple University Press.

Howe, L. 1997. "The AIDS Quilt and Its Traditions." *College Literature* 24, no. 2: 109–25.

Kaplan, F. 2000. Art, Science and Art Therapy. London: Kingsley.

Kretzmann, J., and J. McKnight. 1993. *Building Communities from the Inside Out: A Path toward Finding and Mobilizing a Community's Assets*. Chicago: ACTA.

Kunzle, D. 1995. *The Murals of Revolutionary Nicaragua*. Berkeley: University of California Press.

Laver, S., B. Van den Borne, and G. Kok. 1998. "Using Theory to Design an Intervention for HIV/AIDS Prevention for Farm Workers in Rural Zimbabwe." In *Progress in Preventing AIDS? Dogma, Dissent, and Innovation: Global Perspectives*, edited by D. Buchanan and G. Cernada, 259–72. Amityville, N.Y.: Baywood.

Laver, S., B. Van den Borne, G. Kok, and G. Woelk. 1996–97. "Was the Intervention Implemented As Intended? A Process Evaluation of an AIDS Prevention Intervention in Rural Zimbabwe." *International Quarterly of Community of Health Education* 16: 25–46.

Lippard, L. R. 2000. *Mixed Blessings: New Art in a Multicultural America*. New York: New Press.

Longman, R. 1994. "Creating Art: Your $R_x$ for Health." *American Artist* 58: 68–73.

Lorde, A. 1984. *Sister Outsider*. Freedom, Calif.: Crossing.

Lykes, M. B. 1997. "Activist Participatory Research among Maya of Guatemala: Constructing Meanings from Situated Knowledge." *Journal of Social Issues* 53, no. 4: 725–46.

Mairs, N. 1994. *Voice Lessons*. Boston: Beacon.

McDonald, M. 2000. "Building Communities to Promote Health: Lessons from the Latino Health Outreach Project." Paper presented at a seminar for the Centers for Disease Control and Prevention, Center for Chronic Disease Prevention and Health Promotion, Division of Reproductive Health, Atlanta, March 10.

McDonald, M., G. Antunez, and M. Gottemoeller. 1998–99. "Using the Arts and Literature in Health Education." *International Quarterly of Community Health Education* 18, no. 3: 269–82.

Minkler, M. 1994. "Ten Commitments for Community Health Education." *Health Education Research* 9, no. 4: 527–34.

Minkler, M., and K. Cox. 1980. "Creating Critical Consciousness in Health: Applications of Freire's Philosophy and Methods to a Health Care Setting." *International Journal of Health Services* 10, no. 2: 311–21.

Mokuau, N. 1998. *Responding to Pacific Islanders: Culturally Competent Perspectives for Substance Abuse Prevention*. CSAP Cultural Competence Series. Washington, D.C.: U.S. Department of Health and Human Services.

"Ms.: The Many Faces of Feminism." 1994. *Ms.* (July–August): 5.

NAMES Project Foundation. 1996. *The AIDS Memorial Quilt*. San Francisco: Names Project Foundation.

National Alliance for Hispanic Health (NAHH). 2000. Quality Health Services for Hispanics: The Cultural Competency Component. Washington, D.C.: U.S. Department of Health and Human Services.

———. 2001a. *A Primer for Cultural Proficiency: Towards Quality Health Services for Hispanics*. Washington, D.C.: Estrella.

———. 2001b. A Primer for Cultural Proficiency, Workbook: Tools and Resources for Self-Assessment. Washington, D.C.: Estrella.

National Latino Communications Center (NLCC). 1996. *The Struggle in the Fields: Episode 2, Chicano! History of the Mexican American Civil Rights Movement*. Video. Los Angeles: National Latino Communications Center Educational Media.

Nyswander, D. B. 1956. "Education for Health: Some Principles and Their Application." *Health Education Monographs* 14: 65–70.

Office of Minority Health, Public Health Service. 2000. "Assuring Cultural Competence in Health Care: Recommendations for National Standards and an Outcomes-Focused Research Agenda." Retrieved January 20, 2002. http://www.omhrc.gov/clas/po.htm.

Olsen, T. 1978. *Silences*. New York: Delta.

Ordones, O., and H. Vanolli, eds. 1995. *Violence and Health: Memoirs of the Inter-American Conference on Society, Violence and Health*. Washington, D.C.: Pan American Health Organization.

Perry, C., T. Baranowski, and G. Parcel. 1990. "How Individuals, Environments, and Health Behavior Intersect: Social Learning Theory." In *Health Behavior and Health Educa-*

*tion*, edited by K. Glanz, F. M. Lewis, and B. K. Rimer, 153–78. San Francisco: Jossey-Bass.

Randall, M. 1984. *Risking a Somersault in the Air: Conversations with Nicaraguan Writers*. San Francisco: Solidarity.

———. 1991. *Walking to the Edge: Essays of Resistance*. Boston: South End.

Rich, A. 1993. *What Is Found There: Notebooks on Poetry and Politics*. New York: Norton.

Richardson, L., and V. Taylor, eds. 1994. *Feminist Frontiers III*. New York: McGraw-Hill.

Riley, S. 2001. "Art Therapy with Adolescents." *Western Journal of Medicine* 175, no. 1: 54–57.

Rosen, R. 2000. *The World Split Open: How the Modern Women's Movement Changed America*. New York: Viking Penguin.

Rosenstock, I. 1990. "The Health Belief Model: Explaining Health Behavior through Expectancies." In *Health Behavior and Health Education*, ed. K. Glanz, F. M. Lewis, and B. K. Rimer, 39–62. San Francisco: Jossey-Bass.

Ruiz, V., and E. C. DuBois, eds. 1994. *Unequal Sisters: A Multicultural Reader in U.S. Women's History*, 2d ed. New York: Routledge.

Rukeyser, M. 1996. *The Life of Poetry*. Ashfield, Mass: Paris.

Shaffer, R. 1983. *Beyond the Dispensary*. Nairobi, Kenya: African Medical and Research Foundation.

Smedley, B. D., A. Y. Stith, and A. R. Nelson, eds. 2003. *Unequal Treatment: Confronting Racial and Ethnic Disparities in Health Care*. Washington, D.C.: National Academics Press.

Smith, M. 1995. "Community Outreach Art Program for Hospitalized Children." *School Arts* 94: 21–22.

Spears, L. 1999. "Picturing Concerns: The Idea Is to Take the Messages to Policy Makers and to Produce Change." *Contra Costa Times*, April 11, pp. A27, A32.

Steckler, A., J. P. Allegrante, D. Altman, R. Brown, J. N. Burdine, R. M. Goodman, and C. Jorgensen. 1995. "Health Education Intervention Strategies: Recommendations for Future Research." *Health Education Quarterly* 22, no. 3: 307–28.

Strack, R., and C. Magill. 2004. "Engaging Youth through Photovoice." *Journal of Health Promotion Practice* 5, no. 1: 49–58.

Tolley, E. E., and M. E. Bentley. 1996. "Training Issues for the Use of Participatory Research Methods in Health." In *Participatory Research in Health*, edited by K. De Koning and M. Martin, 50–61. Atlantic Highlands, N.J.: Zed.

Torres, M. I., and G. Cernada, eds. 2003. *Sexual and Reproductive Health Promotion in Latino Populations: Parteras, Promotoras y Poetas*. Amityville, N.Y.: Baywood.

U.S. Department of Health and Human Services (DHHS), Bureau of Primary Health Care. 1998. *Cultural Competence: A Journey*. Bethesda, Md.: Health Resources and Services Administration.

Wallerstein, N. 1999. "Power between Evaluator and Community: Research Relationships within New Mexico's Healthier Communities." *Social Science and Medicine* 49, no. 1: 39–53.

Wallerstein, N., and E. Bernstein. 1988. "Empowerment Education: Freire's Ideas Adapted to Health Education." *Health Education Quarterly* 15: 379–94.

Wallerstein, N., and M. Weinger. 1992. "Empowerment Approaches to Worker Health and Safety Education." *American Journal of Industrial Medicine* 22, no. 5: 619–84.

Wang, C. C. 1999. "Photovoice: A Participatory Action Research Strategy Applied to Women's Health." *Journal of Women's Health* 8, no. 2: 185–92.

———, ed. 2000. *Strength to Be: Community Visions and Voices*. Ann Arbor: University of Michigan Press.

———. 2003. "Using Photovoice As a Participatory Assessment and Issue Selection Tool: A Case Study with the Homeless in Ann Arbor." In *Community Based Participatory Research for Health*, edited by M. Minkler and N. Wallerstein, 179–96. San Francisco: Jossey-Bass.

Wang, C. C, and M. A. Burris. 1994. "Empowerment through Photo Novella: Portraits of Participation." *Health Education Quarterly* 21, no. 2: 171–86.

———. 1997. "Photovoice: Concept, Methodology, and Use for Participatory Needs Assessment." *Health Education and Behavior* 24, no. 3: 369–87.

Wang C. C, M. A. Burris, and Y. P. Xiang. 1996. "Chinese Village Women As Visual Anthropologists: A Participatory Approach to Reaching Policymakers." *Social Science and Medicine* 42, no. 10: 1391–1400.

Wang C. C., J. L. Cash, and L. S. Powers. 2000. "Who Knows the Streets As Well as the Homeless? Promoting Personal and Community Action through Photovoice." *Health Promotion Practice* 1, no. 1: 81–89.

Wang, C. C., S. Morrel-Samuels, P. Hutchison, L. Bell, and R. M. Pestronk. In press. "Flint Photovoice: Community-Building among Youth, Adults, and Policy Makers." *American Journal of Public Health*.

Werner, D., and B. Bower. 1982. *Helping Health Workers Learn*. Palo Alto, Calif.: Hesperian Foundation.

Whitehead, K. 1996. *The Feminist Poetry Movement*. Jackson: University Press of Mississippi.

Wilson, N., M. Minkler, S. Dasho, R. Carrillo, N. Wallerstein, and D. Garcia. In press. "Training Students As Partners in Community Based Participatory Research: The Youth Empowerment Strategies (YES!) Project." *Journal of Community Practice*.

Winkler, M. G. 1993. "The Visual Arts in Medical Education." *Second Opinion* 19: 60–70.

# Part VIII

# Participatory Evaluation and Measuring Community Empowerment

As NOTED in chapter 2, although considerable progress has been made in the past decade, one of the biggest gaps in community organizing and community building practice lies in its frequent failure to adequately address issues of measurement and evaluation. The complex environments in which organizing typically takes place, the fact that community building and community organizing are by definition continually evolving, and the multiple levels on which change is sought all conspire against effective evaluative research (Connell et al. 1995). When we add to this mix severe funding constraints, lack of knowledge about evaluative processes and methods, and the fact that many traditional evaluative techniques are ill-suited to measuring the outcomes of community building and organizing, the forces that mitigate against evaluation appear even more formidable. Yet without adequate evaluations of community organizing and community building projects, we will continue to be hampered in our attempts to assess our strengths and weaknesses, learn from our mistakes, and demonstrate to funders and others the worth of these community practice efforts.

If we are to see improvements in both the quantity and the quality of evaluative research on community organizing and community building, special evaluative techniques and approaches are needed. In particular, we must choose evaluative methods that empower rather than disempower the community, in part by meaningfully involving community members in the design and conduct of the evaluation. An important tool can be found in the philosophy and methodology of participatory evaluation, a body of approaches that emphasizes building community capacity while collecting useful information for project improvement and involving the various stakeholders throughout the process. Bradley Cousins and Elizabeth Whitmore (1998) have identified two streams in participatory evaluation: a *pragmatic stream*, which places its greatest emphasis on program improvement, and an *emancipatory* or *transformative tradition*, grounded in an ideological commitment to reallocating power and promoting social change.

In chapter 20, Chris M. Coombe examines the limitations of traditional research when applied to community organizing and community building efforts, including the tendency to collect knowledge that may be irrelevant or invalid and the fact that such outside-expert approaches can reinforce powerlessness. She then introduces participatory evaluation as an alternative approach and discusses the particular utility of the emancipatory tradition for evaluating community organizing and community health initiatives. She offers a practical framework comprised of a series of steps for incorporating an emancipatory-participatory approach in the evaluation of community organizing and related efforts. Coombe includes practical tips and suggestions with each step and explores the limitations and drawbacks of participatory approaches.

Among the various approaches introduced in chapter 20 is *empowerment evaluation*, which Stephen Fawcett et al. (1996) define as an interactive process in which communities work with a support team to identify their concerns, determine how to address them, measure their progress toward their goals, and use the information gained to increase the viability and success of their efforts. In chapter 21, Kathleen M. Roe, Kevin Roe, Christine Goette Carpenter, and Cindy Berenstein Sibley describe the challenge of evaluating five community planning efforts for HIV prevention. They did not consciously select empowerment evaluation as a strategy but, in their words, backed into it. Looking for an evaluative methodology that would stimulate and nurture community and respect and empower participants, they evolved an approach that, in retrospect, shares many principles, commitments, and processes with empowerment evaluation.

According to Roe and her colleagues, community planning for HIV prevention has the potential to stimulate community organizing and community building through social planning. In their chapter, they choose four of the steps in empowerment evaluation and demonstrate their applicability to this challenging effort. In keeping with the spirit of evaluation that is empowering and respectful of community members, Roe et al. draw on the words, stories, and perceptions of community members to enrich our understanding of what transpired in their unique social planning experiment. As chapter 21 suggests, although planning councils have become less concerned with empowerment as they have become more institutionalized, outside evaluators still can play an important role in fostering capacity building and empowerment in the way in which they approach their work. Although not a pure application of David Fetterman, Shakeh Kaftarian, and Abraham Wandersman's (1996) empowerment evaluation, this fascinating case study and its transformation during the past decade demonstrate the utility of evaluative approaches grounded in a commitment to individual and community empowerment.

## References

Connell, J. P., A. C. Kabisch, L. B. Schorr, and C. H. Weiss, eds. 1995. *New Approaches to Evaluating Community Initiatives: Concepts, Methods, and Contexts*. Washington, D.C.: Aspen Institute.

Cousins, J. B., and E. Whitmore. 1998. "Framing Participatory Evaluation." In *Understanding and Practicing Participatory Evaluation*, edited by E. Whitmore, 5–23. San Francisco: Jossey-Bass.

Fawcett, S. B., A. Paine-Andrews, V. Francisco, J. Schultz, K. Richter, R. Lewis, K. Harris, E. Williams, J. Berkeley, C. Lopez, and J. Fisher. 1996. "Empowering Community Health Initiatives through Evaluation." In *Empowerment Evaluation: Knowledge and Tools for Self-Assessment and Accountability*, edited by D. M. Fetterman, S. J. Kaftarian, and A. Wandersman, 161–87. Thousand Oaks, Calif.: Sage.

Fetterman, D. M., S. J. Kaftarian, and A. Wandersman, eds. 1996. *Empowerment Evaluation: Knowledge and Tools for Self-Assessment and Accountability*. Thousand Oaks, Calif.: Sage.

CHRIS M. COOMBE

*Chapter 20*      Participatory Evaluation

---

*Building Community While*
*Assessing Change*

Eᴠᴀʟᴜᴀᴛɪᴏɴ ɪs ᴏɴᴇ of the most challenging and promising issues in community organizing and community building for health. Over the past twenty years funders have come to expect formal program evaluation of health education efforts. Yet historically, communities organizing to transform social and material conditions have been skeptical of both the usefulness and intent of externally mandated evaluation. Few community organizations have formal evaluation skills and knowledge and must rely on external evaluators. Faced with insufficient funding to address complex and intransigent health and social problems, community practitioners often resist spending scarce resources on what they perceive to be proving rather than improving (Magerison 1987). Organizations that aim to alter existing power relationships or distribution of resources may fear that evaluation results will be used to punish or threaten them with loss of funding.

In addition, key dimensions of community organizing and community building, such as participation, power and empowerment, community competence, and multilevel change (see chapter 2), are difficult to capture using traditional evaluation methods and indicators. These challenges, combined with the emergence and widespread acceptance of collaborative partnerships, comprehensive community initiatives, and community-based participatory research, have led to the development over the past two decades of promising new methods and approaches to evaluation (Connell et al. 1995, Fetterman et al. 1996, Springett 2003, Wallerstein 2002).

Central among them is participatory evaluation, a partnership approach to evaluation that engages those who have a stake in the project, program, or ini-

368

tiative in all aspects of evaluation design and implementation. Findings are applied as they emerge to solve problems and adjust course. Most important for community organizing and community building, participatory evaluation also departs from traditional evaluation by rethinking who owns and controls the process of creating, interpreting, and applying knowledge and to what end. In the emancipatory stream of participatory evaluation, both the process and products of evaluation are used to transform power relations and promote social action and change (Cousins and Whitmore 1998).

This chapter examines how participatory evaluation can be used for not only assessing the merit and effectiveness of community organizing, but also building organizational and community capacity for social change. First, I discuss some limitations of traditional evaluation to establish the rationale for a more participatory approach. Next, I describe the theoretical foundation of participatory evaluation, including its roots in participatory research traditions from several disciplines. Drawing on recent work in participatory evaluation, I suggest a practical framework for incorporating this approach at each step of the evaluation process. The final sections discuss some of the benefits as well as challenges of this approach.

## *Limitations of Traditional Evaluation: A Rationale for Participatory Evaluation*

Until recently, most public health evaluations have been based on the positivist research paradigm of the natural sciences. Conventional program evaluation is characterized by a search for causal relationships between treatments and outcomes, using primarily quantitative methods and carried out by an external researcher-evaluator. The professional evaluator determines what is to be studied, what methods are to be used, and what conclusions may be drawn from the findings. Intended beneficiaries are involved in the evaluation process minimally, if at all; and evaluators are careful to maintain a stance of neutrality and objectivity. Many authors have been critical of this approach, arguing that it promotes the myth of objectivity, oversimplifies social reality, is not conducive to subsequent action to solve social problems, and is elitist (Fals-Borda and Rahman 1991, Hall et al. 1982).

Although inclusion of qualitative methods and community participation has become widespread in recent years, the conventional biomedical paradigm remains the gold standard for evaluation in public health education. Even so, it has become increasingly evident that the traditional program evaluation approach may be neither appropriate nor effective for evaluating community organizing and community building initiatives. Using traditional research approaches to evaluate community change efforts may be counterproductive to promoting community health in at least three ways:

1. The knowledge produced may be irrelevant or invalid.
2. The methods used may reinforce the powerlessness of community members and the power imbalance between experts-professionals and the people.
3. The results often are not applied to solving underlying problems and may indeed be used in ways that are harmful to the community.

### IRRELEVANT OR INVALID KNOWLEDGE

Traditional methods designed to test a few variables under controlled conditions and with a comparison group have been adapted and applied to community settings. But community organizing does not take place in a laboratory. Many sectors are involved in solving complex problems with multiple causes, and the unit of study is a population or group rather than an individual. Theory and hypotheses are seldom explicit when the intervention is designed. Projects use different strategies with different targets over varying time periods, making it difficult to track actions and outcomes, let alone establish links between the two. As a result, it is common for evaluation results to miss the mark or be irrelevant.

Who owns the development of knowledge is another concern. As noted in previous chapters, knowledge has become one of the most important bases of power and control in our society (Maguire 2001) and remains concentrated in the hands of experts and the elite. In modern western society, the most legitimate form of knowledge is technological or scientific, which can be produced only by formally certified experts such as academics, researchers, and evaluators. Ordinary human knowledge is typically seen as invalid (Hall 1979). It is too early to know whether the Internet will truly democratize knowledge or instead widen the chasm between those who are poor and those who are not by escalating the accumulation of knowledge (as opposed to information) at the privileged end.

Participatory research paradigms, described later in this chapter, arose in response to the continued and increasing monopoly of knowledge by the powerful. Three premises underlie these approaches: (1) oppressed people should be involved in the analysis of and solutions to social problems (Hall 1979), (2) social scientists must work in collaboration with the community to identify relevant research questions and accurately understand findings (Hatch 1993, Green and Mercer 2001), and (3) scientific knowledge must be linked with social action (Greenwood et al. 1993). Although some conventional academic research has contributed much to our understanding of oppressed groups, as exemplified in works such as Carol Stack's (1974) classic *All Our Kin*, much researcher-centered investigation has been flawed by theory rooted in the perceptions, biases, and agendas of the external observer.

C. Fletcher (1992) suggests that the knowledge that people themselves produce offers useful counterinformation because it opposes abstract theories about them. Like qualitative methods that attempt to bring popular knowledge to the surface, however, participatory research is still considered by many in medical and public health fields to be biased and unreliable. Fortunately, this attitude is changing, even among government and private funders, who have come to expect authentic community participation in interventions (Minkler et al. 2003).

## REINFORCEMENT OF POWERLESSNESS

In traditional evaluation there is a clear distinction between evaluator and program participants, with the expert evaluator-researcher in charge of designing, implementing, analyzing, and reporting the findings. Although program staff may be involved and consulted, the evaluator is expected to have not only the technical skills but also the insight, knowledge, and objectivity for interpreting the meaning of the data. Program participants are objects of study who in effect depend on the outside agent for interpretation of the reality of their experience. The process of evaluation remains both mystified and external to the organization's own process of planning and development.

The role of empowerment in health promotion and the role of powerlessness as a broad risk factor for disease have been widely discussed (Wallerstein 1992; see also chapters 2 and 12). Central to the empowerment concept is the importance of individuals and communities having influence and control over decisions that affect them (Israel et al. 1994; see appendix 9). Evaluation approaches that maintain the separate and hierarchical relationship between evaluator and community foster dependence and powerlessness and thereby mitigate against empowerment as an outcome. Participatory researchers refute the disempowering notion that an external agent is necessary for the achievement of research objectivity (Chesler 1991, Israel et al. 1998). Perhaps objectivity is gained not through detachment from the setting but through deep involvement in and reflection about the setting.

In addition, traditional approaches reinforce marginalization by viewing health problems as located in individuals and in the community and by judging program success based on narrowly focused indicators. Traditional program evaluation methods are ill-suited to evaluate impact on complex long-term targets of change or to assess the powerful influence of the broader social and physical environments on community health.

## UNAPPLIED OR HARMFUL RESULTS

Traditionally, evaluation has aimed at assessing a program's worth, value, and contribution to knowledge. Evaluators are trained to prove rather than improve and are expected to remain impartial. Using evaluation to improve programs, build community competence, or change policies has fallen under the domain of other professions; researchers-evaluators are seldom trained or expected to be proficient in program, policy, or organizational development.

This approach is counterproductive to promoting community health in at least three ways. First, it is a missed opportunity. Evaluators have information and insights that could help an organization translate evaluation findings into implications for action rather than solely into implications for further study. Second, it perpetuates a condition in which reflection and analysis are activities separate from organizational planning and action rather than necessary, sequential steps in an integrated, collaborative, decision-making process. Third, because action planning is distinct from evaluation, which is perceived as external to the organization, programs and strategies may be less effective because they are not based on all the available data. Practitioners often do not use evaluation results.

But opponents have used evaluation and research findings to justify actions that are harmful to the community or specific segments of it. Community activists and researchers can cite numerous examples in which their evaluation-research findings were used against the constituencies they intended to help. For example, policymakers in New York City dismissed or misused research findings about housing and neighborhood conditions as risk factors for homelessness among pregnant women in favor of personal dysfunction explanations. As a result, punitive policies replaced actions that would have addressed poverty and poor housing conditions (Clayson et al. 1995).

Many evaluators struggle with the tension of competing role demands. On the one hand, they are expected to maintain sufficient professionally prescribed distance and neutrality so that their findings will be credible to policymakers, funders, and other audiences. On the other hand, they want to ensure that the evaluation at least improves organization and program effectiveness and, if possible, generates action to transform the social structures and conditions that oppress communities.

There is ample evidence that social inequalities based on race, gender, and class are at the root of our most persistent public health problems (James et al. 2001, Krieger et al. 1993, Link and Phelan 1995). Given the entrenchment of causes and the complexity of solutions, evaluation has been evolving to become more responsive and relevant to communities. People are demanding much more of evaluation and becoming intolerant of the limited role of the outside expert who has no knowledge or vested interest in their community (Green et al. 1995). Participation, collaboration, and empowerment are becoming requirements—not just recommendations—in many evaluations of community-based efforts. Evaluation has the potential to build a dynamic community of transformative learning, thereby contributing to the empowerment of disenfranchised communities (Fetterman 1996). In the words of the turn-of-the century social reformer Jane Addams (1907), "We slowly learn that life consists of processes as well as results, and that failure may come quite as easily from ignoring the adequacy of one's method as from selfish or ignoble aims."

## What Is Participatory Evaluation?

Participatory evaluation is the systematic assessment of the progress, merit, or significance of a program or effort by those who have a vested interest in it. Interested parties, usually called stakeholders, are engaged as partners in a collaborative process of investigation, education, and action (Cousins and Whitmore 1998). Participatory evaluation is an "educational process through which social groups produce action-oriented knowledge about their reality, clarify and articulate their norms and values, and reach consensus about further action" (Brunner and Guzman 1989, 11).

Bradley Cousins and Elizabeth Whitmore (1998) suggest that participatory evaluation has emerged in two streams distinguished primarily by function. The pragmatic stream emphasizes program improvement as the principle aim of participatory approaches. The transformative or emancipatory stream is based on an explicit ideological commitment to reallocating power and promoting social change. While the streams are not mutually exclusive, the latter is more consistent with community organizing and community building for health and is the focus of this chapter.

A set of guiding principles forms the basis for transformative participatory evaluation (Cousins and Whitmore, 1998):

- Participation and ownership by the community
- A collaborative, co-learning process in which all participants are equitably engaged in and responsible for the evaluation
- Findings that promote action and change on multiple levels
- Power relationships that transform by empowering and building capacity of local community and changing systems

Participatory evaluation arises from a number of research traditions aimed at legitimizing community members' experiential knowledge, acknowledging the role of values in research, empowering community members, democratizing research inquiry, and enhancing the relevance of evaluation data for communities. These research traditions include action research (Lewin 1946, Argyris 1983), popular education (Freire 1970), grounded theory (Glaser and Strauss 1967, Strauss and Corbin 1990), naturalistic inquiry (Lincoln and Guba 1985), participatory research (Hall 1979, Tandon 1981), participatory action research (Fals-Borda and Rahman 1991), feminist research (Maguire 1987, 2001), popular epidemiology (Brown 1992, Wing 1998), community-based participatory research (Israel et al. 1998, Minkler and Wallerstein 2003), and empowerment evaluation (Fetterman et al. 1996).

Participatory action research (PAR) is the approach most influential in the development of participatory evaluation and involves a cyclical process of diagnosing, planning, and then taking action, evaluating outcomes, and identifying the learning that has occurred (Susman and Evered 1978). Like PAR, participatory evaluation involves oppressed people in studying and finding solutions to social problems. It gives the people most affected by the problems control over the evaluation, with the ultimate goal of transforming societal structures to benefit their community. Breaking up the paradigm in which participants are passive objects of study and researchers are the discoverers and creators of knowledge, participatory evaluation establishes a spirit of collaborative inquiry in which community members and evaluators work hand in hand. Participants collect and analyze data; and evaluators actively support planning, organizational development, and action (Cousins and Whitmore 1998, Springett, 2003, Fawcett et al. in press). Participatory evaluation democratizes evaluation by putting community members at the center of defining the evaluation agenda. Outside evaluators and local participants are on a more equal footing than they are in traditional evaluation (Fetterman et al. 1996). Participants help determine what kinds of questions are asked and what issues are investigated. Because local investigators are members of the community, they often have perspectives and experiences that can help shape the inquiry and interpret results (Hancock 1989). Participants' local expertise and contextualized knowledge can also contribute to the development of innovative methods. Evaluators are resources, allies, coaches, facilitators, and advocates, building capacity of local participants to perform credible evaluation. Optimally, both local and external participants are transformed in the process: skills and understanding are deepened; the balance of power shifts; and stronger ties, energy, and commitment are generated.

Like participatory action research and community-based participatory research (CBPR), participatory evaluation goes beyond collecting information and links knowing and doing through a cyclical process of investigation, education, and action. Once information is gathered, it is analyzed, fed back to the community, and applied to the program or organizing effort to improve effectiveness. Scarce resources can be targeted or redirected to strategies that work best. Professional and academic stakeholders can apply their expertise and connections to translate findings into policy or funding opportunities. More information is then gathered on the results of the actions. This process of critical reflection becomes self-generating and builds the capacity of communities for future problem solving, planning, action, and assessment. In this way, both the process and findings of participatory evaluation build community competence.

## A Framework for Using Participatory Evaluation

Participatory evaluation is more an approach than a methodology and uses a mix of both quantitative and qualitative methods along a continuum of degrees of community participation. Decision making remains a joint responsibility throughout the evaluation, although the level of participation of different stakeholders may differ at various stages in the evaluation. Evaluation design, process, and methods are guided by the key principles just described.

Several frameworks have been developed that lay out key steps in participatory evaluation (Fawcett et al. 1996, Springett 2003, Maltrud et al. 1997, Zukoski and Luluquisen 2002). The following eight-step process of participatory evaluation draws from key elements of these frameworks, focusing primarily on aspects that differ from traditional evaluation. Evaluators and community participants work collaboratively to define outcomes and measures, collect process and outcome data, and analyze findings. Regular collection, feedback, and interpretation of information throughout the organizing or initiative process enable participants to keep on track, adjust their course, see evidence of their progress, and report to funders and the community. The evaluation process itself is intended to transform participants and empower communities as co-creators of knowledge. Results are translated into actions, systems, and policies at multiple levels.

## STEP 1: JOINTLY IDENTIFY THE PURPOSE OF THE EVALUATION AND COMMIT TO PARTICIPATORY EVALUATION

Groups and organizations with a vested interest in the organizing effort determine the parameters of the evaluation, including what will be evaluated and the extent and type of stakeholder participation. Important considerations are the project's stage of development; whether or not there is a history of collaboration in the community; past experience with evaluation and participatory research; resources available for evaluation, including time, people, money, and skills; and resources needed such as training and outside expertise. Participants establish a set of guiding principles to facilitate the process (Israel et al. 1998, Wallerstein et al. 2002).

## STEP 2: BUILD AN EVALUATION TEAM

Collaborative partnerships require adequate time to establish and maintain relationships, build trust, and develop the means to understand differences and resolve conflicts. Laying the proper groundwork is critical to success, and there are three key tasks at this stage. First, formally identify who will be involved, the level and nature of participation expected, and what personal and institutional resources each partner brings to the table. Acknowledge existing power relationships and distribution of resources, a process essential to striving toward equity within the team.

Second, identify roles of participants, allowing that participation may change at different stages of evaluation as well as in response to changing conditions in organizations and the community. As already described, the roles of evaluator and community member differ significantly from those in traditional evaluation, and specific needs for training and knowledge are planned early in the evaluation. For example, outside evaluators and funders must gain a deep understanding of the community, context, and program (Wandersman et al. 2003). Community members may need knowledge of standards and methods in evaluation research.

Third, participants should engage their broader constituencies early on to build trust and ownership of the evaluation process, inspire confidence and vision, address concerns, and build a culture of transformatory evaluation and learning.

### STEP 3: CLEARLY ARTICULATE THE ORGANIZING EFFORT'S GOALS AND OBJECTIVES AND IDENTIFY INDICATORS OF CHANGE AND PROGRESS

Community projects are often implemented before assumptions, goals, and targets are clearly identified. In emancipatory participatory evaluation, the community decides what is to be evaluated and how. At this step, professional evaluators facilitate discussion to clarify the community's implicit theory underlying the effort (Weiss 1995). Objectives and evaluation criteria emerge from answering questions such as the following:

- What results would we like to see?
- How will we know if we achieve them?
- What level of change is desirable or acceptable?
- How will we know if we are making progress?
- What changes (intermediate outcomes) could serve as benchmarks or early markers of movement toward our goals?
- How will we assess our process and performance?
- How will we take into account the effects of environmental conditions outside our control?

Community organizing and community building efforts aim for change at multiple levels that may be difficult to specify or may emerge during the process. Include indicators of healthier environments, systems, or policies rather than focus solely on individual behavior change or long-term health outcomes typical of health education program planning models. Consider measures of collaboration (Sofaer 2001), empowerment and community control (Israel et al. 1994; see appendix 9), and community competence (Eng and Parker 1994, Aspen Institute 1996), consistent with the underlying premises of community organizing. Nina Wallerstein and her colleagues (2002) have developed a three-level framework for identifying process, people-population, and system indicators. Logic models linking actions to outcomes have gained increasing acceptance as a tool for program planning and evaluation and may be useful for community organizing (Milstein and Chapel 2002). Finally, there is a large body of practice on developing community-level indicators (see chapter 8).

## STEP 4: SELECT, DEVELOP, AND TEST METHODS FOR
## TRACKING PROGRESS AND DOCUMENTING CHANGE

The participatory evaluation team develops monitoring and evaluation systems that are realistic and make the best use of community resources while ensuring that results are valid and methods are free enough from bias to be credible to interested audiences. Identify methods that (1) are appropriate to the community and the issue, (2) build community competence through training and data sharing, (3) expand use of technology, and (4) are potentially sustainable. Take advantage of existing resources such as data collection by other CBPR projects or youth empowerment organizations (Community Network for Youth Development 1995).

There has been a rapid growth in creative participatory assessment and research techniques in the past decade, and ideas are widely available on the web and through publications (http://ctb.ke.edu, www.ids.ac.uk/ids/bokshop/briefs/brief12.html, www.dec.org/pdf_docs/pnabs539.pdf, Fetterman et al. 1996, Minkler and Wallerstein 2003).

## STEP 5: COLLECT DATA AND TRACK PROGRESS

Participatory evaluation involves community members to the extent feasible in documenting the organizing effort and its effects. Train selected evaluation team and other community members in data collection methods such as interviewing, conducting focus groups, or mapping communities (see chapter 9). Systems for recording activities and events as they unfold should be developed closely with those who will be using them. Consolidating efforts and information with partner organizations and others doing similar research, such as adding questions to an existing survey, can maximize existing resources, strengthen links among projects, and build ongoing community capacity to collect and use data (Zukoski and Luluquisen 2002). Technology, such as Internet-based supports (Fawcett et al. in press) or handheld computers for recording data in the field, can expand the community's ability to create and use knowledge.

## STEP 6: ANALYZE AND INTERPRET DATA COLLECTIVELY

Making sense of the data is a collaborative effort that combines technical expertise, experiential knowledge, and deep understanding of the community. Organize and integrate different types of data into a common body of information that participants can work with and discuss. Build consensus on findings and incorporate preliminary implications and recommendations with the results to set the stage for moving from knowledge to action. View results in the larger context, examining environmental factors that are out of the control of the initiative or organizing project. Frame findings in terms of community strengths rather than deficits.

STEP 7: COMMUNICATE RESULTS TO RELEVANT AUDIENCES

Unlike more conventional approaches, participatory evaluation communicates findings to key stakeholders as information emerges. Using evaluation data, engage participants and the community at large in reflection, interpretation of meaning, and problem solving to improve the project or take advantage of new opportunities. Share achievements as they occur to energize the community and build trust and commitment to the project. Support can be garnered from prospective funders, new constituencies, and neighboring communities.

Teamwork and mutual learning are critical. Professional evaluators share expertise in compiling and presenting data in both written and visual form, while community evaluation team members contribute expertise in communicating with diverse constituencies in understandable and meaningful ways. For sharing results, use creative media, such as a video, a calendar, or a poster; they get the word out more effectively than reports and presentations do alone. Data can be presented in terms of strengths and resilience rather than deficits. For example, in the Harlem Birth Project, team members presented data on percent employed rather than percent unemployed (Mullings and Wali 2001). Convey project outcomes to interested parties outside the community as well, thereby contributing to other empowerment efforts, building networks beyond the local level, and setting the agenda for future research and action. Professional evaluators take a more active role in helping communities effect social change by using their expertise and connections in academic, funding, and policy arenas.

### STEP 8: TRANSLATE FINDINGS INTO
### ACTIONS, SYSTEMS, OR POLICIES

Evaluation findings must be acted on to be useful to the community. In this step the group determines how to use the lessons learned to strengthen or expand organizing efforts, institutionalize changes, and plan future actions. Valuable information about how the process worked in relation to outcomes may lead the project to redefine objectives, adjust strategies, redirect scarce resources, or modify methods.

External evaluators use organizational development, facilitation, and training skills to help the project strengthen its leadership and structure, integrate evaluation into ongoing operations, and seek out new funding resources. Participatory evaluation is a process of learning, creating knowledge, and building relationships that is an important outcome in itself.

## Benefits of Participatory Evaluation

In addition to the benefits already described, participatory evaluation has the potential to advance the field of evaluation and increase its effectiveness. First, it can help overcome resistance to and suspicion of evaluation, demystify the process, and institutionalize evaluation methods in communities (Cousins and Whitmore 1998, Springett 2003). When the community shares ownership of goals, process, and skills, evaluation becomes an integral part of organizing for change. Being responsible for evaluation can also push an organization to examine its assumptions and make implicit theory explicit, thus contributing to the development of local theory.

Second, participatory evaluation can enhance the integration of qualitative and quantitative methods (Fawcett et al. 1996). Complex interventions such as community organizing efforts and broad-based health initiatives involve multiple factors. Integration of qualitative information with quantitative data on accomplishments can increase understanding of which factors contribute to the functioning of the initiative or organizing effort and in what ways.

Third, such evaluation can adapt, evolve, and invent evaluation methods, indicators, and instruments. Community participation in evaluation can be a rich source of innovation in the development of methods. For example, because associational networks play a crucial role in community organizing and other community-wide change efforts, participatory evaluation teams may develop better methods for measuring social networks and identifying both informal and formal community institutions and links (Hollister and Hill 1995).

Fourth, participatory evaluation can enhance the ability of communities to do systematic data collection (Hollister and Hill 1995). Participatory evaluation can provide an incentive for local organizations to maintain their records in relatively common formats so that records data can be pulled together to create a community data base. Community members of the evaluation team can gather new data of their own to give clout and credibility to advocacy efforts, using methods ranging from mapping conditions of the physical environment to conducting household surveys.

Fifth, participatory evaluation can creatively link community investigators and outside evaluators in a mutual learning partnership (Fawcett et al. 1996). Training, facilitation, and technical assistance enable community stakeholders to understand and apply evaluation methods within the field's standards for validity and rigor. The experiential wisdom of community leadership can ensure that evaluation questions are important, data collection methods realistic, and findings relevant and applicable within the local cultural context. Evaluators can help ensure that policymakers and other audiences hear community voices. Funders and institutional participants can gain deeper understanding of the critical role of the macrolevel context in the success of community efforts, influencing allocation of resources.

## Challenges of Using Participatory Evaluation

There are a number of philosophical and practical challenges to the emerging practice of participatory evaluation. First, as noted, participatory evaluation frameworks may conflict with traditional assumptions about objectivity and distance. Charges of bias, conflict of interest, and misuse can undermine the credibility of the evaluation, thereby lessening its clout. This may be particularly critical in policy and funding arenas. Yet even though the goal of any evaluation is usually improvement, what is not always clear is improvement for whom and at what price. Evaluation has never been neutral, and participatory evaluation simply makes explicit the importance of community self-determination.

Participatory evaluation must meet the field's standards for propriety and accuracy as well as utility and feasibility (Joint Committee on Educational Evaluation 1994). Evaluators can increase accuracy and propriety by exploring ways to minimize participant bias and including multiple methods, measures, and data sources in the evaluation design. Qualitative researchers have developed a number of strategies for addressing concerns of validity and reliability (see Fawcett et al. 1996, Hollister and Hill 1995, Brown 1995, Lincoln and Guba 1985).

Because of the paradigm shift that participatory evaluation involves, it can be challenging for traditional evaluators. As a process of co-discovery (Mayer 1996), it models the learning process and is quite fluid. Investigators must continually sample a changing environment and evaluate situations by degrees rather than as absolutes. Like grounded theory in qualitative methods (Glaser and Strauss 1967, Strauss and Corbin 1990), the logic is often drawn directly from the data.

Second, both professional evaluators and community members on the evaluation team must develop new skills and understanding for empowerment to occur. Outside evaluators must be able to work hands-on with community investigators in areas such as organizational development, program planning, implementation, grant writing, and advocacy. Community evaluators will need training in evaluation methods to ensure rigor. Group process skills such as team building, collaborative problem solving, negotiation, conflict resolution, and consensus building may not be part of the everyday repertoire of many community members or evaluators and must be learned. As Paul Light (2002) of the Brookings Institution has said, "We've got a bunch of evaluators who do program evaluation; we've got a very small number of evaluators who do capacity-building evaluation."

As outsiders, professional evaluators must be particularly sensitive to the history of the community, the local ethnic and political culture, and the aims of the project. They must be able to address power and resource differences openly; understand empowerment and collaboration as outcomes as well as processes; and talk with, not down to, the community. Above all, diverse players must operate under principles of ongoing mutual learning, collaboration, and respect.

Third, participatory evaluation takes a great deal of time, effort, and personal commitment, which both evaluators and community members may find difficult to make. They may feel that the process is diverting precious resources away from the "real work," be it the evaluation or the community organizing. Ironically, what to enthusiastic researchers may seem like an opportunity for capacity building may seem to participants like yet another unfunded mandate that places too much responsibility on the community for fixing a problem (Fetterman 1996, Israel et al. 1998). Evaluation must be feasible and practical, balancing the interests of both evaluators and community members.

Fourth, the greatest strength of this emerging approach is also one of its greatest hurdles: being responsive to rapid and unexpected shifts in program design and operation. To be effective, community organizing and community-based health initiatives must be flexible, developmental, and responsive to changing local needs and conditions (Brown 1995). This requires continual collection, description, reflection, and feedback of information about a group or an organization in all its complexity (and chaos). Besides being time-consuming, such a process conflicts with conventional notions of scientific rigor, which preclude constant tampering with the intervention.

A final challenge is related to indicators and measurement. Community organizing, community building, and comprehensive community initiatives typically address complex problems with multiple causes affecting different constituencies in interrelated ways. Traditional evaluation focuses on long-term changes in health or social indicators that go beyond project time frames and are difficult to assess. Participation, collaboration, empowerment, and community competence are challenging to conceptualize and measure as both process and outcomes (Israel et al. 1994, Eng and Parker 1994, Connell et al. 1995, Fulbright-Anderson et al. 1998, Parker et al. 2001, Wallerstein 2002; see appendix 9). Little is understood about the relationship between individual and community empowerment; and it is difficult to attribute empowerment outcomes to specific interventions, including participatory evaluation itself. Analysis at ecological levels or across levels is both conceptually and methodologically challenging.

## Conclusion

Participatory evaluation can be a powerful tool for community organizing efforts and community-based initiatives that have capacity building and social change as goals. The evaluation process itself can strengthen participation and ownership, build community competence, and reveal important outcomes that might be overlooked in conventional evaluations.

Participatory evaluation pays attention to the real voices of real people, demystifying and democratizing the process of developing knowledge. Working as a team, evaluators and community members learn from each other and increase their abilities to have an impact on conditions affecting the community. Participatory evaluation has the potential for transformation.

Finally, participatory evaluation is both an art and a science, requiring changes in philosophy and practice by professional evaluators, community investigators, and funders. It requires new skills, new relationships, and a fair amount of faith. Given the enormity of the problems facing impoverished and disenfranchised communities, it is an investment we need to make. Participatory evaluation can make an important contribution to building healthy, competent, and self-determined communities.

## References

Addams, J. 1907. *Social Ethics.* Cambridge, Mass.: Belknap.

Argyris, C. 1983. "Action Science and Intervention." *Journal of Applied Behavioral Science* 19, no. 2: 115–40.

Aspen Institute. 1996. *Measuring Community Capacity Building: A Workbook in Progress for Rural Communities.* Aspen, Colo.: Aspen Institute Rural Economic Policy Program.

Brown, Ph. 1992. "Popular Epidemiology and Toxic Waste Contamination: Lay and Professional Ways of Knowing." *Journal of Health and Social Behavior* 33, no. 3: 267–81.

Brown, Pr. 1995. "The Role of the Evaluator in Comprehensive Community Initiatives." In *New Approaches to Evaluating Community Initiatives: Concepts, Methods, and Contexts,* edited by J. P. Connell, A. C. Kubisch, L. B. Schorr, and C. J. Weiss, 201–25. Washington, D.C.: Aspen Institute.

Brunner, I., and A. Guzman. 1989. "Participatory Evaluation: A Tool to Assess Projects and Empower People." In *International Innovations in Evaluation Methodology,* edited by R. F. Conner and M. Hendricks, 9–17. San Francisco: Jossey-Bass.

Chesler, M. A. 1991. "Participatory Action Research with Self-Help Groups: An Alternative Paradigm for Inquiry and Action." *American Journal of Community Psychology* 19, no. 5: 757–68.

Clayson, Z., B. Weitzman, J. McGuire, and N. Freudenberg. 1995. "Politics of Community-Based Research: Accountability and Action." Workshop presented at the annual meeting of the American Public Health Association, San Diego, November.

Community Network for Youth Development. 1995. *Assessment and Evaluation That Empower.* Redwood City, Calif.: Community Network for Youth Development.

Connell, J. P., A. C. Kubisch, L. B. Schorr, and C. H. Weiss, eds. 1995. *New Approaches to Evaluating Community Initiatives.* Vol. 1, *Concepts, Methods, and Contexts.* Washington, D.C.: Aspen Institute.

Cousins, J. B., and E. Whitmore. 1998. "Framing Participatory Evaluation." In *Understanding and Practicing Participatory Evaluation,* edited by E. Whitmore, 5–23. San Francisco: Jossey-Bass.

Eng, E., and E. Parker. 1994. "Measuring Community Competence in the Mississippi Delta." *Health Education Quarterly* 21, no. 2: 199–220.

Fals-Borda, O., and M. A. Rahman, eds. 1991. *Action and Knowledge: Breaking the Monopoly with Participatory Action Research.* New York: Apex.

Fawcett, S. B., R. I. Boothroyd, J. A. Schultz, V. T. Francisco, V. Carson, and R. Bremby. In press. "Building Capacity for Participatory Evaluation within Community Initiatives." *Journal of Prevention and Intervention in the Community.*

Fawcett, S. B., A. Paine-Andrews, V. Francisco, J. Schultz, K. Richter, R. Lewis, K. Harris, E. Williams, J. Berkeley, C. Lopez, and J. Fisher. 1996. "Empowering Community

Health Initiatives through Evaluation." In *Empowerment Evaluation: Knowledge and Tools for Self-Assessment and Accountability*, edited by D. M. Fetterman, S. J. Kaftarian, and A. Wandersman, 161–87. Thousand Oaks, Calif.: Sage.

Fetterman, D. M. 1996. "Empowerment Evaluation: An Introduction to Theory and Practice." In *Empowerment Evaluation: Knowledge and Tools for Self-Assessment and Accountability*, edited by D. M. Fetterman, S. J. Kaftarian, and A. Wandersman, 3–46. Thousand Oaks, Calif.: Sage.

Fetterman, D. M., S. J. Kaftarian, and A. Wandersman, eds. 1996. *Empowerment Evaluation: Knowledge and Tools for Self-Assessment and Accountability*. Thousand Oaks, Calif.: Sage.

Fletcher, C. 1992. "Issues for Participatory Research in Europe." In *Participatory Research for Community Development: An Annotated Bibliography*, edited by H. Van Vlaederen. Grahamstown, South Africa: Rhodes University, Institute of Social and Economic Research.

Freire, P. 1970. *Pedagogy of the Oppressed*, translated by M. B. Ramos. New York: Seabury.

Fulbright-Anderson, K., A. C. Kubisch, and J. P. Connell. 1998. *New Approaches to Evaluating Community Initiatives*. Vol. 2, *Theory, Measurement, and Analysis*. Washington, D.C.: Aspen Institute.

Glaser, B. G., and A. L. Strauss. 1967. *The Discovery of Grounded Theory: Strategies for Qualitative Research*. Chicago: Aldine.

Green, L. W., and S. L. Mercer. 2001. "Can Public Health Researchers and Agencies Reconcile the Push from Funding Bodies and the Pull from Communities?" *American Journal of Public Health* 91, no. 12: 1926–29.

Greenwood D. J., W. F. Whyte, and I. Harkavy. 1993. "Participatory Action Research as a Process and as a Goal." *Human Relations* 46, no. 2: 175–91.

Hall, B. L. 1979. "Knowledge As a Commodity and Participatory Research." *Prospects* 9, no. 4: 4–20.

Hall, B. L., A. Gillette, and R. Tandon, eds. 1982. *Creating Knowledge: A Monopoly? Participatory Research in Development*. New Delhi, India: Society for Participatory Research in Asia.

Hancock, T. 1989. "Information for Health at the Local Level: Community Stories and Healthy City Indicators." Unpublished paper.

Hatch, J. 1993. "Community Research: Partnership in Black Communities." *American Journal of Preventive Medicine* 9, no. 6: 27–31.

Hollister, R. G., and J. Hill. 1995. "Problems in the Evaluation of Communitywide Initiatives." In *New Approaches to Evaluating Community Initiatives: Concepts, Methods, and Contexts*, edited by J. P. Connell, A. C. Kubisch, L. B. Schorr, and C. H. Weiss, 127–71. Washington, D.C.: Aspen Institute.

Israel, B. A., B. Checkoway, A. Schultz, and M. Zimmerman. 1994. "Health Education and Community Empowerment: Conceptualizing and Measuring Perceptions of Individual, Organizational, and Community Control." *Health Education Quarterly* 21, no. 2: 149–70.

Israel, B. A., A. Schulz, E. Parker, and A. Becker. 1998. "Review of Community-Based Research: Assessing Partnership Approaches to Improve Public Health." *Annual Review of Public Health* 19: 173–202.

James, S. A., A. Schulz, and J. van Olphen. 2001. "Social Capital, Poverty and Community Health: An Exploration of Linkages." In *Social Capital and Poor Communities*, edited by S. Saegert, J. P. Thompson, and M. R. Warren, 165–88. New York: Sage Foundation.

Joint Committee on Educational Evaluation. 1994. *The Program Evaluation Standards: How to Assess Evaluations of Educational Programs*. Thousand Oaks, Calif.: Sage.

Krieger, N., D. L. Rowley, A. A. Herman, B. Avery, and M. T. Phillips. 1993. "Racism, Sexism, and Social Class: Implications for Studies of Health, Disease, and Well-Being." *American Journal of Preventive Medicine* 9, supp. 6: 82–122.

Lewin, K. 1946. "Action Research and Minority Problems." *Journal of Social Issues* 2: 34–46.

Light, P. 2002. "A Conversation with Paul Light." *Evaluation Exchange, Harvard Family Research Project* 8, no. 2: 10–11.

Lincoln, Y., and E. Guba. 1985. *Naturalistic Inquiry.* Beverly Hills, Calif.: Sage.

Link, B. G., and J. C. Phelan. 1995. "Social Conditions As Fundamental Causes of Disease." *Journal of Health and Social Behavior* 35, extra issue: 80–94.

Magerison, C. J. 1987. "Integrating Action Research and Action Learning in Organizational Development." *Organizational Development*, pp. 88–91.

Maguire, P. 1987. *Doing Participatory Research: A Feminist Approach.* Amherst: University of Massachusetts, Center for International Education.

———. 2001. "Uneven Ground: Feminisms and Action Research." In *Handbook of Action Research: Participative Inquiry and Practice*, edited by P. Reason and H. Bradbury, 59–69. Thousand Oaks, Calif.: Sage.

Maltrud, K., M. Polacsek, and N. Wallerstein. 1997. *Participatory Evaluation Workbook for Community Initiatives.* Albuquerque: University of New Mexico, Masters Program in Public Health Education.

Mayer, S. E. 1996. "Building Community Capacity with Evaluation Activities That Empower." In *Empowerment Evaluation: Knowledge and Tools for Self-Assessment and Accountability*, edited by D. M. Fetterman, S. J. Kaftarian, and A. Wandersman. Thousand Oaks, Calif.: Sage.

Milstein, B., and T. Chapel. 2002. "Developing a Logic Model or Theory of Change. In *Community Tool Box.* http://ctb.ke.edu.

Minkler, M., A. G. Blackwell, M. Thompson, and H. Tamir. 2003. "Community-Based Participatory Research: Implications for Public Health Funding." *American Journal of Public Health* 93, no. 8: 1210–13.

Minkler, M., and N. Wallerstein, eds. 2003. *Community Based Participatory Research for Health.* San Francisco: Jossey-Bass.

Mullings, L., and A. Wali. 2001. *Stress and Resilience: The Social Context of Reproduction in Central Harlem.* New York: Kluwer Academic.

Parker, E. A., R. L. Lichtenstein, A. J. Schulz, B. A. Israel, M. A. Schork, K. J. Steinman, and S. A. James. 2001. "Disentangling Measures of Individual Perceptions of Community Social Dynamics: Results of a Community Survey." *Health Education and Behavior* 28, no. 4: 462–86.

Sofaer, S. 2001. *Working Together, Moving Ahead: A Manual to Support Effective Community Health Coalitions.* New York: Baruch College, School of Public Affairs.

Springett, J. 2003. "Issues in Participatory Evaluation." In *Community Based Participatory Research for Health*, edited by M. Minkler and N. Wallerstein, 263–88. San Francisco: Jossey-Bass.

Stack, C. B. 1974. *All Our Kin: Strategies for Survival in a Black Community.* New York: Harper and Row.

Strauss, A. L., and J. Corbin. 1990. *Basics of Qualitative Research: Grounded Theory Procedures and Techniques.* Newbury Park, Calif.: Sage.

Susman, G. F., and R. D. Evered. 1978. "An Assessment of the Scientific Merits of Action Research." *Administrative Science Quarterly* 23, no. 4: 582–603.

Tandon, R. 1981. "Participatory Research in the Empowerment of People." *Convergence* 24, no. 3: 20–29.

Wallerstein, N. 1992. "Powerlessness, Empowerment, and Health: Implications for Health Promotion Programs." *American Journal of Health Promotion* 6, no. 3: 197–205.

Wallerstein, N., M. Polascek, and K. Maltrud. 2002. "Participatory Evaluation Model for Coalitions: The Development of Systems Indicators." *Health Promotion Practice* 3, no. 3: 361–73.

Wandersman, A., D. C. Keener, J. Snell-Johns, R. L. Miller, P. Flahspohler, M. Livet-Dye, J. Mendez, T. Behrens, B. Bolson, and L. V. Robinson. 2003. "Participatory Evaluation: Principles and Action. In *Participatory Community Research: Theories and Methods in Action*, edited by L. A. Jason, C. B. Keys, Y. Suarez-Balcazar, R. R. Taylor, M. Davis, J. Durlack, and D. Isenberg. Washington, D.C.: American Psychological Association.

Weiss, C. H. 1995. "Nothing As Practical As Good Theory: Exploring Theory-Based Evaluation in Comprehensive Community Initiatives." In *New Approaches to Evaluating Community Initiatives: Concepts, Methods, and Contexts*, edited by J. P. Connell, A. C. Kubisch, L. B. Schorr, and C. H. Weiss, 65–92. Washington, D.C.: Aspen Institute.

Wing, S. 1998. "Whose Epidemiology, Whose Health?" *International Journal of Health Services* 28, no. 2: 241–52.

Zukoski, A., and M. Luluquisen. 2002. "Participatory Evaluation: What Is It? Why Do It? What Are the Challenges?" In *Community-Based Public Health Policy Practice*. Retrieved January 30, 2004. http://www.partnershipph.org/col4/policy/apr02.pdf.

KATHLEEN M. ROE
KEVIN ROE
CHRISTINA GOETTE CARPENTER
CINDY BERENSTEIN SIBLEY

Chapter 21

# Community Building through Empowering Evaluation

## A Case Study of Community Planning for HIV Prevention

Aʟᴍᴏsᴛ sɪxᴛʏ ʏᴇᴀʀs ᴀɢᴏ, poet Edna St. Vincent Millay (1988) wrote of the "dark hour" of her "gifted age." For many of us, the AIDS epidemic has been among the darkest hours of our time. Although we have made important strides, the global epidemic has nevertheless infected more than 42 million people (UNAIDS 2002). While AIDS in countries such as the United States has been transformed from an acute to a chronic disease, effective treatment remains beyond the reach of many people in this country and most people worldwide. More than two decades of loss, remembrance, research, and activism have made clear what we always knew: effective prevention must be community-based, ecologically dispersed, locally relevant, adequately funded, responsive to change, and sustained over time. Yet the complex epidemiology of HIV in the United States, the fiscal struggles of public health departments and community-based organizations, and the social barriers to frank discussion of drug use and sexual behaviors make effective primary prevention of HIV/AIDS uniquely and continually challenging.

Ten years into the U.S. epidemic, without a meaningful national prevention policy, the CDC mandated community planning for HIV prevention. This social planning initiative required that local groups work together to establish comprehensive, community-based HIV prevention plans. To support a federally mandated, locally implemented community planning process, the architects of the initiative drew from the tradition of citizen participation established in the 1960s; the multisectoral planning movement of the 1970s and 1980s, particularly Healthy Cities; and experience gained from substance abuse prevention community partnerships in the 1980s. The required outcome was the development

386

of five-year, evidence-based HIV prevention plans tailored to the needs, strengths, and resources of individual states and local communities. A decade later, community planning groups (CPGs) for both HIV prevention and health services are present in all fifty states, nine cities, and countless counties across the nation, albeit in a social, political, and epidemiological environment significantly different from that of the early 1990s. Although now institutionalized and considerably less novel than they used to be, CPGs, particularly prevention planning groups, continue to operate as uniquely inclusive vehicles for addressing prevention issues on a community level. As such, they retain an inherent potential for community building, enhancing community capacity and recommitment to participatory democracy.

This chapter describes community planning as a method of community organizing and demonstrates the ways in which an empowering approach to evaluation can enhance even a formal planning model's community building potential. Specific examples are drawn from our evaluations of five community planning efforts for HIV prevention and our long-term involvement with one group in particular. We conclude with a discussion of the challenges that arise at the juncture of social planning and community organizing, the varying roles and relative priority of community building at different points in the planning process, and some of the skills we drew on as we used evaluation as a community capacity–building tool.

## Community Organization through Social Planning

In January 1994, the CDC awarded sixty-five grants (to all fifty states as well as fifteen directly funded jurisdictions) for the specific purpose of creating community-wide planning processes for HIV prevention. The grants specified that recipients must seek significant and meaningful involvement of their communities in developing comprehensive five-year HIV prevention plans. The community plans would then form the basis of each jurisdiction's future cooperative agreement applications. With this initiative, sixty-five CPGs began operating across the United States.

The planning initiative was based on the conviction that a participatory process would offer the best means for making decisions about HIV prevention programming. As defined in the CDC's (1995) guide for planning grantees, community planning was to be an ongoing process in which public health agencies would share responsibility with community representatives, nongovernmental organizations, and other state and local agencies for identifying needs, determining priorities, and developing comprehensive HIV prevention plans. Community planning was envisioned as a new, ongoing process catalyzed by the 1994 planning grants and continuing in local areas as the prevention plans were implemented.

Grantees were allowed considerable flexibility in the design and operation of their planning groups. The CDC did, however, specify that all community planning efforts were to be evidence-based and encompass six core elements: (1) an epidemiological profile of HIV in the relevant service area, (2) an assessment of service needs for HIV prevention, (3) identification and prioritization of groups to be served, (4) development of criteria for selecting prevention strategies, (5) identification of prevention providers' technical assistance needs, and (6) evaluation of the community planning process. Some planning groups extended their mandate to include developing resource allocation protocols and monitoring implementation of the plans. Draft prevention plans were due nine months after funding began, with final plans due three months later. The high expectations and short time line generated considerable attention and organizing activity in communities and subcommunities around the country.

In an effort to guarantee meaningful community participation, CDC extended the traditional social planning framework by establishing requirements for the design and dynamics of the planning group. CPGs were to be organized around the principles of parity, inclusion, and representation. *Parity* was defined as an equal opportunity for input and participation and an equal vote in decision making among all members of the planning body. *Inclusion* was defined as meaningful representation and involvement of all affected communities. *Representation* required those who were nominated and selected to represent a specific affected community to reflect that community's values, norms, and behaviors. These terms were specified in the formal community planning guidance and described in detail in a user-friendly handbook (Academy for Educational Development 1995) made available to all grantees.

The specification of parity, inclusion, and representation immediately mobilized subcommunity organizing in several ways. Many organized internally to nominate members for the local planning body and sent additional members to observe the open planning meetings. Key subcommunities were contacted by early planning group leaders, who invited participation or sought guidance. In addition, many affected communities and stakeholder groups (that is, people with AIDS, youth advocates, sex industry workers, sero-dischordant or magnetic couples (in which one partner is HIV-positive and the other negative), immigrant rights activists, faith community leaders, and members of the activist group ACT-UP) organized for public comment and participation. Their involvement in hearings, focus groups, needs assessments, and subcommittees meant that diverse marginalized groups had a voice in the process. Once preliminary population and resource priorities were established, communities organized again to register their reactions and, if necessary, advocate for changes in the plans, priorities, or resource recommendations.

Within this flurry of overlapping, sometimes proactive, most often reactive community and subcommunity organizing were the planning participants—

typically a core council of fifteen to forty-five members representing the epidemic and key stakeholders; health department personnel who staffed the process; and, depending on local resources, consultants to support the planning process through specific facilitation, training, research, writing, or evaluation tasks. The centrality of parity, inclusion, and representation to the planning effort brought these players into unprecedented partnership. It also created a unique opportunity in many local states and areas for the development of a new community of HIV-prevention leaders with roots and influence in previously underrepresented communities.

As community planning got underway, most people acknowledged that the stakes were high. Many warned that community planning would be disastrous, bringing unequal players to an uneven table to participate, yet again, in pre-determined decision making about population priorities and woefully inadequate resources and furthering the divide among stakeholders. Others hoped that community planning might break new ground, stimulating community building and broader organizing and capacity development based on the unique intersection of shared task, heightened respect and camaraderie, skill building, broad networks, and sound decisions that could arise from these historic working groups. Tensions and enthusiasm ran high around both the group process and the scope of work. Recognizing the volatility and the potential of what had been catalyzed, CDC assigned high priority to a collaborative process evaluation of the community planning process.

## Evaluation as a Tool for Community Building

Our experience with community planning evaluation began with an invitation to serve as evaluators of a very large state planning effort. We immediately saw the opportunity for community impact and were intrigued by the challenge of finding an evaluation approach that would meet the core objectives while enhancing the community organizing and capacity building potential of the community planning initiative. Although standard social planning evaluation methods would have been sufficient to meet the contract requirements, we were committed to using the evaluation process to enhance and facilitate individual and community empowerment. Our health education training and a commitment to doing our part in the fight against AIDS led us to the approach now known as empowerment evaluation (Fetterman et al. 1996).

We actually backed into empowerment evaluation by embracing principles and methods based on respect, practical utility, and empowerment. We defined evaluation as a continuous, emergent process that creates reality (Guba and Lincoln 1989). While we endorsed the notion that evaluation can be a joyful and exhilarating process for all involved (Patton 2001), we were ever mindful of other ways in which evaluation has been experienced, including victimization (Butler 1992) and intellectual theft (Fleming 1992). If evaluation could create reality, then evaluation could certainly stimulate and nurture community. In this context, the ability of the evaluation process to foster community development and capacity depended on the empowering characteristics of the process.

We used these working definitions and our shared values as health educators to articulate a set of assumptions about evaluating community planning. First, evaluation should enhance the group's capacity for planning. Second, it would be done with people, not to them. Third, evaluation would never be mysterious. Fourth, goals, methods, and emerging findings would always be available to everyone involved. Fifth, our work would bring forward the voices of every person involved in community planning. Sixth, the methods and findings would be based on respect for the dignity and validity of multiple perspectives. We also agreed that one of the ways in which we could contribute to stopping the spread of AIDS, the ultimate goal of our evaluation, was by contributing to the development of a community of planning participants who would take their new insights and experiences back to the communities they represented, thus extending the impact of community building and capacity development achieved during the planning process.

Unaware as yet of the emerging model of empowerment evaluation, we chose an eclectic and ever-expanding tool kit of approaches and techniques to create what we called empowering evaluations of community planning. We used traditional evaluation methods, including triangulation of methods, pre- and post-testing, surveys, archival review, key contact interviews, and process monitoring. We experimented with less traditional methods, such as participant observation, training, coaching, and facilitating. We also imported methods from the principles of applied anthropology and qualitative research as well as from rapid rural appraisal (Schoonmaker-Freudenberger 1993), including offsetting of biases, triangulation of investigators, appropriate imprecision, and self-critical awareness and responsibility.

Together, these assumptions, principles, goals, and methods provided a fertile base from which to craft an empowering evaluation process, which we eventually applied to five different planning groups across a combined total of fourteen community planning years. Our evaluation designs were structured to incorporate new developments and emerging group dynamics. They were capable of identifying and illuminating significant moments and unanticipated outcomes of community planning for HIV prevention. Particularly in the early years, we watched evaluation stimulate and nurture community building among those at the planning table, enhancing their individual and collective capacities for the tasks at hand as well as their broader community organizing goals. Community planning helped us understand the profound power and potential of evaluation.

## Empowering Evaluation in Action

Our experiments with empowering evaluation strategies paralleled the emergence of the empowerment evaluation model (Fetterman 1996). The two broad goals of empowerment evaluation are (1) *illumination*, the ability to see things differently, and (2) *liberation*, the ability to act in new ways, free from previous constraints (Fetterman 1996). Although our own evaluation designs were not based on this model, they shared similar goals. The four development steps of the empowerment evaluation model (taking stock, setting goals, developing strategies, documenting the process) provide a useful framework for discussing some of the specific methods we used to stimulate community building through evaluation of a social planning process.

### STEP 1: TAKING STOCK

In the first step of empowerment evaluation, the evaluator helps program participants take stock of the status, resources, capacities, and challenges of the community, the staff, and the program. This type of preliminary analysis is familiar territory to social planning evaluators, whose traditional methods include review of an array of documents, including budgets, organizational charts, annual reports, previous assessments or plans, reports of previous planning efforts, and the requirements of the new planning initiative. These archival methods, possibly supplemented with observations or key contact interviews, provide useful, fact-based snapshots of the planning task at given points in time. Implications for community building or organizing can be drawn from these methods, but they are likely to provide little insight into the development of community identity or the nuances of emerging community capacity.

From an empowering perspective, taking stock is a process full of possibility. We saw opportunities to take stock repeatedly in evaluations of community planning for HIV prevention and to use both the process and the results to facilitate a sense of community among planning participants. Defining *community* as a group with shared identity and collective resources, our evaluation team looked for opportunities to expand the ways in which planning participants knew and thought about each other. Particularly in the formative stages of community planning, our goal was to enhance participants' immediate capacity for sound planning and their long-term enthusiasm for future community organization.

Planning meetings often begin with an icebreaker question, and the participants' responses are data for an empowerment-oriented process evaluator: "tell us about something you're really proud of," "the best part of your day so far," or even "your hair at sixteen." Such icebreakers provide glimpses of the history and experiences of individual members. Reframed as a collective set or organized by themes, these seemingly insignificant opening moments of a planning meeting vividly portray characteristics of an emerging community. Through focused survey and interview questions, we expanded our process evaluation to engage participants in additional ways of taking stock, including sharing their greatest personal challenges during community planning and their own contributions to the process, articulating their own experiences of community planning, and monitoring their own commitments to the planning process.

One of the most empowering ways of taking stock with newly formed groups was to assess background experiences. Process evaluators often use surveys of background experiences to take stock of the resources and potential needs of a group. When constructed and implemented with an eye to empowerment potential, these assessments can identify and validate an astonishingly wide range of assets and often surprising similarities and important differences among participants. We found that careful treatment of the resulting data can provide a particularly valuable resource for stimulating, fostering, or reinforcing community ties, particularly in new planning groups.

For example, one group quickly divided along lines separating researchers and community service providers, with a deepening gulf of misunderstanding and resentment between them. A sense of community among planning participants had never taken hold in this group. Indeed, participants were increasingly vested in and bitter about the differences they perceived among themselves. Some stopped attending meetings, others attended in increasingly bitter silence, and still others were frustrated and angry that all council members were "not actively participating" or "holding up their end."

The linear and incremental nature of planning enabled even a divided group to continue making task progress despite these process dynamics. But our evaluation team was concerned about the extended impact on future community building and organizing efforts that might result from entrenched alienation among people involved in HIV prevention in a relatively small geographic area. We wondered if process evaluation could help dissolve the barriers.

Strategic selection of questions to be included in an otherwise standard background experiences inventory enabled our team to show members of the group that, despite articulated differences in education, professional experience, status, recognition, agendas, culture, and values, and despite the broader dynamics of racism and sexism that they felt entrapped their interactions, planning group members shared something that had profound implications for each member's life course. What they shared was the experience of deep and personal losses to AIDS. In this 1995 planning group, everyone had lost someone to the epidemic. More than two-thirds reported "a lot" or "a great deal" of experience in losing not only acquaintances to AIDS but also colleagues, friends, and people they loved. Only three of the twenty-three who were surveyed reported just a few of these experiences to date, including the youngest member, who qualified many of his responses with a somber "not yet."

Strong communities know their history, understand how they are different from others, and find ways to honor their shared paths. Eliciting and sharing this type of evaluation data during planning or program work can help group members step back from the intensity of the tasks at hand and take stock of who they are and what they share. In the community planning groups for HIV prevention, the exercise frequently revealed previously unrecognized common history, which, in turn, fostered a positive identity grounded in broader shared experiences. Hard planning decisions with enormous community implications still had to be made, but the groups were better able to approach the tasks or reflect on the experience with the added asset of shared history.

### STEP 2: SETTING GOALS

In the second step of empowerment evaluation, the evaluator helps group members identify where they want to go and what kind of evaluation they want to create. This step represents a bit of a departure for traditional social planning evaluators, who most often inherit explicit, objective-driven evaluation requirements. Evaluators commonly request group discussion of core evaluation questions or the parameters of the inquiry, provide in-progress reports, or invite periodic feedback as ways of ensuring that at least key stakeholders are getting the kind of evaluation they want.

The community planning guidance provided by the CDC established core objectives and final outcomes for both planning and evaluation, but we saw community planning as much more. Although articulating shared vision or identifying broad organizing goals was not incorporated into the work plans of the groups we evaluated, our team felt that these activities, woven into process evaluation, might provide opportunities for community building and lay a foundation for later capacity development.

As planning groups formed, our team began listening for common vision and broad goals, making them explicit whenever possible. We felt strongly that hopeful communities are able to dream and are willing to share their visions and articulate what they want and do not want. The intense time pressures of the community planning assignment precluded lengthy group discussions of potential planning or evaluation goals. But we stretched our process evaluation to encompass an assessment of what people wanted and why, and we routinely re-presented the results to the group. Specific evaluation questions included asking individual members about their visions for an effective planning process; their understanding of the ultimate goals of community planning; and the goals for participation for themselves, their organizations, and the communities they represented. We also constantly revisited our own evaluation goals, both as a team and with planning participants, adjusting our activities as needed to better serve emerging group goals.

One of the most fruitful ways of eliciting unspoken goals was to listen carefully for personal dreams and perspectives shared during other evaluation moments. The empowering visions that brought individuals to the planning table and the dreams that kept them there, particularly in the turbulent formative stages of group development, were eloquent testimony to the commitment of community planning participants. When combined across common themes and re-presented to the group, the resonance among visions began to merge into the beginnings of group goals. Often, this was a seminal moment in community building.

We are not suggesting that common goals emerged easily. Indeed, the planning groups we have worked with often experience a tension between at least two competing visions of the community planning process. One vision, grounded in the assumptions and culture of service delivery, assumes that the primary task of community planning is to divide resources in the most rational, cost-effective manner. From this perspective, planning should proceed through objective, sequential deliberations governed by rules of order, time, and procedure. The short-term goal is sound decisions; the long-term goal is stopping the spread of HIV/AIDS within the existing service delivery structure. In the words of a CPG member, the broader goal of community planning is "finding a framework that will remove the politics and enable sound planning to proceed."

The other vision, grounded in advocacy, assumes that the primary task of community planning could be to radically change the way in which HIV/AIDS prevention is conceptualized. From this perspective, existing data are unreliable, old paradigms too narrow, and standard rules of time and order too controlling to address the urgency of the epidemic and draw out the diversity of voices and wisdom that must be brought into any real discussion about stopping the spread of AIDS. From this perspective, community planning is seen as calling on both heart and mind; and explicit, passionate values are an asset rather than a liability. "Getting professionals to act like advocates, with urgency and passion" was a typical goal from this perspective.

Although planning group facilitators never directly addressed the conflict-encounter between the two cultures, it was easy as evaluators to observe the two cultures as they met in the context of community planning. Standard evaluation protocol would require only that we monitor the influence of each in the unfolding process and outcome of the planning effort. We felt, however, that the unacknowledged coexistence of two compelling and competing perspectives created faultlines within the planning group that precluded the trust so necessary for the emergence of collective vision beyond the required core objectives. The group's ability to understand its internal differences and respectfully work with them was, to us, an important indicator of short- and long-term community capacity.

Careful participant observation enabled our evaluation team to sound out the depth and strength of the competing perspectives. Once we had a sense of the situated details of each, we were able to present the scenario to the planning group as a potential explanation for the recurring frustrations among members. We knew we had accurately captured the passions, motivations, and visions of each perspective when members saw themselves in one depiction ("They got that from me," members could be heard to say) and saw colleagues in a new light in the other ("That's how that feels?"). The illumination of these previously obscured perspectives led to group commitment to a broader goal of respectful engagement, a term introduced by a planning group member. This vision, shared by members from both perspectives, became a compass that the group could rely on as it wrestled with the often difficult analysis of priority needs and resource allocation for their community.

### STEP 3: DEVELOPING STRATEGIES

In the third step of empowerment evaluation, the evaluator works with the program group or staff to help them develop strategies to meet their goals based on information gathered through the evaluation. Again, this is familiar terrain for collaborative process evaluators, who might systematically monitor program objectives, administer formative surveys, analyze special initiatives, and provide in-progress reports and consultation to assist in the success of social planning efforts.

Involvement in strategy development is essential for evaluators working from an empowering perspective because it provides an opportunity to constantly infuse the effort with community and capacity building possibilities. A resilient community develops strategies, takes action, gauges reactions, and makes modifications in a constantly reflexive cycle. Empowered members know that their ideas are important and their experiences are valid, and they can see their contributions in the next round of innovation. As a result, we tailored all of our process evaluation queries to include opportunities for feedback and suggestions for change and made certain to attribute innovations and insight that led to new ways of thinking or working together.

One of the planning groups we worked with struggled with difficult group dynamics exacerbated by uneven facilitation and inexperienced staff. The project was underfunded to begin with and quickly over budget. Staff, consultants, and planning council members were chronically frustrated and behind. Our evaluation strategies stretched to include considerable staff and consultant coaching.

With a change of this magnitude in our role and influence, we had to ground our strategy recommendations in the experience of planning participants. A group that is floundering still has insight and ideas, but they emerge with less frequency as the collective spirit falters. Thus, one of our tasks became to look for, nurture, and sustain the group's wisdom and then anchor the eventual resolution of its processual problems in its own recommendations and capabilities.

This group's structural problems were so obvious and seemingly intractable that it was easy for group members to slide into a passive, resentful relationship with staff, consultants, and eventually each other. Our evaluation team addressed the structural issues through intensive individual coaching but also felt it was important to shift the group's focus from complaining about the problems and personalities to actively proposing and participating in realistic solutions. Toward that end, and in an effort to draw out the insight of individual participants, we added strategically selected and sequenced questions to the standard meeting evaluation survey. The new questions were designed to bring forward the broadest possible view of what was going wrong and generate a varied and grounded list of suggestions for change.

For example, our team actively worked against the trend of disengagement and disempowerment by asking participants to name the biggest hassle of community planning ("people that complain," "people who don't listen," "uneven workload") and identify what they particularly appreciated in each of the other players ("commitment," "hard work," "respect for differences"). We also invited each participant to specify something that he or she would like the other key players (council colleagues, consultants, staff, evaluators) to try ("be there when you say you're going to be there," "take care of more of the details before the meetings," "smile," "stop bickering," "stay focused"). Finally, we asked each participant to identify something he or she could do to help the group function more smoothly ("be more understanding," "listen," "be better prepared for meetings," "remember we're here to fight AIDS, not each other"). Our team collected and organized the written responses, forwarding the relevant set of uplifts and requests to each of the key players within a few days and presenting the full set of responses at the next council meeting. We also facilitated a lively and productive group discussion among meeting participants about hassles, uplifts, and ways of changing course.

This simple approach to diagnosing process problems and developing strategies provided a role for everyone and generated insight and ideas within the vocabulary and priorities of group members. Our team may have been able to help solve the worst of the organizational problems through coaching alone. But we felt that an empowering opportunity would be lost if we did not honor and amplify the self-correcting capacity of this fragile and troubled community. Indeed, by the end of the planning period, new and more productive group norms and relationships had emerged, with clear roots in the things that participants had offered to do and asked each other to try.

## STEP 4: DOCUMENTING THE PROCESS

The final step in the empowerment evaluation model is documenting the process. In this step, evaluators have the responsibility to keep a written record of what occurred and why in a format accessible to all interested parties. Evaluators of social planning projects invariably produce written documents, often supplemented by executive summaries and other abridged versions of key findings.

Documenting the process takes on additional dimensions when viewed from an empowering perspective. Our evaluation team found many ways in which the responsibility for documentation gave us opportunities for community building beyond the initial evaluation mandate. Based on our belief that evaluation should never be mysterious (see also chapter 20), for example, we regularly shared our methods, data, framework, and interpretations so that participants would know what we were doing, how, and why. We consciously modeled enthusiasm for evaluation, enjoyment of the many tasks it involved, and appreciation for the lessons in the data. We hoped that our love of what we do would encourage others to embrace and enjoy evaluation as well. We further hoped that our skills would be assumed and extended by those we worked with in their own community-based efforts beyond the community planning process.

In addition to generating required reports, our team regularly produced written summaries of evaluation feedback, which we distributed to all participants. We searched for a presentation style and a narrative voice that were both professional and accessible, adjusting fonts, titles, and layout to fit the tone of the different planning groups we worked with. All of our reports contained verbatim quotations from respondents, and we privately checked to make sure that something from every single participant was included. Our goal was to make our written documents inviting and interesting to read; we wanted them to validate lived experience and inspire continued community work.

An empowering approach to evaluation led our team to help groups monitor their own progress through the rocky and predictable challenges of community-based planning. Particularly in the early phases of community planning, we looked for opportunities to chart or support group progress through the goals and symbols indigenous to each individual CPG. Because much of the community planning vocabulary, time lines, and specific assignments was imposed on the groups from outside, we used evaluation surveys, discussion, and consultation to encourage participants to identify or recall their own fixed stars and milestones. This collective wisdom could then be used to reinvigorate a struggling process or document progress against landmarks familiar and meaningful to planning participants.

One of the most affirming examples of the empowering potential of collaborative evaluation occurred during one of the darkest moments of a community planning process. After working together for nearly a year, the planning group, on a three-day retreat, faced a crucial set of decisions with statewide implications. Behind-the-scenes maneuvering and miscommunication since the last meeting, combined with recent fracturing of long-standing alliances, had left group members suddenly wary, suspicious, and very angry with each other and the staff as they approached this watershed moment. As evaluators, we knew that a vote could proceed; but as community organizers, we knew that the conditions under which the decisions were about to be made were disempowering and dangerous to broader community building.

Using our standing invitation from the leaders to address the group at key process points, we asked the facilitators for time on the agenda before the vote was taken. Far from our offices but close to our voluminous portable files, we found some data we had collected after an icebreaker exercise nearly a year before. In this exercise, the facilitators had asked participants to write down and then share their personal mottoes or messages to the world. We had retrieved these data after they had been used and discarded, sensing that they might be important later. Using a laptop computer and the one copy store in town, we quickly compiled and organized these messages, printed them, and had them ready to distribute within an hour.

We used our time on the agenda to remind planning group members of the importance of the vote they were about to take and the historic progress they had made up to this moment. We then passed out the list of personal mottoes and messages and asked each participant to read aloud from the list as we went around the table:

> My friends are dying. . . . If we don't, who will? . . . One second at a
> time . . . Enjoy yourself; it's later than you think. . . . Be compassionate
> and kind towards each other. . . . Never lose your self-confidence. . . .
> Share your wealth. . . . Where will you be when they come for you? . . .
> Live in peace and be good to the earth. . . . Do something you'll be
> proud of. . . . It all pays the same. . . . Speak up; I can't hear you! . . .
> Never take a day for granted. . . . Never grow up. . . . Be kind, be
> flexible, be understanding. . . . Life is complex; being alive is simple. . . .
> Show up; tell the truth. . . . Faith is stepping out on nothing and
> believing until something is there. . . . Give back. . . . ¡Si, se puede! . . .
> Get over it; life goes on. . . . Protect our children. . . . Do what you can
> with where you are and what you have. . . . Live life like you mean it. . . .
> Never give up hope. . . . We've got to stop throwing each other away—
> each and every human being is valuable. . . . Adelante caminante. . . .
> If not now, when? . . . Keep moving forward. . . . We are one. . . .
> T-minus 50 cells and counting down. Kindly cooperate in stopping
> this disease.

The mood in the room shifted completely by the end of the reading. Although names were not attributed to individual members, everyone knew that the last message read had been written by a well-respected member who had died of AIDS just a few months before. Hearing his words and their own firmly rerooted the planning group in its collective wisdom. Once again mindful of shared commitments, group members were ready to vote with a unified spirit.

This example demonstrates what we have seen repeatedly in our work with community planning groups. An empowering approach to our evaluation tasks gave us insight and called us to action. Holding the group's records, caring about its progress, and watching for the empowering moment at every turn in the road provides opportunities to transform the potentially dry task of documenting the progress of social planning into a vibrant moment of community building and renewal.

## Combining Evaluation, Empowerment, and Community Building with Planning

Social planning and empowerment evaluation are not natural partners. Traditional social planning is about reform and system improvement; empowerment evaluation is about illumination and liberation. In our ten years of involvement with community planning for HIV prevention, we have found timing, context, and staff support to be crucial contributors to the success of the partnership.

### TIMING AND CONTEXT

Planning initiatives invariably struggle with rigorous time lines for needs assessment, data collection, strategy development, priority setting, decision making, and final reports. Widely held assumptions about sound planning further contribute to an environment of focused and linear deliberations. In most cases, evaluation is to be unobtrusive and follow the planning process rather than actively contribute to its direction, tone, and dynamics. Staff, other planning participants, and funders may not appreciate or desire evaluation methods with an expanded agenda.

During the past ten years, we have found that timing is critical. Participants are particularly eager for proactive, "transformative evaluation" (Cousins and Whitmore 1998) during the early stages of community planning. In the state and local groups we worked with, enthusiasm for evaluators as process stewards was high. Our contracts called for considerable staff and member involvement, including coaching, interviewing, and regular reporting. Role delineation was less of a concern from all parties than the widely shared commitment to breaking old barriers and establishing a new planning culture. We found that the exercises, discussions, and reflections that an empowering approach to process evaluation can elicit were particularly helpful when groups had an enthusiastic commitment to doing something new, doing it right, and making history.

As welcome as empowering evaluation approaches may be during the early stages of a planning process, we have found that evaluators need to be sensitive to changing priorities of the group or its leadership. As the planning process becomes an ongoing part of a community's HIV prevention infrastructure, its radical energy is invariably challenged by the calmer rhythm of institutionalized programs. We have learned, not always quickly enough, that the methods and demeanor of empowerment-oriented evaluators need to shift as a new initiative matures and changes. During this period, empowering methods and results are quieter, less obtrusive, and more carefully offered. First and foremost, evaluators need to be reflective and self-aware, able to shift gears gracefully and assist the group in meeting its planning objectives. At the same time, they must continue to nurture emerging community building skills or momentum. Institutionalized social planning may not be the center of transformative action; but it can be the context for new alliances, the emergence of common dreams, skill development and dissemination, and demystification of previous barriers to change. An empowering process evaluation is sensitive to the grand potential in even the quietest planning moments.

## STAFF SUPPORT

We have been extremely fortunate to work with staff who endorsed our approach to evaluation. Indeed, empowering evaluation is not possible without it. In the early days of community planning, our staff partners encouraged us to participate actively in a process that was new, highly visible, and extremely challenging for both the community and the health departments charged with implementation. We have worked with research and facilitation consultants who understood that they, too, were part of the process and, as such, were willing to be evaluated as part of our broadly cast inquiry. As HIV prevention planning has become routine in many communities, we have found that we need to be even more sensitive to the needs and experiences of the staff. Without the rush of early expectations and community interest, a truly inclusive, dynamic, and analytical community process can be difficult to sustain. As evaluators, our field of vision changes as the process and context change. During some periods, our focus has been the growth and development of the leadership; at other points, our priority has been staff support. These ways of working require a lighter touch and a less visible presence. They challenge but never obscure our commitment to empowering evaluation and our vision of the potential and importance of community planning.

## THE EMPOWERING EVALUATORS' SKILL SET

Although the HIV/AIDS epidemic has changed dramatically since CDC's 1994 community planning mandate, participatory process evaluation remains a valuable mechanism for nurturing and documenting the planning groups' progress and their outcomes. Our experience with very different community planning groups has led us to appreciate the specific skills and talents necessary for evaluating social planning from an empowering perspective. We close this chapter by offering our own priority list, knowing that other evaluators might draw on different skills or strategies to foster community empowerment through evaluation.

Evaluators who facilitate empowerment must have excellent traditional evaluation skills. Even though the underlying assumptions may be quite different from those of empowerment evaluation, traditional methods provide a kind of data and point of observation that can be usefully triangulated with other data and perspectives. Additionally, solid traditional skills enhance the credibility of evaluators who are about to stretch the purpose and scope of a planning evaluation.

We have also found that teamwork is best when planning is evaluated from an empowerment perspective. Although the lead evaluator remained the same on all five projects, a team was created for each site that reflected the diversity of planning participants. CDC guidance required planning groups to represent the diversity of the epidemic in the local area. We extended that requirement to our own team. As a result, our evaluators reflected the diversity of gender, race-ethnicity, sexual orientation, and HIV status of each group with which we worked. The multiple perspectives that we brought to our work greatly enhanced our ability to elicit sound data from participants and interpret what they offered.

Most important, empowering evaluation requires an additional set of professional skills. Evaluators must be flexible, quick-thinking, self-critical, optimistic, and truly interested in the groups they work with and the potential of community. Collecting this type of data requires the ability to engender trust, coax out stories, process qualitative information, and re-present heartfelt experiences, all within the more traditional framework of a social planning model. This takes time, energy, and a keen eye for the phrase or the moment that may move a group forward. Evaluators must have affection for the communities they work with while always maintaining an internal distance from which to observe process and explore empowering strategies.

Our community planning evaluations have validated our belief in the potential of collaborative evaluation to stimulate community development and capacity building. The formulation of the empowerment evaluation model and related participatory and capacity building evaluation approaches (Springett 2003, Stockdill et al. 2002; see also chapter 20) provide a welcome structure, rationale, and vocabulary for this kind of work. A product of this gifted age, participatory, empowering evaluation offers a sensitive and resonant framework within which evaluation can not only document but also stimulate and reinforce community building and community organization.

### Acknowledgments

We wish to thank the community planning participants we worked with on the evaluations referenced in this chapter—in particular, Tracey Packer, Valerie Rose, Steven Tierney, Wendy Hussey, Chata Ashley, Ellen Goldstein, Israel Nieves-Rivero, Gwen Smith, Lyn Paleo, Dara Coan, and Chuck Darrah.

### References

Academy for Educational Development. 1995. *Handbook for HIV Prevention Community Planning*. Washington, D.C.: Academy for Educational Development.

Butler, J. 1992. "Of Kindred Minds: The Ties That Bind." In *Cultural Competence for Evaluators: A Guide for Alcohol and Other Drug Abuse Prevention Practitioners Working with Ethnic/Racial Communities*, edited by M. I. Orlandi, 23–54. Rockville, Md.: U.S. Department of Health and Human Services.

Centers for Disease Control and Prevention (CDC). 1995. "Guidance for Community Planning Grantees." Unpublished document.

Cousins, J. B., and E. Whitmore. 1998. "Framing Participatory Evaluation." In *New Directions for Evaluation: Understanding and Practicing Participatory Evaluation*, edited by E. Whitmore, 5–23. San Francisco: Jossey-Bass.

Fetterman, D. M. 1996. "Empowerment Evaluation: An Introduction to Theory and Practice." In *Empowerment Evaluation: Knowledge and Tools for Self-Assessment and Accountability*, edited by D. M. Fetterman, S. J. Kaftarian, and A. Wandersman, 3–46. Thousand Oaks, Calif.: Sage.

Fetterman, D. M., S. J. Kaftarian, and A. Wandersman, eds. 1996. *Empowerment Evaluation: Knowledge and Tools for Self-Assessment and Accountability*. Thousand Oaks, Calif.: Sage.

Fleming, C. M. 1992. "American Indians and Alaska Natives: Changing Societies Past and Present." In *Cultural Competence for Evaluators: A Guide for Alcohol and Other Drug Abuse Prevention Practitioners Working with Ethnic/Racial Communities*, edited by M. I. Orlandi, 147–71. Rockville, Md.: U.S. Department of Health and Human Services.

Guba, E. G., and Y. S. Lincoln. 1989. *Fourth-Generation Evaluation*. Newbury Park, Calif.: Sage.

Millay, E.S.V. 1988. *Collected Sonnets of Edna St. Vincent Millay*. Revised and expanded edition. New York: Harper and Row.

Patton, M. Q. 2001. *Qualitative Evaluation and Research Methods*. 3d ed. Newbury Park, Calif.: Sage.

Schoonmaker-Freudenberger, K. 1993. "Rapid Rural Appraisal." Unpublished paper.

Springett, J. 2003. "Issues in Participatory Evaluation." In *Community Based Participatory Research for Health*, edited by M. Minkler and N. Wallerstein, 263–88. San Francisco: Jossey-Bass.

Stockdill, S. H., M. Baizerman, and D. W. Compton. 2002. "Toward a Definition of the ECB Process: A Conversation with the ECB Literature." In *New Directions in Evaluation*, vol. 93, 7–25. San Francisco: Jossey-Bass.

World Health Organization and Joint United Nations Program on HIV/AIDS (UNAIDS). 2002. Statement. Retrieved August 17, 2003. http://www.unaids.org/worldaidsday/2002/press/Epiupdate.html.

# Influencing Policy through Community Organizing and Media Advocacy

*Part IX*

WITH ITS EMPHASIS on community mobilization to bring about change, influencing the policy process would seem to be a logical area of concern for community organizers in fields such as health education and social welfare and the communities with which they are engaged. Yet for many community residents, policy seems to be abstract and confusing; and as Toby Citrin (2000) has pointed out, many professionals also shy away from policy advocacy, deeming it too time-consuming and risky. As a result, they may lose valuable opportunities for potentially influencing the lives of large numbers of people (Themba and Minkler 2003).

In part 9, we turn our attention to the often neglected area of policy and policy advocacy. In chapter 22, Angela Glover Blackwell, Meredith Minkler, and Mildred Thompson summarize Beaufort Longest's (2001) conceptual framework for understanding the U.S. policymaking process as well as the steps in the process that Alan Steckler and his colleagues (1987) delineate. The authors then elaborate on each step, paying particular attention to the roles that community organizations and their professional allies can play at different stages. The bulk of the chapter is devoted to four case studies, each of which demonstrates the powerful role that community organizing can play in advocating for policy enactment, change, or implementation. Two of the case studies specifically deal with youth: one illustrates their involvement in successfully crafting and advocating for anti-smoking ordinances in Minnesota; the other follows a strong cadre of youth leaders being trained to work for youth-driven, local and state policy change in New Mexico. Another case study looks at the work of Champaign County [Illinois] Health Care Consumers (CCHCC), a direct-action organizing project that creates citizens' task forces to deal with issues such as women's health and Medicare and then works for relevant policy change. Finally, the authors explore the work of West Harlem Environmental Action (WE ACT), which has fought to reduce bus-related pollution, joined partnerships to study community exposures and health outcomes such as asthma, and used the findings to influence policy. In conclusion, the chapter calls for the application of community building principles to policy design (see appendix 2) so that our policies reflect a commitment to high-level community participation and civic engagement.

Previous chapters have applied a variety of techniques and approaches to influencing policy, among them line activism (chapter 18) and photovoice (chapter 19). Chapter 23 describes and vividly demonstrates another tool with tremendous potential for community organizing: media advocacy. Written by Lawrence Wallack, who is widely regarded as the foremost architect of this approach, chapter 23 views media advocacy as rooted in the broader area of community advocacy. It defines *media advocacy* as "the strategic use of mass media to advance a social or public policy initiative." Whereas traditional media approaches try to fill the "knowledge gap," Wallack sees media advocacy as concerned instead with filling the power gap by highlighting alternative definitions of problems and policy-level approaches to solutions. Its strategies include working with community groups to harness the media's power to change the environment in which a problem occurs.

As Wallack suggests, communities of color and other groups have increasingly used media advocacy to transform how their issues and concerns are portrayed and handled by mass media. By shifting the focus from the personal to the social and from individual behavior to the policy and environmental contexts that shape individual behavior, media advocacy demonstrates immense potential for community organizing and social change.

## References

Citrin, T. 2000. "Policy Issues in a Community-Based Approach." In *Community-Based Public Health: A Partnership Model*, edited by T. A. Bruce and S. Uranga McKane, 83–90. Washington, D.C.: American Public Health Association.

Longest, B. B. 2001. "The Process of Public Policy Making: A Conceptual Model." In *The Nation's Health*, 6th ed., edited by P. R. Lee and C. L. Estes, 109–15. Sudbury, Mass.: Jones and Bartlett.

Themba, M. N., and M. Minkler. 2003. "Influencing Policy through Community Based Participatory Research." In *Community Based Participatory Research*, edited by M. Minkler and N. Wallerstein, 349–70. San Francisco: Jossey-Bass.

Steckler, A., L. Dawson, R. M. Goodman, and N. Epstein. 1987. "Policy Advocacy: Three Merging Roles for Health Education." In *Advances in Health Education and Promotion*, edited by W. B. Ward, 2:5–27. Greenwich, Conn.: JAI.

ANGELA GLOVER BLACKWELL
MEREDITH MINKLER
MILDRED THOMPSON

# Using Community Organizing and Community Building to Influence Policy

*Chapter 22*

COMMUNITY ORGANIZING and community building in health and related fields are committed to action and social change. Although such action may take many forms, community builders and organizers are increasingly turning to policy approaches as potent ways to affect the health and well-being of communities.

The rationale for an emphasis on policy has been well documented. Throughout the past century, dramatic declines in U.S. mortality rates can be attributed in large part to policy-related changes in sanitation, water supply, and food quality (McKinlay and McKinlay 1977, Brownson et al. 1997). More recently, community organizing and the subsequent development of social movements surrounding issues such as women's health, HIV/AIDS, and environmental justice have played a crucial role in changing policies on local and national levels. Successful efforts to ban smoking in public places and to curb the sale of hand guns, the fast tracking of new drugs for the treatment of HIV/AIDS, the enactment of legislation (albeit inadequate) to clean up toxic waste, and new federal policies mandating a far greater emphasis on women's health issues are among the many policy-related victories rooted in local community organizing and community building efforts. On a global level, the Healthy Cities/Healthy Communities movement has, since its inception, focused on broad policy-level changes as a way to help communities realize their visions of healthy places in which to live (Brownson et al. 1997; see also chapter 8).

For many community residents, however, "public policy has become unfamiliar and irrelevant, complicated, inaccessible and confusing" (Blackwell and Colmenar 2000, 162). And even those who believe in the importance of public policy often feel unable to influence major decisions affecting their lives. Similarly, professionals in health, social welfare, and related fields who work on the community level sometimes have been reluctant to focus on policy-related activity, which in their eyes takes place primarily "out there" on the state and national levels, far removed from day-to-day community organizing efforts (Themba and Minkler 2003).

As this and other chapters suggest, however, health professionals and their community partners, as well as policymakers themselves, are beginning to recognize that community organizing and community building are critical strategies for influencing healthy public policy. Indeed, as Angela Glover Blackwell and Raymond Colmenar (2000) point out, "If community building principles are fully embraced, policy making itself becomes a community building process because community residents will be involved in every step, from framing the issues to interpreting the data and discussing the options" (163).

We begin this chapter by offering a conceptual framework for understanding policy and policy advocacy from a community organizing and community building perspective, including a look at the key steps involved in the process. We then offer several examples from around the United States to demonstrate some of the many ways in which local community organizing and community building efforts have worked to influence the policymaking process. We conclude by broadening our gaze to examine how the application of community building and community organizing principles can make a difference in policy design. Using as a model the Federal Healthy Start Program to reduce infant mortality, we suggest that large-scale policy initiatives that build on lessons from day-to-day community work and incorporate community involvement and community building in their design and implementation can make a real difference in eliminating health disparities and growing healthy communities and a healthier, more just society in the twenty-first century.

## Conceptual Framework

For the purposes of this chapter, *policies* are defined as "those laws, regulations, formal and informal rules and understandings that are adopted on a collective basis to guide individual and collective behavior" (Schmid et al. 1995, 1207).

From the vantage point of health, "The intent is to achieve a more acceptable state of affairs and, from a public health perspective, a more health-promoting society" (Milio 1998, 15).

Many models of the policymaking process are relevant to community organizing and community building (see, for example, Brownson et al. 1997, Longest 1998, Milio 1998, Steckler et al. 1987). Most of these models emphasize the cyclical nature of the process; its sociopolitical contexts; and a series of steps through which the process typically progresses, albeit with many loops and detours along the way (Milio 1998, Themba and Minkler 2003). Finally, models of the policy-making process often stress a "window of opportunity [that] opens when there is a favorable confluence of problems, possible solutions, and political circum-stances" (Longest 1998, 110).

In this chapter, we use a conceptual framework drawn from both Alan Steck-ler and his colleagues' (1987) model of the policymaking process and Makani Themba's (1999) suggested roles for advocates and organizers at each stage:

- *Problem awareness and identification.* Policymakers and advocates interested in influencing policy identify problems or issues to be addressed in future legislation. Advocates and community organizers test the waters at this stage, working with community members and conducting research to identify a shared problem or vision.
- *Problem refinement.* Participants hone these problems or issues and choose priorities. Community input and organizing opportunities help shape the problem-refining process.
- *Policy objectives.* Clear policy objectives are identified based on the problem reframing process. A SWOT analysis may be conducted to help community members visualize the strengths and weaknesses internal to their case and the opportunities in and threats from the larger environment (Barry 1997).
- *Alternative courses of action.* In this "marketplace stage," participants discuss competing interests and compromises. Advocates, organizers, and community members assess the likelihood of winning with their initial proposal and discuss necessary alternatives.
- *Consequences of alternative actions.* Participants discuss competing policies, their content, implementation processes, and funding levels. Advocates and organizers often must compromise at this stage, negotiating about specifics while maintaining community priorities.
- *Victory and defense.* Although they are not typically listed in policy process models, community celebrations of victories and attaining media exposure for these wins are important parts of the process from a community organizing and community building perspective. At the same time, however, participants must anticipate and prepare for legal and other challenges (Themba 1999).
- *Implementation responsibility.* Decision makers identify the agency or unit with responsibility (and ideally the resources) for implementation; community groups work to ensure that enforcement takes place and that oversight mechanisms are in place.
- *Evaluation.* Formal mechanisms assess policy impact and outcomes. Ideally, from a community building and community organizing perspective, participatory evaluation (Maltrud et al. 1997) is used throughout the process to enable community members to play active roles in evaluation (see chapters 20 and 21).

As suggested, this process is dynamic and frequently circuitous rather than strictly linear. Further, we should not underestimate the often substantial role of private interest groups and political considerations. Almost a century ago, Honoré Mirabeau warned, "Laws are like sausages. You should never watch them being made." Yet despite its messiness, involvement in policymaking is increasingly important for those concerned with community building and improving public health, as the following case studies demonstrate.

## Case Examples

### ORGANIZING TO CHANGE POLICIES THAT SUPPORT ENVIRONMENTAL RACISM IN HARLEM

The asthma morbidity and mortality rates in New York City's Northern Manhattan neighborhoods are among the highest in the nation; recent studies find that one-quarter of central Harlem children are afflicted (Perez-Pena 2003, Shepard 2000). Compounding the problem, the air quality of Northern Manhattan (comprised of East, West, and Central Harlem and Washington Heights) has historically been degraded by pollution. The area houses one-third of New York City's 4,200 diesel bus fleet as well as the Port Authority's 650 diesel buses; and numbers of them idle on streets, in depots, and in makeshift parking lots—a situation that residents and researchers have long suspected to be related to the area's high asthma rates (Shepard 2000). The neighborhoods are home to more than 600,000 African American and Latino residents who, in addition to the buses, share 7.4 square miles with two sewage treatment plants, two hundred sanitation trucks that line up to dump garbage for barging, and 75 million truck crossings per year on two heavily trafficked bridges and highways, thus compounding an already bad situation (Shepard 2000).

Founded in 1988 to improve environmental health and protection and secure environmental justice in communities of color, West Harlem Environmental Action (WE ACT) has been a key community-based player in the fight to reduce bus-related pollution through use of alternative fuels. It has also formed partnerships with Harlem Hospital and Columbia University's Mailman School of Public Health to (1) study the relationship between community-level environmental exposures and environmental health outcomes and (2) translate those findings into policy changes that create equity in environmental decision making and environmental protection. Having defined one problem as excessive exposure to diesel fumes (which the U.S. Environmental Protection Agency [EPA] considers carcinogenic), WE ACT began organizing and educating community residents and policymakers through a broad-based public awareness campaign using the motto "If You Live Uptown, Breathe at Your Own Risk," which appeared in seventy-five bilingual bus shelter ads as well as on posters and buttons and in 15,000 brochures.

The organization then moved to the setting of a policy objective and the selection of a strategy for achieving it. Consistent with Themba's (1999) reminder to begin by identifying the individuals or institutions with the power to solve or ameliorate the problem and address the community's demands, WE ACT began by targeting government entities with the power to make relevant policy change: the Metropolitan Transit Authority (MTA), the governor, and a state legislative oversight committee. Because WE ACT's repeated efforts to meet and negotiate with MTA were unsuccessful, the group and its environmental allies focused on persuading the governor and the legislative oversight committee to purchase three hundred natural-gas buses and convert the largest depot in Northern Manhattan to natural gas. Residents signed and sent thousands of post-cards to the governor and MTA's chair. But years of budget cuts and MTA's decision to pursue hybrid diesel technology interfered with any commitment to natural gas. Thus, WE ACT needed to think creatively about yet more alternative approaches.

As Themba (1999) has pointed out, well-framed legal actions, such as law-suits and other court actions, may be risky and time-consuming; but they should not be ignored as a policy strategy, particularly if other approaches are unsuccessful (also see Themba and Minkler 2003). When they failed to convince the governor to take their concerns seriously, WE ACT and its partners decided to go through legal channels. With two civil rights attorneys, they filed a formal complaint with the U.S. Department of Transportation under Title VI of the Civil Rights Act, which bars federal funding of any program that discriminates on the basis of race. Plaintiffs alleged that locating six diesel bus depots and parking lots in a geographic area largely comprised of communities of color was excessive and unfair and effectively used the Civil Rights Act to bolster their case (Shepard 2000, Thompson et al., 2002) As of this writing, the case is still pending, although Congressman Charles Rangel has sent a letter of consternation to the secretary of transportation. That letter appears to have jolted MTA into playing a bus shell game: they made plans to close a depot downtown to make way for a park, reopen a rebuilt depot in East Harlem, and close one in West Harlem, all on the same day in the fall of 2003! (personal communication, Peggy Shepard, August 4, 2003).

Meanwhile, WE ACT and its community partners have followed other avenues, strengthening their arguments by collecting air-quality data in affected neighborhoods. WE ACT staff members recruited and trained local youth to collect and test these air samples. Involving youth in this phase of the process was particularly effective: the teenagers wore air monitors to school to collect samples on busy thoroughfares, and their participation in the data collection process brought additional media attention to the issue (see http://www.weact.org).

Successful policy advocacy often involves enlisting the support of new allies. In addition to gaining strong local media coverage, WE ACT found a critical ally in the EPA, which was convinced to conduct air quality tests of its own. When these studies showed the existence of fine particulates in the air exceeding proposed federal standards by more than 200 percent, advocates had a powerful new piece of ammunition; and the EPA bolstered its promulgation of a new fine-particulate standard, which is now being phased in. A co-chair of the Northeast Environmental Justice Network, WE ACT mobilized network members to come to New York to testify at the EPA's regional hearing on the standard, which, though hotly contested by industry, has finally withstood all legal appeals.

This combination of strategies may prove to be effective. In addition to the complaint filing, the EPA data, and a newly adopted New York State environmental justice policy that WE ACT helped initiate, WE ACT's partners at the Columbia Children's Environmental Health Center have recently found that pollutants in diesel are causing low birth weight and small head size in African American children in northern Manhattan (Perera et al. 2003). Along with consistent, high-level resident mobilization around this issue and visibility in local media, these strategies and findings suggest that Northern Manhattan neighborhoods may finally be poised for real change.

## CHAMPAIGN, ILLINOIS'S, CONSUMER ORGANIZING
## FOR IMPROVED HEALTH CARE ACCESS

Because more than 40 million Americans are now uninsured (CDC 2002), community groups around the nation and their professional allies in the health professions have mobilized to help change this situation. Key among them is the Illinois-based group known as Champaign County Health Care Consumers (CCHCC), also known simply as Health Care Consumers. CCHCC is a grassroots, nonprofit organization founded on the belief that access to health care is a basic human right and must be accompanied by a recognized right to a decent standard of living and a safe community in which to live. Central to CCHCC's mission and organizing work is the conviction that "meaningful reforms in the health care system will only come with the active involvement of consumers," and coalition building has been a key strategy in its work (http://www.prairenet. org/cchcc/mision.html).

Health Care Consumers uses a direct-action organizing approach (see chapters 3 and 11) to give people a sense of their own power to make change, help them win concrete victories, and alter power relations in communities. As community members bring new issues to CCHCC's attention through either its hotline or its board of directors, the organization sets up citizen task forces to help bring about needed policy change.

Health Care Consumers was instrumental in establishing the Women's Health Task Force (WHTF), a coalition comprised of health care, labor, and women's organizations. Among WHTF's early policy objectives was expanding employer health insurance coverage to include contraceptive care. Consistent with Saul Alinsky's (1972) admonition to choose a target that is visible, local, and capable of responding, the coalition decided to press one of the county's largest employers, the University of Illinois, to include contraceptives under its employee insurance plans (http://www.prairenet.org/cchcc/whtf.htm).

Like WE ACT, WHTF's policy efforts received an early boost from federal civil rights legislation (Title VII of the Civil Rights Act), which in this instance was used to support the argument that employers who failed to provide contraceptive coverage were guilty of gender discrimination. Rather than file a lawsuit, however, WHTF used direct-action strategies to organize hundreds of employees and dozens of organizations, who in turn contacted the university chancellor or signed petitions indicating their support of this policy change. The task force also garnered considerable media coverage. In response, the chancellor agreed to meet with the task force and begin providing contraceptives to thousands of employees through the university health center.

Although WHTF had won a significant victory, and one that merited celebration (Themba 1999), their success was only partial because the university stopped short of including contraceptives in employees' health insurance plans. Therefore, WHTF has moved into the next phase of its campaign, marshalling evidence to help them achieve their broader policy objective—for example, demonstrating that the $1.43 contraceptive price tag per woman per month is far less than the cost of paying for unwanted pregnancies (http://www.prairenet.org/cchcc/whtf.htm). As in the previous campaign, an emphasis on consumer involvement in the process and on giving community members a sense of their own power rather than simply advocating for change on their behalf remains a core organizing principle behind this and related work.

## ORGANIZING TO ENACT ORDINANCES IN MINNESOTA CURBING YOUTH ACCESS TO TOBACCO

Therese Blaine and her colleagues (1997) have detailed the development and implementation of a project in seven Minnesota communities known as Tobacco Policy Options for Prevention (TPOP), giving us a particularly clear account of the use of direct-action organizing to achieve the passage and enforcement of a healthy public policy initiative. Part of a broader action research study, this ambitious effort followed the steps in the policymaking process that we have already listed, beginning with extensive information gathering and efforts to raise community awareness of the issue through multiple channels. In each of the seven communities, local organizing teams conducted one-on-one interviews with an average of nearly one hundred residents and other stakeholders. The teams were made up of teens, educators, and others in the neighborhood with a personal commitment to both the issue of tobacco access and the use of policy approaches to address the problem. In addition to building a broad base of relationships, these initial interviews were designed to uncover needed information about socioeconomics and power relationships in each community (Blaine et al. 1997).

To build their capacity for active involvement in the community awareness phase of the campaign, TPOP team members received training in group work, strategic planning, tactical decision making, teen advocacy, and the role of data in the policymaking process. Through presentations to civic, professional, and community groups and a variety of youth-focused activities, such as tobacco forums and poster contests, they considerably broadened their base of support. Local underaged youth also were engaged in a critical data-gathering phase of the project: they attempted to buy cigarettes from local merchants and reported their results. This effort served multiple purposes—for example, providing graphic evidence of the problem for use in media advocacy and testimonials and countering the claims of many local merchants that their stores did not sell to minors (Blaine et al. 1997).

In each community, the policy teams then moved toward crafting a tobacco control ordinance. Following the Alinsky (1972) dictum to do your homework by finding out what other communities have done, TPOP members collected and studied model youth access ordinances and used them to fashion ordinances that might have the best chances for success in their own local social, economic, and political landscapes. They also met with local political figures, city attorneys, and other key stakeholders to garner early support for the proposed initiatives (Blaine et al. 1997).

Team members worked to frame their message for the local media, practiced countering opposing arguments, and built a large and vocal base of support for upcoming city council hearings. In light of the policymaking importance of understanding and potentially negotiating with those who hold alternative positions, TPOP members also met with local merchants to assess their beliefs about youth tobacco sales, determine their receptivity to change, and identify those likely to strongly oppose the proposed legislation. Finally, targeted mass mailings, strategic use of radio and newspaper coverage, and another round of meetings with city council members and other key stakeholders shored up support for the ordinances.

As a result of this painstaking approach to policy advocacy, coupled with the window of opportunity opened by growing anti-tobacco sentiment in the 1990s, each of the seven communities successfully passed a youth tobacco prevention ordinance. In every case, advocates made minor compromises in the initial proposal during the hearing phase, largely to decrease merchant opposition; but in no case was the crux of the ordinance seriously compromised.

A critical and sometimes forgotten role for organizers in the policymaking process involves working "to ensure that their hard won legislation is enforced, and that there are mechanisms for oversight" (Themba and Minkler 2003). Although three of the communities had strong law enforcement commitment to compliance and other efforts to ensure oversight, the remaining four were less fortunate. In these communities, the TPOP team continued to engage decision makers and to apply local pressure to ensure that compliance was in fact checked. Finally, in keeping with the organizing dictum that each issue campaign should be part of a larger overall mission or agenda, TPOP's victories with the local ordinance campaigns were seen as paving the way for subsequent related work in their communities (Blaine et al. 1997).

## BUILDING YOUTH CAPACITY TO ORGANIZE
## FOR POLICY CHANGE IN NEW MEXICO

In the Minnesota case study just described, community organizers and community builders provided training and capacity building for community members involved in organizing for policy change. All too often, however, community members are asked to turn out for rallies or city council meetings, conduct door-to-door canvassing, or gather petition signatures without having learned to develop the tools they need to truly understand the policymaking process.

New Mexico's Youth Link is a statewide effort to build a strong cadre of youth leaders who can be actively involved in making youth-driven policy change on local and state levels. According to consultant Nina Wallerstein (2002), the mission of this ambitious project is "to create opportunities for youth, who are traditionally disenfranchised, to organize with adult support so that their voices, their needs and their strengths will be heard by policy makers" (75).

Youth Link's primary mechanism of action has been the Community Action Teams (CATs) that operate throughout the state and are comprised of both youth (ages twelve and up) and adults concerned about developing action plans and policies to address community-identified needs. Although the fourteen CATs initially limited their work to local activities, such as decreasing underaged drinking and creating meeting places for teens in rural areas, preparation for a statewide youth town hall meeting helped young people recalibrate their dreams to include true state-level policy activity.

Through focus groups held around the state, youth brought to the surface a number of collective concerns for the town hall meeting, among them violence, substance abuse, teen pregnancy, and school-related issues. Nearly 150 youth and 20 adults then came together during the three-day meeting to translate these concerns into concrete principles and corresponding policy suggestions, including the following (Wallerstein 2002):

• Youth representation on school boards and implementation of
  in-school suspensions to combat dropout problems

- Reality-based sex education and school distribution of condoms, particularly in rural areas, to combat teen pregnancy
- Increased youth activities, drug-free safe places, more jobs for youth, and increased outreach to former youth gang members to curb violence and crime
- Lowering the voting age to sixteen to demonstrate respect for youth and increase their involvement in decision making

To translate such recommendations into action, several CATs developed study bills (memorials) for the state legislature, requesting, for example, the state departments of health and education to study the relationship between school sex education and teen pregnancy rates as well as alternatives to student expulsion and suspension. As Themba (1999) has pointed out, formally calling for such studies can itself be a powerful policy tool, drawing attention to an issue and proposed means of addressing it and catalyzing future action.

Youth Link's voice was heard. The state legislature called for a memorial to study suspension and expulsion policies and their effects on dropout rates and the like and charged the Legislative Education Study Committee to undertake this research. Although a report with recommendations for action was completed in 2000–2001, lack of political will has thus far prevented follow-up.

Because of a move from foundation funding to state prevention grants, Youth Link recently circumscribed its advocacy activities. Although state grants do allow for work in advocacy and legislative education, their categorical mandate limits this work to particular areas such as tobacco and alcohol, preventing critical follow-up on some of the concerns previously identified by Youth Link leaders and participants. Yet even within these narrower parameters, the organization has been effective in achieving a number of policy victories. Ninety youth throughout New Mexico joined adult coalition members on a visit to the state capital, where they educated legislators on the need for continued funding of youth prevention projects through tobacco settlement monies. Although the state had been seriously considering major budget cuts to transfer money into other areas, it maintained its prior funding level for youth-focused prevention programs; and Youth Link participants were credited with having played a major role in the legislature's decision (personal communication, Stephanie Gabriel, Youth Link project director, June 17, 2003).

Youth Link has also achieved local victories. Young people in both Albuquerque and Santa Fe joined adult coalitions to help secure the passage of citywide smoke-free ordinances, and in Santa Fe they played a key role in passing an ordinance on tobacco product placement.

Another important outcome of Youth Link's seven years of organizing and advocacy has been an increased sense of collective efficacy (Bandura 1997) and per-

ceived control among young people. As focus groups and the project's formal evaluation have suggested (Wallerstein et al. 2000), youths' honing of skills in critical analysis and participation in developing youth bills, delivering testimony, and
related activities appear to have contributed to the development of a cadre of young
people prepared to engage actively in the policymaking process. Further, as project director Stephanie Gabriel points out, adult advocates and policymakers in
the state increasingly see Youth Link as not simply a voice for youth but a full partner in efforts to promote healthy and youth-focused public policy (personal communication, June 17, 2003).

## The Next Step: Grounding Public Policy in Community Organizing and Community Building

As this chapter has shown, community organizing and community building strategies can help us achieve a wide array of healthy public policies. These efforts are
critical and offer an important counter to weakened forms of civic engagement
that are part of our social landscape (Putnam 2000). But for community building
and community organizing to reach their full potential in a democratic society,
policymaking must itself be transformed so that local residents are involved in every
stage of the process. "Approaching policy in this way could bring isolated and fragmented movements for change to scale, moving results from years of experimentation and innovation into policies" (Blackwell and Colmenar 2000, 163).
Community building principles (see appendix 2) should also be applied to policy
design so that the policies enacted themselves encourage and ideally mandate high-
level community involvement in devising solutions to complex health and social
problems.

For example, consider the federal Healthy Start Program to reduce infant mortality. Launched in 1991 in fifteen demonstration sites and including more than
ninety sites around the country today, the program was mandated to incorporate
community involvement as a centerpiece of its operation (HRSA 1991). At
each site, community consortia comprised of program participants, providers,
community leaders, and other stakeholders were to have major roles in planning
and decision making, with the assumption that such community-driven approaches
would lead to better, more culturally relevant programs (Minkler et al. 2002, Thompson et al. 2000).

Dramatic shifts in population in many of the Healthy Start sites and the difficulty of detecting health status changes "in a form attributable to a particular intervention" (Kreuter and Lezin 1998, ix) make it difficult to determine the extent
to which this program has contributed to declining infant mortality, which fell
by 21.7 percent nationally from 1990 to 1997 (Moreno et al. 2000). Yet an in-depth
evaluation of the community involvement component of the program at nine sites

(Thompson et al. 2000, Minkler et al. 2001) did suggest its effectiveness in reaching the interim goals of creating sustainable, community-driven structures; building leadership; and in other ways enhancing local assets and problem-solving ability. Resident organizing to oppose a toxic waste incinerator at a local hospital in Cleveland and successful efforts by the consortium in Chicago to mobilize for the prevention of mandated Medicaid managed care are among many examples of successful community involvement efforts to address shared concerns through the Healthy Start program. Policies that create programs such as Healthy Start, which include community involvement and community building as a central organizing feature, may provide an important means of enhancing the community capacity and civic engagement that are central to the creation of healthy communities.

## Conclusion

Although efforts to influence policy are time-consuming and fraught with difficulties, they are critical avenues for improving public health and therefore should be important parts of the community organizer's and community builder's tool kit. By intentionally focusing on the policy level, professionals and community residents can help translate community concerns into concrete action (Themba and Minkler 2003) and influence decision making by democratizing knowledge and access.

At the same time, community involvement in the policymaking process can enhance community capacity building and contribute to a more engaged populace. To promote such community involvement, however, the very nature of our policies should be reconsidered: community building should become central to how policies are shaped and what they look like. Only through such reorientation can oft-repeated phrases such as "civic engagement," "empowered communities," and indeed "community building" itself have any real power or meaning.

### Acknowledgments

The authors are grateful to Makani Themba for her wonderful collaboration on related earlier work and to Peggy Shepard for her helpful comments and editing of a previous draft of the WE ACT case study presented in this chapter.

### References

Alinsky, S. D. 1972. *Rules for Radicals*. New York: Vintage.
Bandura, A. 1997. *Self-Efficacy: The Exercise of Control*. New York: Freeman.
Barry, B. W. 1997. *Strategic Planning Workbook for Nonprofit Organizations*. St. Paul, Minn.: Wilder Foundation.
Blackwell, A. G., and R. Colmenar. 2000. "Community-Building: From Local Wisdom to Public Policy." *Public Health Reports* 115, nos. 2–3: 161–66.

Blaine, T. M., J. L. Forster, D. Hennrikus, S. O'Neil, M. Wolfson, and H. Pham. 1997. "Creating Tobacco Control Policy at the Local Level: Implementation of a Direct Action Approach." *Health Education and Behavior* 24, no. 5: 640–51.

Brownson, R. C., C. J. Newschaffer, and F. Ali-barghoui. 1997. "Policy Research for Disease Prevention: Challenges and Practical Recommendations." *American Journal of Public Health* 87, no. 5: 735–39.

Centers for Disease Control and Prevention (CDC). 2002. *Health, United States, 2002*. Washington, D.C.: National Center for Health Statistics.

Health Resources and Services Administration (HRSA). 1991. "Guidance for the Healthy Start Program." Unpublished document.

Kreuter, M., and N. Lezin. 1998. "Are Consortia/Collaboratives Effective in Changing Health Status and Health Systems?" Paper prepared for the Health Resources and Services Administration, Atlanta, January 9.

Longest, B. 1998. *Health Policymaking in the United States*. 2d ed. Chicago: Health Administration Press.

Maltrud, K., M. Polacsek, and N. Wallerstein. 1997. *Participatory Evaluation Workbook for Community Initiatives*. Albuquerque: New Mexico Department of Health, Public Health Division, Healthier Communities Unit.

McKinlay, J. B., and S. M. McKinlay. 1977. "Medical Measures and the Decline of Mortality." *Milbank Memorial Fund Quarterly* (summer): 405–28.

Milio, N. 1998. "Priorities and Strategies for Promoting Community-Based Prevention Policies." *Journal of Public Health Management Practice* 4, no. 3: 14–28.

Minkler, M., M. Thompson, J. Bell, and K. Rose. 2001. "Contributions of Community Involvement to Organizational Level Empowerment: The Federal Healthy Start Experience." *Health Education and Behavior* 28, no. 6: 783–807.

Minkler, M., M. Thompson, J. Bell, K. Rose, and D. Redman. 2002. "Using Community Involvement Strategies in the Fight against Infant Mortality: Lessons from a Multisite Study of the National Healthy Start Experience." *Health Promotion Practice* 3, no. 2: 176–87.

Moreno, L., B. Davaney, D. Chu, and M. Seeley. 2000. *Effects of Healthy Start on Infant Mortality and Birth Outcomes*. Final report prepared for U.S. Department of Health and Human Services, Health Resources and Services Administration. Princeton, N.J.: Mathematica Policy Research.

Perera, F. P., V. Rauh, W. Y. Tsai, P. Kinney, D. Camann, D. Barr, T. Bernet, R. Garfinkel, Y. H. Tu, D. Diaz, J. Dietrich, and R. M. Whyatt. 2003. "Effects of Transplacental Exposure to Environmental Pollutants on Birth Outcomes in a Multiethnic Population." *Environmental Health Perspectives* 111, no. 2: 201–5.

Perez-Pena, R. 2003. "Study Finds Asthma in 25% of Children in Central Harlem." *New York Times*, April 19, p. A1.

Putnam, R. D. 2000. *Bowling Alone: The Collapse and Revival of American Community*. New York: Simon and Schuster.

Schmid, T. L., M. Pratt, and E. Howe. 1995. "Policy As Intervention: Environmental and Policy Approaches to the Prevention of Cardiovascular Disease." *American Journal of Public Health* 85, no. 9: 1207–11.

Shepard, P. M. 2000. "Achieving Environmental Objectives and Reducing Health Disparities through Community-Based Participatory Research and Interventions." In *Successful Models of Community-Based Participatory Research: Final Report*, edited by L. R. O'Fallon, F. L. Tyson, and A. Dearry, 30–34. Washington, D.C.: National Institute of Environmental Health Sciences.

Steckler, A., L. Dawson, R. Goodman, and N. Epstein. 1987. "Policy Advocacy: Three Emerging Roles for Health Education." In *Advances in Health Education and Promotion*, edited by W. B. Ward, 2:5–27. Greenwich, Conn.: JAI.

Themba, M. N. 1999. *Making Policy, Making Change: How Communities Are Taking Law into Their Own Hands*. San Francisco: Jossey-Bass.

Themba, M. N., and M. Minkler. 2003. "Influencing Policy through Community Based Participatory Research." In *Community Based Participatory Research*, edited by M. Minkler and N. Wallerstein, 349–70. San Francisco: Jossey-Bass.

Thompson, M., M. Minkler, Z. Allen, J. D. Bell, J. Bell, A. G. Blackwell, M. Carpenter, K. Rose, and H. B. Tamir. 2000. *Community Involvement in the Federal Healthy Start Program: A Report from PolicyLink*. Oakland, Calif.: PolicyLink.

Thompson, M., R. Phillips, and J. Bell. 2002. *Fighting Childhood Asthma: How Communities Can Win*. Oakland, Calif.: PolicyLink.

Wallerstein, N. 2002. "Empowerment to Reduce Health Disparities." *Scandinavian Journal of Public Health* 30, supp. 59: 72–77.

Wallerstein, N., M. Larson-Bright, A. R. Adams, and R. M. Rael. 2000. "Youth Link: A Youth Policy Leadership Program in New Mexico." Paper presented at a meeting of the American Public Health Association, Boston, November 14.

| *Chapter 23* | Media Advocacy |
|---|---|

## A Strategy for Empowering
## People and Communities

*If you don't exist in the media, for all practical purposes,*
*you don't exist.*

— DANIEL SCHORR

AN EIGHTH-GRADE GIRL in Pojoaque, New Mexico; a family physician in Davis, California; a network of tobacco control advocates around the country all share a strong belief in the power of the media to promote public health goals. Each took on powerful "manufacturers of illness" (McKinlay 2000), and each, with creative use of mass media, was able to achieve his or her objectives. In Pojoaque, a school substance abuse project turned into a battle to remove alcohol billboards from the immediate area of the school. The combination of community organizing and the power of the press made a young girl into a giant-killer and brought the billboards down. In Davis, a physician concerned about children inadvertently killing other children with easily available handguns that often were mistaken for toy guns combined scientific research with a topic the media could not resist to focus attention on the need for policy change. One short-term outcome is the difficulty of finding certain kinds of toy guns in California stores. Tobacco control advocates successfully developed a media strategy to counter the Philip Morris "Bill of Rights Tour." The cigarette maker's public relations dream turned into a nightmare when advocates successfully reframed the issue in the media and made it a health story.

The experience of these people is part of the foundation of a creative and innovative approach to use mass media as an advocacy tool. What they learned, and what people are learning in communities across the country, is that the power of the press can be claimed by advocacy groups and used to promote changes in the social environment. In breaking from traditional public education campaigns that convey health messages, they developed a "voice" to wield power. Media advocacy can be a significant force for influencing public debate, speaking directly to those with influence, and putting pressure on decisionmakers (Wallack et al. 1999). Media advocacy is a tactic for community groups to communicate their own story in their own words to promote social change. It is a hybrid tool combining advocacy approaches with the strategic and innovative use of media to better pressure decisionmakers to support changes for healthy public policies.

Historically, the mass media have tended to present health issues in medical terms, with a focus on personal health habits, medical miracles, physician heroics, or technological breakthroughs (Turow and Coe 1985; Gerbner et al. 1981; Wallack et al. 1993, 1999; Turow 1989; Wallack and Dorfman 1992). High tech curative treatment and low tech preventive behavior change have been the primary focus. Social, economic, and political determinants of health have been largely ignored by the most pervasive media. Media advocacy tries to change this by emphasizing the social and economic, rather than individual and behavioral, roots of the problem.

The research base in public health strongly suggests that while a balance of initiatives are necessary, policy change is a key factor in promoting public health goals. Current research in public health and mass communication clearly indicates that it is time to shift the balance of our efforts in using the mass media from individual change to social change, from promoting health information to promoting health policies, from giving people a message about their personal health to giving communities a voice in defining and acting on public health issues. Certainly the provision of clear, accurate information about risk factors and personal behavior change through public information campaigns must be a constant part of the media environment. However, the research indicates that it is appropriate and necessary for public health to move from the public affairs desk to the news and opinion desks.

Health advocates are attracting news attention more and more frequently on issues such as violence, alcohol, tobacco, and HIV infection (Wallack et al. 1993). Public health issues are newsworthy because they can link personal stories with broader social and political concerns. Community initiatives have provided solid evidence that local groups can gain access to media, reframe issues to focus on policy, and advance community initiatives for policy change.

## The Information Gap versus the Power Gap

Traditional forms of mass media interventions emphasize the "information gap," which suggests health problems are caused by a lack of information in individuals with the problem or at risk for the problem. Public education campaigns provide information to fill that gap. Media advocacy, on the other hand, focuses on the "power gap," where health problems are viewed as a lack of power to define the problem and create social change. The target of media advocacy is the power gap. It attempts to motivate broad social and political involvement rather than changes in personal health behavior (Wallack et al. 1999).

The mass media regularly reinforce the view that health matters are personal problems rather than social or community concerns (Wallack 1990, Iyengar 1991). The definition of the problem at the personal level leads to solutions designed for and directed to the individual. In this "information gap" model the person is seen as lacking some key information, and it is this lack of information which is the problem. When people have the information and "know the facts," it is assumed they will then act accordingly and the problem will be solved. If every individual gets the right information and makes the right decision, then the community's problem will be eliminated. The role of the media is to deliver the solution (knowledge) to the millions of individuals who need it.

The information gap model sees the context in which the problem exists only as a place to deliver a message. It accounts for the pressures and demands of daily life only in determining how to deliver the message. It assumes people have adequate available resources for meeting those demands. Family, school, community, and social variables are seen as less important than having the "right information."

A classic example of using the media to fill the information gap is the Partnership for a Drug Free America. This program is based on the idea that "if only people really knew how bad and uncool drugs were, they wouldn't use them." Many of these ads are memorable, but their strong statements generally do not take a public health approach. Instead, they focus almost exclusively on individual behavior and personal responsibility. The partnership ads insist that "the drug problem is your problem, not the government's. The ads never question budget allocations or the administration's emphasis on [law] enforcement over treatment. . . . If there are mitigating reasons for drug use—poverty, family turmoil, self-medication, curiosity—you'd never know it from the Partnership ads" (Blow 1991, 31–32). The partnership ads laud volunteerism, self-discipline, and individualism (Miller 1988, 34), precisely the values that resonate with the American people. And the partnership strategies meet with little political resistance because they are consistent with a victim-blaming orientation toward public health (Ryan 1976).

The partnership campaigns, like virtually all public information efforts, assume that information is the magic bullet which inoculates people against drugs. Social conditions that form the context of the problem, such as alienation, poor housing, poor education, and lack of economic opportunity, are ignored. Because the context of the problem is part of the problem, any solution that does not take the context into account inevitably will be inadequate. In fact, the partnership's public service advertisements, despite their intent to improve the public's health, ultimately may do more harm than good by undermining support for more effective health promotion efforts that focus upstream on power relationships and social conditions. The ads occupy valuable media time with compelling messages that reinforce a downstream, victim-blaming approach.

Media advocacy emphasizes the power gap by highlighting alternative definitions of problems and policy level approaches to addressing the problem. In the tradition of sociologist C. Wright Mills (1959), media advocacy takes personal problems and translates them into social issues. A primary strategy of media advocacy is to work with individuals and groups to claim power from the media to change the context or environment in which the problem occurs.

The focus on policy addresses determinants of health which are external to the individual. These determinants include variables such as basic housing, employment, education, health care, and personal security and might be considered under the general rubric of social justice issues. A second set of determinants focus more closely on immediate marketing variables associated with health-compromising products such as alcohol, tobacco, high fat foods, and other dangerous products. These marketing variables include advertising and promotion, pricing, product development, and product availability. For example, alcohol activists are concerned about advertising and promotion of alcohol at events or in media which attract large youth audiences. In addition, the pricing of alcohol so that it is competitive with soft drinks coupled with its easy availability contributes to an environment that is conducive to problematic use of the product. Store owners who indiscriminately sell malt liquor to children or companies that develop new products such as wine coolers which target youth further contribute to the seductive environment. These are all potential focal points for media advocates.

## The Practice of Media Advocacy

Media advocacy is the strategic use of mass media to advance a social or public policy initiative (U.S. Department of Health and Human Services 1989). It uses a range of media and advocacy strategies to define the problem and stimulate broad-based coverage. Media advocacy attempts to reframe and shape public discussion to increase support for and advance healthy public policies. Fundamental to media advocacy is knowing what policy goals you want to accomplish. Thus, the first step is to establish what your group's policy goal is—what do you want to happen? The second step is to decide who your target is—to whom do you want to speak? Does this person, group, or organization have the power to make the change you want to see happen? The third step is to frame your issue and construct your message. The fourth step is to construct an overall media advocacy plan for delivering your message and creating pressure for change. Finally, you want to evaluate how well you have done what you set out to do.

To illustrate the planning process, consider a coalition that is seeking to reduce deadly violence among youth. They decide on three local policy goals: limit handgun availability, limit alcohol availability, and increase employment opportunities for youth. They decide their primary audience is the city council, with community opinion leaders as a secondary audience. The general message they decide to use is that violence is a public health issue, is predictable, and can be prevented. They frame their message to emphasize the social and economic aspects of violence among youth. They develop a media strategy to reach their audience with the message and to promote their policy initiatives. In their media strategy they consider methods for creating news, taking advantage of existing news opportunities (e.g., localizing a national story), and buying media time and space to speak directly to their audience. All through the process they institute feedback mechanisms to get a sense of how they are doing.

The process and success of media advocacy, however, are linked to how well the advocacy is rooted in the community. Local media outlets feel a legal and civic responsibility to their communities. They are concerned about what the community wants. The more support and participation at the local level for media initiatives, the more likely journalists will define the issue as relevant and newsworthy. As Tuchman (1978, 92) notes, "The more members, the more legitimate their spokesperson." Media advocacy, then, really combines the separate functions of mass communication with community advocacy.

Traditional public health communication strategies tend to see individuals and groups as part of an audience to be addressed in a one-way communication. At best if the "audience" is included in the planning, it is after major boundaries of the issue have been set. Media advocacy treats the individual or group as potential advocates who can use their energy, skills, and other resources to influence what issue is addressed and what solutions are put forth. While traditional campaigns seek to convince individuals to change their health habits, media advocacy initiatives create pressure to change the environment which, in large part, determines these habits.

## The Functions of Media Advocacy

*Mass media are like the beam of a searchlight that moves restlessly about, bringing one episode and then another out of darkness into vision.*
—Walter Lippmann (1922)

The three functions of media advocacy can be thought of in terms of Lippmann's classic image of the mass media. First, media advocacy uses the media to place attention on an issue by bringing it to light. This is the process of agenda setting. Substantial evidence suggests that the media agenda determines the public agenda:

what's on people's minds reflects what is in the media (e.g., McCombs and Shaw 1972, Rogers and Dearing 1988, Dearing and Rogers 1992). Second, media advocacy holds the spotlight on the issue and focuses in on "upstream" causes. This is the process of framing. Recent research from the political science field suggests that the way that social issues are framed in the news media is associated with who or what is seen as primarily responsible for addressing the problem (Iyengar 1991). Third, media advocacy seeks to advance a social or public policy initiative(s) as a primary approach to the problem. Changes in the social environment through the development of healthy public policies are viewed as the means for improving public health.

## SETTING THE AGENDA: FRAMING FOR ACCESS

A local news program in the San Francisco Bay Area used billboards and television commercials to tell people, "If it goes on here, it goes on [Channel] 4 at 10." The implication was that if you do not see it on the news, then an event has not happened. When AIDS was not covered by the New York Times, it did not make it on the nation's policy agenda either. If the press does not cover your demonstration to highlight a contradiction in health policy, it might as well as have not taken place as far as the broader community (and probably the person with the power to make the change you want) is concerned. Daniel Schorr, National Public Radio commentator and longtime journalist, says, "If you don't exist in the media, for all practical purposes, you don't exist." Gaining access to the media is the first step for media advocates who want to set the agenda.

Gaining access is important for two reasons. First, the public agenda setting process is linked to the level of media coverage and thus the broad visibility of an issue. The media alert people about what to think about, and the more coverage a topic receives in the media, the more likely it is to be a concern of the general public (Cohen 1963, Iyengar and Kinder 1987, McCombs and Shaw 1972, Rogers and Dearing 1988). Second, media are a vehicle for gaining access to specific opinion leaders. Politicians, government regulators, community leaders, and corporate executives are people you might want to reach specifically. In successful media advocacy both objectives will be met. For example, recent efforts to remove PowerMaster malt liquor from the market were able to get the problem out in the media, which helped to make it a public issue (Wallack et al. 1993). At the same time, specific politicians and government regulators at the Bureau of Alcohol, Tobacco, and Firearms were exposed to media reports which gave them a greater sensitivity to the issue and a greater expectancy that others around them would be aware of the issue. Journalists themselves put pressure on bureaucrats just by doing the story, apart from what might happen with public opinion after the story is broadcast. With tape rolling, officials had to answer for their actions. Consequently, advocates were able to muster enough public and regulatory pressure to prevent the product from staying on the market.

NEWSWORTHINESS. None of us is the president of the United States or an editor for the New York Times, so how can we get access to the media? Media advocates gain access by interpreting their issue in terms of newsworthiness. In a variety of ways, media advocates take advantage of how news is constructed and what its objectives are. Their issue will be covered only to the extent that they are timely, relevant, defined to be in the public's interest, and/or meets a number of other news criteria. Shoemaker with Mayfield (1987) present an extensive list of factors that go into determining newsworthiness. Criteria for selecting news "include sensation, conflict, mystery, celebrity, deviance, tragedy, and proximity." To that list Dearing and Rogers (1992, 174) add "the 'breaking quality' of a news issue, how new information can be molded to recast old issues in a new way, and the degree to which new information can be fit into existing constructs." "Human interest," which focuses on people overcoming difficult odds; or helping others; or unusualness is also an important variable.

Very few social problems are new. Alcohol problems, teen pregnancy, drugs, and poverty have been around for a long time and are periodically rediscovered. Gaining access for a particular issue may depend on where it falls in a cyclic media attention span. Anthony Downs (1972) has identified a well ordered "issue-attention cycle" for many domestic problems. His first stage is the preproblem stage. At this stage the problem fully exists and can be quite bad, but it is yet to be discovered and seen as a problem by the broad public. The April 1992 civil unrest in Los Angeles brought to light basic problems of racism, poverty, and alienation that have long existed but were below the threshold of mainstream public attention. The uprising provided the basis for the second stage of the cycle: "alarmed discovery and euphoric enthusiasm" by the media and the mainstream public. Many thought that racism was no longer a problem in our society; the uprising brought home the fact that conditions remained, in fact, quite bad. Fundamental to the American character is a basic optimism that even the most intractable problems can be solved. Soon the media enthusiasm moved from the horrors of the violent disturbances to the "road to recovery," highlighting how volunteers from many different areas were pitching in to clean up the devastation. The media pictures and descriptions of people joining together to clean up reinforced the idea that through diverse people working together, the problem can be solved.

Downs's third stage involves a realization of the cost of making significant progress. Most important here is the awareness that change will require sacrifice and that better off groups may have to bear a burden to help those who are less well off. However, from this stage it is a short trip to a decline in public interest and pessimism about whether change can take place at all. Next is the postproblem stage, which is a kind of twilight where the problem continues to exist but gets little public or media attention. The trail in Los Angeles from Watts of 1965 to South Central of 1992 illustrates two complete cycles of the media attention process.

When the media spotlight fades, attention recedes, and often we return to prior arrangements and prior levels of concern. The shift of the media away from a problem is a curious form of both cause and effect of public perceptions. It is a cause of attention fading because without the media spotlight, issues will gradually fall out of public discussion and will lose a sense of legitimacy as a problem and urgency as a concern. It is an effect because the media will shift only after they sense that people are bored with the issue or that some new, more pressing problem has emerged. The media, after all, are in the business of attracting large audiences, and if they bore or threaten people because the solutions are complex or call for personal sacrifice, they will lose their audience and diminish their economic base (i.e., audience for advertisers).

### SHAPING THE DEBATE: FRAMING FOR CONTENT

Gaining access to the media is an important first step, but it is only a first step in influencing the public and policy agenda. After access, the next barrier that media advocacy seeks to overcome is the definition of health issues in the media as primarily individual problems. As Henrik Blum (1980, 49), a well-known health planner, notes, "There is little doubt that how a society views major problems . . . will be critical in how it acts on the problems." If we alter the definition of problems, then the response also changes (Powles 1979, Watzlawick et al. 1974). Problem definition is a battle to determine which group and which perspective will gain primary "ownership" of the solution to the problem.

The tendency in the U.S. is to attempt to develop clear and concise definitions of problems to facilitate concrete, commonsense-type solutions. This is a very pragmatic approach with strong appeal. Oftentimes, however, problems of health and social well-being are difficult to define, much less solve, and increasing levels of problem complexity are highly correlated with rising degrees of disagreement in definition. Our tendency is to simplify the problem by breaking it down into basic elements which are easier to manage. In most cases this is either a biological unit and the solution is medical or an information unit where the solution is education.

This misguided pragmatism about problem-solving reduces society's drug problem, an enormously complex issue that involves every level of society, to an inability of the individual to "just say no" and resist the temptation to take drugs. Generally diseases are reduced to cognitive, behavioral, or genetic elements. Public and private institutions end up allocating significant resources to identifying the gene for alcoholism while leaving the activities of the alcoholic beverage industry largely unexamined. Even though 30 percent of all cancer deaths and 87 percent of lung cancer deaths are attributed to tobacco use (World Health Organization 1997), the main focus of cancer research is not on the behavior of the tobacco industry but on the biochemical and genetic interactions of cells.

The alternative is to see problems as part of a larger context. Tobacco use, for example, rather than being seen as a bad habit or a stupid thing to do, can be seen as a function of a corporate enterprise which actively promotes the use of a health-compromising product. Decisions at the individual level about whether to smoke could be seen as inextricably linked to decisions of a relatively few people at the corporate level regarding production, marketing, and widespread promotion. Smoking, in this larger context, is seen as a property of a larger system in which a smoker or potential smoker is one part, rather than simply as a property of individual decisions. The same could be applied to automobile safety, nutrition, alcohol, and other issues. This type of analysis takes the problem definition upstream. The key for media advocates is to frame their issue in terms of upstream problem definitions.

THE ENVIRONMENTAL PERSPECTIVE. In public health, a new environmental perspective has evolved that directs attention to the role of policy and community-level factors in health promotion. This environmental perspective includes both a physical and a social element. For example, policies and practices that support product availability and marketing of alcohol and tobacco, both of which help cultivate positive social perceptions about these products, are primary targets for change. Thus, tobacco control advocates have shifted the focus from the behavior of the smoker to the behavior of the tobacco industry and to the policies that support advertising and general marketing activities contributing to excess mortality. Limiting billboard advertising, vending machines, and sponsorship of community activities while also promoting clean indoor air legislation are key targets of the tobacco control movement.

The focus on the immediate marketing and community-level environment is important but still fails to address the most significant variable regarding health status. An extensive body of literature clearly indicates that social class may well be the single most important determinant of health (Kawachi et al. 1999, Marmot and Wilkinson 1999, Wilkinson 1996). Virtually every disease shows an association with measures of social class (Auerbach and Krimgold 2001, Marmot and Wilkinson 1999). This is not the result of a simple rich-poor dichotomy but a graded response that can be seen even in the upper quadrant of society (e.g., Marmot and Wilkinson 1999, Wilkinson 1996). Research suggests that the most important factor within the social class construction may be level of education (Winkleby et al. 1992). Also, in cross-cultural comparisons, it appears that a society's health status is not linked solely to per capita income, but to income variability and therefore the extent of relative deprivation and discrepancy within a society (Wilkinson 1996). The United States, for example, fares poorly on a number of key health indicators when compared to some countries that are less affluent but also show less variability in income across social strata. Successful health promotion thus relies less on our ability to disseminate health information and more on our efforts to establish a fairer and more just society.

There are two important reasons for emphasizing the environment. First, as the history of public health amply demonstrates, prevention that is population-based and focused on social conditions is more effective than efforts aimed primarily at treating individuals (e.g., Amick et al. 1995, Dubos 1959, McKeown 1978). It is the policies that define the environment in which people make choices about health that appear to have the greatest potential to improve health. Second, public health research points to the importance of equality and social justice as the foundation for action. Environmentally oriented solutions try to address the underlying conditions that give rise to and sustain disease and thus promise long term change.

## ADVANCING THE POLICY

The ultimate goal of media advocacy is to create changes in policies that improve health chances for communities. This requires clarity about the policy being advanced, appropriate framing of the issue and consistency in the messages about the policy, and the ability to capitalize on opportunities in the media to advance the policy. Mass media can be used to put pressure on policymakers and influentials, but the pressure is not automatic. The media coverage must be carefully crafted and reflect broad-based support. There are many examples of how this can work, and a series of ten brief case studies have been presented by Wallack and his colleagues (1993).

In many cases media access is relatively easy, but shaping the story and focusing it on policy goals can be quite difficult. Consider a typical, and tragic, example from a major city in California. Early in the evening, on her way home from work, a young woman was kidnapped on the way to her car from public transportation. Her abductors put her in the trunk of her own car, robbed, raped, and murdered her.

The tragedy received tremendous coverage on television and in the local papers. Community members were horrified, frightened, and desperate to do something about public safety. A local church held a candlelight vigil for the woman, and more than five hundred community members attended her funeral.

Several community-based organizations (CBOs) were involved in organizing the vigil, which they anticipated would attract significant media attention. It did. Nevertheless, members of the CBOs were frustrated with the type of coverage the woman's death and the vigil received. They blamed the reporters for focusing too much attention on the drama of the event rather than on the issues of importance for safety and well-being in the community.

Indeed, news reports that discussed safety emphasized what individuals should do to protect themselves. Articles quoted mass transit officials giving advice such as:

- Observe all posted parking regulations and park in designated areas.
- Before leaving, check your headlights, lock your car, and do not leave valuables or packages where they can be seen.
- Carry your keys in your hands.
- When at stations at night, be aware of your surroundings, and stand in the center of the platform. If you need help, call station police.
- If you do not feel safe walking to your parked car, go back to the station.

While all of this is good advice, it places almost total responsibility for safety on the rider. This is important. However, who is asking the question "What would it take to make the environment safe, regardless of what various individual passengers do?" The stories did not focus on environmental factors such as lighting in the station area, cutbacks in station security personnel, or the much larger issue of violence against women.

The responsibility for news coverage does not rest solely with journalists. While members of the CBOs were unsatisfied with the coverage, they also had not clearly articulated the solutions they desired in terms the media could easily use. Access, in this case, was abundant. The work, from the media advocacy perspective, needed to be done to frame for content in order to articulate the solution and move a policy forward.

One of the key goals of media advocacy is to advance a policy or approach to address the problem. Getting the media's attention and having stories air or appear in print are often the easy part of the job. The difficult part occurs when advocates have to put their issues and approaches in the media and in front of the people they want to reach.

The important work of media advocacy is really done in the planning stage before calling the media. Advocates need to know how they will advance their approach, what symbols to use, what issues to link it with, what voices to provide, and what messages to communicate. The issue can be reexplored in terms of media opportunities. Strategies can then be developed to frame for access and frame for content. Framing for access and framing for content force advocates to think in terms of the media and its needs.

In reality, most CBOs do not have the resources or training to use mass media effectively. In this example, the CBOs were in a reactive position. Community groups can anticipate similar situations and prepare their policy solutions and how they want them framed in media coverage. Articulating this vision is the hard work of media advocacy. Media advocacy can then effectively be used to help communities claim the power and confidence they need to better tell their story.

## Conclusion

*For advocates, the press is a grand piano waiting for a player. Strike the chords through a news story, a guest column, or an editorial and thousands will hear. Working in concert, unbiased reporters and smart advocates can make music together.*
                              —Susan Wilson, New Jersey Network for
                              Family Life (in Duncan et al. 1990)

Since the late 1980s media advocacy has become an increasingly popular approach to using mass media to promote public health goals. This approach seeks to enhance the visibility, legitimacy, and power of community groups. Media advocacy represents more than just a different way of using mass media to promote health. It is an effort to fundamentally shift power back to the community by cultivating skills that can enhance and amplify the community's voice. Instead of giving individuals a message about personal health behaviors, it gives groups the ability to broadly present approaches to healthy public policy. It is based on the premise that real improvements in health status will not come so much from increases in personal health knowledge as from improvements in social conditions. It is the power gap, rather than the knowledge gap, which is the primary focus of media advocacy.

Media advocacy reflects a public health approach that explicitly recognizes the importance of the social and political environment and defines health problems as matters of public policy, not just individual behavior. Media advocacy attempts to help individuals claim power by providing knowledge and skills to better enable them to participate in efforts to change the social and political factors that contribute to the health status of all. The health of the community, not necessarily the convenience of the individual, is the primary focus. Active participation in the political process is the mechanism for health promotion.

Social and health programs generally tend to focus on giving people skills to beat the odds to overcome the structural barriers to successful and healthy lives. In the long run it makes more sense to change the odds so that more people have a wider and more accessible range of healthy choices (Schorr 1988). Media advocacy helps to emphasize the importance of changing social conditions to improve the odds. Media advocacy can be instrumental in escaping a traditional, limited focus on disease conditions and instead promote a greater understanding of the conditions that will support and improve the public's health.

## Acknowledgments

Reprinted from *Journal of Public Health Policy* 15, no. 4 (1994): 420–36, by permission of the author and the publisher.

## References

Amick, B. C., III, S. Levine, A. R. Tarlov, and D. C. Walsh, eds. 1995. *Society and Health*. New York: Oxford University Press.

Auerbach, J. A., and B. K. Krimgold, eds. 2001. *Income, Socioeconomic Status, and Health: Exploring the Relationships*. Washington: National Policy Association, Academy for Health Services Research and Health Policy.

Blow, R. 1991. "How to Decode the Hidden Agenda of the Partnership's Madison Avenue Propagandists." *Washington City Paper* 11: 29–35.

Blum, H. 1980. "Social Perspective Risk Reduction." *Family and Community Health* 3: 41–61.

Cohen, B. 1963. *The Press and Foreign Policy*. Princeton, N.J.: Princeton University Press.

Dearing, J., and E. Rogers. 1992. "AIDS and the Media Agenda." In *AIDS: A Communication Perspective*, edited by T. Edgar, M. A. Fitzpatrick, and V. S. Freimuth, 173–94. Hillsdale, N.J.: Erlbaum.

Downs, A. 1972. "Up and Down with Ecology." *Public Interest* 28 (summer): 38–50.

Dubos, R. 1959. *Mirage of Health*. New York: Harper and Row.

Duncan, C., D. Rivlin, and M. Williams. 1990. *An Advocate's Guide to the Media*. Washington, D.C.: Children's Defense Fund.

Gerbner, G., M. Morgan, and N. Signorielli. 1981. "Health and Medicine on Television." *New England Journal of Medicine* 305, no. 15: 901–4.

Iyengar, S. 1991. *Is Anyone Responsible? How Television Frames Political Issues*. Chicago: University of Chicago Press.

Iyengar, S., and D. R. Kinder. 1987. *News That Matters*. Chicago: University of Chicago Press.

Kawachi, I., B. P. Kennedy, and R. G. Wilkinson. 1999. *The Society and Population Health Reader*. Vol. 1, *Income Inequality and Health*. New York: New Press.

Lippmann, W. 1922. *Public Opinion*. New York: Harcourt Brace.

Marmot, M., and R. G. Wilkinson. 1999. *Social Determinants of Health*. Oxford: Oxford University Press.

McCombs, M., and D. Shaw. 1972. "The Agenda-Setting Function of Mass Media." *Public Opinion Quarterly* 36, no. 2: 176–87.

McKeown, T. 1978. "Determinants of Health." *Human Nature* 1, no. 4: 60–67.

McKinlay, J. 2000. "A Case for Refocusing Upstream: The Political Economy of Illness." In *The Sociology of Health and Illness*, 6th ed., edited by P. Conrad. London: Worth.

Miller, M. 1988. "Death Grip." *Propaganda Review* (winter): 34–35.

Mills, C. W. 1959. *The Sociological Imagination*. New York: Oxford University Press.

Powles, J. 1979. "On the Limitations of Modern Medicine." In *Ways of Health: Holistic Approaches to Ancient and Contemporary Medicine*, edited by D. Sobel. New York: Harcourt Brace Jovanovich.

Rogers, E., and J. Dearing. 1988. "Agenda-Setting Research: Where Has It Been, and Where Is It Going?" In *Communication Yearbook*, edited by J. A. Anderson, 555–94. Beverly Hills, Calif.: Sage.

Ryan, W. 1976. *Blaming the Victim*. New York: Vintage.

Schorr, L. 1988. *Within Our Reach: Breaking the Cycle of Disadvantage*. Garden City, N.Y.: Anchor.

Shoemaker, P., and E. Mayfield. 1987. "Building a Theory of News Content: A Synthesis of Current Approaches." *Journalism Monographs* no. 103, pp. 1–36.

Tuchman, G. 1978. *Making News: A Study in the Construction of Reality*. New York: Free Press.

Turow, J. 1989. *Playing Doctor: Television, Storytelling, and Medical Power*. New York: Oxford University Press.

Turow, J., and L. Coe. 1985. "Curing Television's Ills: The Portrayal of Health Care." *Journal of Communication* 34: 36–51.

U.S. Department of Health and Human Services. 1989. *Media Strategies for Smoking Control: Guidelines*. Washington, D.C.: U.S. Department of Health and Human Services.

Wallack, L. 1990. "Mass Communication and Health Promotion: A Critical Perspective." In *Public Communication Campaigns*, edited by R. Rice and C. Atkin, 353–68. Newbury Park, Calif.: Sage.

Wallack, L., and L. Dorfman. 1992. "Television News, Hegemony, and Health." *American Journal of Public Health* 82, no. 1: 125–26.

Wallack, L., L. Dorfman, D. Jernigan, and M. Themba. 1993. *Media Advocacy and Public Health: Power for Prevention*. Newbury Park, Calif.: Sage.

Wallack, L., K. Woodruff, L. Dorfman, and I. Diaz. 1999. *News for a Change: An Advocate's Guide to Working with the Media*. Thousand Oaks, Calif.: Sage.

Watzlawick, P., J. Weakland, and R. Fisch. 1974. *Change: Principles of Problem Formation and Problem Resolution*. New York: Norton.

Wilkinson, R. 1996. *Unhealthy Societies: The Afflictions of Inequality*. New York: Routledge.

Winkleby, M., D. Jatulis, E. Frank, and S. Fortmann. 1992. "Socioeconomic Status and Health: How Education, Income, and Occupation Contribute to Risk Factors for Cardiovascular Disease." *American Journal of Public Health* 82, no. 6: 816–20.

World Health Organization. 1997. *Tobacco or Health: A Global Status Report*. Geneva: World Health Organization.

EUGENIA ENG
LYNN BLANCHARD

# Action-Oriented
# Community Diagnosis

## *Appendix 1*
## Procedure

*Editor's note:* Eugenia Eng and Lynn Blanchard developed the tool in this appendix over several years. Its emphasis on assessing and contributing to community competence rather than merely identifying needs amply illustrates chapter 9's perspective on community assessment. Additionally, the broad range of assessment techniques incorporated in this procedure underscores the utility of triangulation (the use of multiple methods) to provide the richest possible database for analysis.

I.  Specify the target population and determine its component parts using social and demographic characteristics that may identify commonalities among groups of people.
    A.  Race or ethnicity
    B.  Religion
    C.  Income level
    D.  Occupation
    E.  Age

II. Review secondary data sources, and identify possible subpopulations of interest and geographic locations.
    A.  County and townships
    B.  Church, school, and fire districts
    C.  Towns
    D.  Agency service delivery areas

    E. Industries and other major employers
    F. Transportation arteries and services
    G. Health and other vital statistics

III. Conduct windshield tours of targeted areas, and note daily living conditions, resources, and evidence of problems.
    A. Housing types and conditions
    B. Recreational and commercial facilities
    C. Private and public sector services
    D. Social and civic activities
    E. Identifiable neighborhoods or residential clusters
    F. Conditions of roads and distances people must travel
    G. Maintenance of buildings, grounds, and yards

IV. Contact and interview local agency providers serving targeted areas.
    A. What are the communities most in need, and why?
    B. Which communities have histories of meeting their own needs, and how?
    C. What services are being provided by agencies or other organized groups? Which are utilized, and which are underutilized?
    D. What, in their opinion, are the major problems still facing communities they serve?
    E. Where do they recommend finding additional information to document needs?
      — Referrals to other service providers
      — Referrals to leaders of community organizations
      — Referrals to informed members of communities

V. Select a community, and contact and interview community informants most frequently cited in provider interviews.
    A. What is the name their community is most commonly known as?
    B. Describe a time when there was a problem in their community that they tried to resolve.
      — How was the need determined?
      — How did the community organize themselves?
      — Who were the influential people involved?
    C. In their opinion, what are the present needs in their community?
    D. Who would have to be involved to get things done in their community?
    E. What outside services or resources do people in their community know and use to meet their needs?

F.  What other people like themselves who know about their community do they recommend being contacted?

G.  Would they be interested in attending a meeting to find out the results from these interviews? And what do they suggest as times and places to hold such a meeting?

VI. Tabulate the results from the secondary data, the provider interviews, and the community informant interviews, and analyze the degree of convergence among the needs identified.

A.  Determine the extent of agreement/disagreement across the three lists of needs on how each identified need is defined.

B.  Determine the extent of agreement/disagreement across the three lists of needs on the priority accorded to each identified need.

VII. Present the findings in meetings with community informants interviewed and other influential community members frequently cited by the providers and community informants.

A.  Assess the validity of the definitions for each need, and redefine them, if necessary, according to how they are manifested in this community.

B.  Determine a priority listing of needs according to interest in undertaking a solution.

C.  Select a need with high priority, and determine questions that need to be answered, such as:

— Who suffers from this problem?

— When is this problem most prevalent?

— How severe are the short- and long-term consequences from this problem?

— What are the possible causes of this problem?

— What is the range of solutions for reducing or controlling this problem?

— What are the available resources and additional resources required for each possible solution?

D.  Plan the next steps for finding answers to the questions.

ANGELA GLOVER BLACKWELL
RAYMOND A. COLMENAR

Appendix 2

# Principles of Community Building

## A Policy Perspective

*Editor's note:* As this book has shown, the term *community building* can be used in a variety of ways—for example, as communities' efforts to increase a sense of identity and cohesion or as an orientation to practice that puts community at the center of the discussion (see chapter 4). Yet community building may also refer to more macro- and multilevel efforts, often in poor neighborhoods, to build social capital and address poverty and related problems through partnership and policy approaches. The following list of community building principles reflects this broader orientation.

Community building may be defined as "continuous, self renewing efforts by residents and professionals to engage in collective action, aimed at problem solving and enrichment, that creates new or strengthened social networks, new capacities for group action and support, and new standards and expectations for the life of the community" (Blackwell 1997, ii). Central to community building are developing a strategic vision and building the capacity to solve not only the problem at hand but also new ones as they arise.

From a policy perspective, community building means policies that reinvest in communities, are sensitive to the particularities of place, build and sustain social capital, promote community participation, and strengthen families and neighborhoods. These are the basic tenets of community building:

- *Strengthen communities holistically.* In other words, support all aspects of community living, including economic opportunity, affordable housing,

Reprinted from A. G. Blackwell and R. A. Colmenar, 2000, "Community Building: From Local Wisdom to Public Policy," *Public Health Reports* 115, nos. 2 and 3: 161–66, by permission of Oxford University Press.

safety and security, youth development, transportation and utility industries, health care, early childhood services, and education, rather than target bits and pieces of the community puzzle.

- *Build local capacity for problem solving and build relationships between communities and resource institutions.* Community organizing is at the heart of community building. Policies should encourage organizational development and create linkages and partnerships between community organizations and other institutions. They should recognize the value of community assets, strengthen these, and invest in building more.

- *Foster community participation in policy development and implementation.* This can be done through community planning, alternative governance structures, and new financing methods that allow local authorities and even neighborhoods to have a say in the deployment of resources.

- *Deal explicitly with issues of "race" and ethnicity and their role in creating social and economic deprivation.* The face of poverty remains disproportionately African American and Latina(o). Community-building efforts seek to level the playing field and create equitable outcomes for all groups.

- *Break down the isolation of poor communities.* Community improvement should be viewed in the context of the broader region. Neighborhoods must be linked to the larger context of regional development.

- *Tailor programs to local conditions.* The most effective solutions to local problems come from within the community itself, and steps must be taken to engage the community in local problem-solving.

- *Build accountability mechanisms so that efforts are tied to community standards.* This enables communities to maintain improvements and monitor the progress they are making toward achieving a better quality of life.

### References

Blackwell, A. G. 1999. Forward. In *Stories of Renewal: Community Building and the Future of Urban America*, by J. Walsh. New York: Rockefeller Foundation.

# Appendix 3          Coalition Checklist

### Getting Started

1. Has at least one of these catalysts generated interest in forming
   a coalition:

   a significantly committed individual          __ yes __ no
   a disturbing or dramatic event                __ yes __ no
   detailed, timely information about the issue   __ yes __ no

2. Is there enough time to decisively affect policies related to
   the issue chosen by the coalition?            __ yes __ no

3. Will a coalition help potential members achieve goals they
   cannot achieve alone?                         __ yes __ no

4. Is each potential member adequately organized?  __ yes __ no

5. Are there adequate leadership links between potential
   coalition members?                            __ yes __ no

6. Is there adequate funding?                     __ yes __ no

### Building a Constituency

1. Has a list been made up of who is affected by the issue?   __ yes __ no

2. Has it been determined which groups have already done
   work on the issue?                            __ yes __ no

Reprinted from C. R. Brown, 1984, *The Art of Coalition Building: A Guide for Community Leaders* (New York: American Jewish Center), by permission of the author.

3. Is it known which groups will benefit from action
   on the issue? ___ yes ___ no

4. Is there an outline of separate strategies to attract each
   group to join the coalition? ___ yes ___ no

5. Does each group that is considering joining the coalition
   have an acceptable image in the community? ___ yes ___ no

6. Is there an outline of resources (e.g., staff time, money,
   publicity) expected from each member organization? ___ yes ___ no

7. Do the bylaws of each member group permit participation
   in the work of the coalition? ___ yes ___ no

8. Does the person representing each organization have the
   power to act on behalf of that organization? ___ yes ___ no

9. Will certain organizations need incentives (e.g., veto rights)
   to join the coalition? ___ yes ___ no

10. Has it been determined who agrees with the issue, who
    disagrees, and who might agree if more information were
    provided? ___ yes ___ no

### Joining a Coalition: What Groups Should Consider

1. Will the member organization gain visibility? ___ yes ___ no

2. Will membership potential be increased? ___ yes ___ no

3. Will links be created with other important organizations? ___ yes ___ no

4. Does the potential member have the resources to contribute:
   - staff time ___ yes ___ no
   - money ___ yes ___ no
   - office space ___ yes ___ no
   - new allies ___ yes ___ no
   - research capabilities ___ yes ___ no
   - a better reputation in the community ___ yes ___ no
   - media and press coverage ___ yes ___ no
   - a broader constituency ___ yes ___ no

5. Do the individual members' decisionmaking processes fit in
   with the coalition's decisionmaking structure? ___ yes ___ no

6. Are the member organization's ideological principles
   compatible with those of the coalition?                 __ yes __ no

### Mapping Out Coalition Strategy

1. Are invitations to join the coalition being extended to
   concerned organizations early enough for them to contribute
   to the formulation of strategy?                         __ yes __ no

2. Is the issue broad enough to include the larger human needs
   of all the member groups?                               __ yes __ no

3. Have inflammatory rhetoric and moral posturing been
   excluded from the coalition's statements and slogans?   __ yes __ no

4. Have the positions of groups that may be reluctant to join
   the coalition been carefully checked to see if differences of
   opinion can be bridged?                                 __ yes __ no

5. Is there an arrangement for groups that might come to
   the coalition with other urgent issues to find a forum
   for those issues?                                       __ yes __ no

6. Is there an agreement to focus on the key issue around which
   the coalition was formed and to refrain from adding other
   issues that may be important to other member groups?    __ yes __ no

7. Have controversial positions on which there is no
   consensus been put into nonbinding statements
   rather than trying to force an agreement?               __ yes __ no

8. Has a special evening been arranged at which each member
   organization can present its agenda and attract new support
   in the community?                                       __ yes __ no

### Determining Coalition Goals

1. Have the following been determined:
   the ideal situation                                     __ yes __ no
   the present reality                                     __ yes __ no
   the differences between the ideal and the reality       __ yes __ no

2. Have the following kinds of changes been considered?
   changes in consciousness                                __ yes __ no
   changes in policy                                       __ yes __ no

### Building Internal Commitment

1. Have special resources been developed for member groups within the coalition?     __ yes __ no

2. Have special parties, cultural events, or celebrations been planned to help member groups feel more included?     __ yes __ no

### Coalition Leadership

1. Has each person been approached by the leader in order to build a one-to-one relationship?     __ yes __ no

2. Has personal support been built for the leader by:
   encouraging personal responsibility     __ yes __ no
   arranging time for self-estimation     __ yes __ no
   arranging time for appreciations     __ yes __ no

3. Is the leader able to elicit every member's thinking, to consult widely among members, and then to draw the thinking into a concrete program?     __ yes __ no

4. Does the leader acknowledge and correct mistakes?     __ yes __ no

5. Can the leader help the coalition move forward after defeats and, in times of discouragement, recognize the success it has achieved?     __ yes __ no

6. Have one or more replacements been selected for leadership training?     __ yes __ no

7. Does the leader understand the reasons behind attacks and effectively respond to criticism?     __ yes __ no

8. Is the leader willing to disband the coalition when it has outlived its usefulness?     __ yes __ no

### The Coalition's Internal Functions

1. Is it clear which member organizations will contribute staff or, if none, where the staff will come from?     __ yes __ no

2. Is there an explicit agreement about the role of staff in coalition decisions?     __ yes __ no

### Decisionmaking

1. Has the coalition decided who will speak for it in public? __ yes __ no

2. Have any of these procedures been agreed upon for making coalition decisions:

   consensus __ yes __ no
   democratic voting __ yes __ no
   working consensus __ yes __ no
   organizational vetoes __ yes __ no
   weighted decisions __ yes __ no
   other __ yes __ no

### Fund-raising

1. Does the coalition have a procedure that avoids competition for funding among member organizations? __ yes __ no

### Maintaining Commitment

1. Does the coalition leadership allow multiple levels of organization on the part of member organizations? __ yes __ no

2. Does the coalition develop resources (e.g., newspapers, position papers, etc.) to nurture coalition members? __ yes __ no

3. Have parties, cultural sharing, and coalition celebrations been planned to increase member participation? __ yes __ no

### Managing Negotiations

1. Has the coalition assessed its bargaining power in dealing with a negotiating partner and made plans to increase it? __ yes __ no

2. Has the coalition determined its bottom line in negotiation?__ yes __ no

3. Has the negotiation team thoroughly studied the interests, goals, and positions of the other parties? __ yes __ no

4. Have roles been assigned to each person who will participate in the negotiation? __ yes __ no

5. Are the negotiating partners proceeding through each of the six stages of negotiations: rhetoric, issue definition, exploring positions, exploring underlying interests, developing parameters for a settlement, and formalizing an agreement? __ yes __ no

6. Has the negotiating team taken into account cultural differences between itself and the other negotiating team(s)?__ yes __ no

7. Have the negotiating partners identified overlapping objectives? __ yes __ no

8. Has each side attempted to understand how the other perceives it? __ yes __ no

9. Have the issues that can be resolved the most easily been dealt with first? __ yes __ no

10. Has someone been chosen to take on the role of mediator? __ yes __ no

11. Has each side taken care to adopt a problem-solving attitude in the negotiation? __ yes __ no

### Bridging Culture, Ethnicity, and Class Issues

1. Have ways been developed to reach out to diverse kinds of groups through

   symbols __ yes __ no

   quotations __ yes __ no

   religious teachings and rituals __ yes __ no

2. Is the coalition sensitive to the needs of religious groups when it establishes meeting times and locations and provides food? __ yes __ no

3. Are opportunities for cultural sharing built into the coalition's ongoing activities? __ yes __ no

4. Have members of the coalition been offered training in dealing with stereotypes and intergroup tensions? __ yes __ no

5. Have group caucuses been used to facilitate intergroup negotiations and otherwise improve meetings? __ yes __ no

MEREDITH MINKLER
CHRIS M. COOMBE

*Appendix 4*

# Using Force Field and SWOT Analysis as Strategic Tools in Community Organizing

MORE THAN FIFTY years ago, German social psychologist Kurt Lewin (1947) developed force field analysis as a way of understanding social situations and promoting change. Half a century later, health and social service professionals and community groups are applying a related tool, SWOT analysis, as a technique for strategic planning, mapping out the "strengths, weaknesses, opportunities and threats" that relate to their organizations (Barry 1997). Although neither tool was designed with community organizers in mind, both have been used effectively in community organizing practice.

### Force Field Analysis

Lewin (1947) argued that social situations exist in a state of "quasi-stationary social equilibria" caused by driving and resisting forces that work in opposition to one another. When the forces are weighted most heavily on the driving side, change is likely to take place. When the resisting or restraining forces are most powerful, no change is likely. Strengthening existing driving forces or adding new ones increases the likelihood of change, as does removing or weakening resisting forces. Of the two, however, the latter is most likely to enable lasting change.

Force field analysis has been used to help participants think through the challenges facing a local HIV/AIDS prevention and organizing project at a difficult time in its history (Wohlfeiler 1997), nutritionists and their community partners plan their fight against food vending machines in school cafeterias, and health department staff assess the forces working for and against community involvement in passing a local antismoking ordinance (Ellis et al. 1995). To conduct a force field analysis as part of a community organizing, follow these simple steps:

444

1. On a large chalkboard or a piece of butcher-block paper, write the desired change in the middle of the space, above a line that runs down the center of the board or paper. On one side of the line, have group members list forces working for the change—for example, buy-in from the president of the board or other key players, likely positive media attention, and so on.

2. On the other side of the line, list forces likely to work against the change—for example, fiscal costs, opposition of a key coalition or other community group, the labor required, and so on.

3. Beneath each listed force, draw an arrow whose thickness illustrates the factor's relative strength.

4. Brainstorm about which resisting forces can most easily be removed or weakened and how; a note taker should keep track of the ideas generated. During the discussion, remove arrows or change their thickness as necessary.

5. Repeat this process for the driving forces, in this case looking at which forces can be strengthened and what new ones might be added to increase your chances of success.

6. Decide on next steps: which strategies will you use in what order, and who will be responsible for follow-up on each of the action steps involved?

### SWOT Analysis

Although SWOT analysis is most often used in business as part of corporate strategic planning, it has become a common planning approach in community organizations and can be a powerful tool for developing organizing strategies. Also called environmental scanning or situation analysis, SWOT is a process in which participants assess where they are by identifying strengths and weaknesses internal to their organizations and opportunities and threats in the external environment that will influence the effectiveness of potential organizing efforts. The group then develops strategies that maximize strengths and take advantage of opportunities while overcoming weaknesses and avoiding threats. Although there are a number of ways to conduct a SWOT analysis, the following works well in a community setting:

1. Place four large sheets of butcher-block paper on the wall labeled, at the top, *Strengths*, *Weaknesses*, *Opportunities*, and *Threats*, respectively.

2. Explain to the group that strengths and weaknesses refer to factors internal to their organization or agency and thus ideally within their control; opportunities and threats refer to forces in the external environment, such as a budget cut or a new, community-friendly mayor or city council that may influence the organizing issue at hand.

3. Give all participants several blank Post-it notes in each of four colors, using a different color for each of the four categories. Have participants think of important SWOT factors and write them on individual notes— for example, a strength on yellow, a weakness on blue, and so forth.

4. Have team members place these Post-its on the appropriate sheets of chart paper.

5. As a group, look for common themes in each area and cluster items together by moving the Post-its around as needed. Add any new factors that come up and identify urgent or high-priority issues.

6. Stepping back, look at all four areas to identify strategic or critical issues that emerge from the discussion. A critical issue is typically a challenge, dynamic tension, or conflict around which change needs to occur. For example, your environmental justice organization has just received a grant for neighborhood organizing (strength), a new incinerator is being proposed for a high-asthma neighborhood (threat), and a key planning commission official has been exposed for accepting bribes from the industry backing the incinerator (an opportunity).

7. Look for a fit between different forces and your core issue. Prioritize strategic issues by importance and timing, decide what area to focus on, and brainstorm possible scenarios.

The Berkeley Media Studies Group (1995) developed a variation of SWOT analysis specifically for advocates and organizers building "a coordinated strategy toward policy goals" (1). Called the ACTION framework for strategic planning, it involves group brainstorming around factors that can advance or block the group's policy goals, the new information or intelligence needed (which might include polls, media monitoring, and so on), and the most important next steps necessary to advance the overall policy goal. The acronym ACTION captures these various elements:

Assets and strengths
Challenges, barriers, or liabilities
Threats (external)
Information needs
Opportunities
Next steps

Whether using force field analysis, the SWOT tool, or variations such as ACTION, such approaches to environmental analysis lay a foundation for generating potential organizing and policy advocacy strategies and provide criteria for making informed planning decisions.

## References

Barry, B. W. 1997. *Strategic Planning Workbook for Nonprofit Organizations*. St. Paul, Minn.: Wilder Foundation.

Berkeley Media Studies Group. 1995. *ACTION Framework for Strategic Planning*. Berkeley, Calif.: Berkeley Media Studies Group.

Ellis, G. A., D. F. Reed, and H. Scheider. 1995. "Mobilizing a Low-Income African-American Community around Tobacco Control: A Force Field Analysis." *Health Education Quarterly* 22, no. 4: 443–57.

Lewin, K. 1947. "Quasi-Stationary Social Equilibria and the Problem of Social Change." In *Readings in Social Psychology*, edited by T. M. Newcomb and E. L. Hartley, 340–44. New York: Holt, Rinehart, and Winston.

Wohlfeiler, D. 1997. "Community Organizing and Community Building among Gay and Bisexual Men: The Stop AIDS Project." In *Community Organizing and Community Building for Health*, 1st ed., edited by M. Minkler, 230–43. New Brunswick, N.J.: Rutgers University Press.

# Appendix 5    Inclusivity Checklist

CULTURAL DIFFERENCES can either enrich or impede coalition functioning. Creating multicultural coalitions challenges us to deal with differences and use them to strengthen our common work. Awareness of sensitive issues and dynamics can help you to detect potential obstacles and develop approaches to address them—either before problems arise or after they occur.

Building effective multicultural coalitions involves:

- Articulating a vision
- Conducting strategic outreach and membership development
- Setting ground rules that maintain a safe and nurturing atmosphere
- Establishing a structure and operating procedures that reinforce equity
- Practicing new modes of communication
- Creating leadership opportunities for everyone, especially people of color and women
- Engaging in activities that are culturally sensitive or that directly fight oppression

Reprinted from B. Rosenthal, 1995, *From the Ground Up: A Workbook on Coalition Building and Community Development*, edited by T. Wolff and G. Kaye (Amherst, Mass.: AHEC/Community Partners), 54–55, 69, by permission of the author and editors.

## Checklist

*Instructions:* Use this Inclusivity Checklist to measure how prepared your coalition is for multicultural work and to identify areas for improvement. Place a check mark in the box next to each statement that applies to your group. If you cannot put a check in the box, this may indicate an area for change.

❑ The leadership of our coalition is multiracial and multicultural.

❑ We make special efforts to cultivate new leaders, particularly women and people of color.

❑ Our mission, operations, and products reflect the contributions of diverse cultural and social groups.

❑ We are committed to fighting social oppression within the coalition and in our work with the community.

❑ Members of diverse cultural and social groups are full participants in all aspects of our coalition's work.

❑ Meetings are not dominated by speakers from any one group.

❑ All segments of our community are represented in decisionmaking.

❑ There are sensitivity and awareness regarding different religious and cultural holidays, customs, recreational and food preferences.

❑ We communicate clearly, and people of different cultures feel comfortable sharing their opinions and participating in meetings.

❑ We prohibit the use of stereotypes and prejudicial comments.

❑ Ethnic, racial, and sexual slurs or jokes are not welcome.

JOSH KIRSCHENBAUM
LISA RUSS

*Appendix 6*

# Community Mapping and Geographic Information Systems

## Tools for Organizers

C OUNTLESS QUESTIONS about socioeconomic conditions, health, development opportunities, and neighborhood change can be answered by community mapping. Mapping is the visual representation of data by geography or location, linking information to place to support social and economic change on a community level. Mapping is a powerful tool for two reasons: (1) it makes patterns based on place much easier to identify and analyze, and (2) it provides a visual way of communicating those patterns to a broad audience, quickly and dramatically. The central value of a map is that it tells a story about what is happening in our communities. This understanding supports decision making and consensus building and translates into improved program design, policy development, organizing, and advocacy.

### Community Mapping: A Visual Narrative

*Community mapping is a vibrant way of telling a neighborhood's story. It can highlight the rich array of community assets, display the concentration of childhood asthma, analyze the relationship between income and the location of services, or document vacant lots and buildings.*

The products of community mapping can take several forms. *Context maps* represent one or a few variables by a broad unit of geography (for example, income level by census tract). *Display maps* are more complex, illustrating single or multiple variables by smaller units of geography (such as the condition of individual properties at the parcel level). Analytical maps are the most complex, layering and analyzing multiple variables by various levels of geography. An analytical map might combine income at the census-tract level and condition of individual properties at the parcel level and highlight how the two variables relate to each other.

Community maps can be hand-drawn or computer-generated. Some complex computer-generated maps are also interactive, using Internet technologies that allow participants to analyze data and create other maps based on the locations and kinds of data that interest them. Increasingly, community practitioners are using computer software such as geographic information systems (GIS) for creating maps and analyzing data. As defined by the U.S. Geological Survey, GIS are "computer system(s) capable of assembling, storing, manipulating, and displaying geographically referenced information—data identified according to location" (U.S. Geological Survey 2003). GIS are not just tools for making maps or visually displaying data; they are used for analyzing many layers of data, allowing users to see information in new ways. They can illustrate data for a single point in time or show changes over time. The term *GIS* usually refers to the type of software used, while *GIS application* describes how a particular organization uses that software to analyze and map its own data.

### How to Use Community Mapping

Community mapping involves five broad steps, some of which can be implemented simultaneously. The process begins and ends with local communities, and each step builds on the information obtained in a previous step.

#### STEP 1: IDENTIFY COMMUNITY ISSUES AND BUILD A COMMUNITY MAPPING COLLABORATIVE

All community mapping efforts start with community-based organizations and residents and their in-depth understanding of community conditions, assets, and problems. Community knowledge is used to identify issues and problems; set benchmarks, goals, and outcomes; locate opportunities for revitalization; frame data-gathering efforts; determine the appropriate types of geography and maps; and use maps for community-building purposes. By designing and leading the mapping process, community residents and organizations are better positioned to ensure that the maps offer community benefits and accurately reflect community needs. Community leadership also promotes community values in the mapping process and better equips community groups to use the resulting maps for advocacy and organizing purposes.

#### STEP 2: DETERMINE THE APPROPRIATE GEOGRAPHY

Selecting the appropriate geographies is one of the first decisions in the mapping process. Community mapping projects can use a range of geographic units for mapping, ranging from individual parcels to census tracts to entire neighborhoods. Most initiatives will include several different geographies, from parcels to census tracts. The smaller the geography, the more detailed the data, but the more difficult it is to acquire.

### STEP 3: COLLECT DATA

Community mapping initiatives are only as strong as the data on which the maps are built. Maps that are most useful in a community context will likely consist of information from many sources. There are four major data types used in community mapping projects: public statistics, commercial data, administrative data, and survey data.

*Public statistics.* Census data are the primary source of public data for community mapping. They can be categorized into five major groups: demographics, socioeconomic characteristics, housing, business and economy, and transportation. The American Factfinder (http://factfinder.census.gov/servlet/BasicFactsServlet) is particularly useful for creating thematic maps and setting the geographic area and the specific census characteristics to be mapped.

*Administrative data.* Administrative data collected by state and local government agencies (such as tax assessors, police departments, city agencies, zoning offices, and school districts) are key inputs for community mapping projects. These data are usually available for small levels of geography (smaller than census tracts) and often for parcel-level mapping.

*Commercial data.* Data are available for sale from companies such as DataQuick and Dun and Bradstreet, and real estate brokers and others seeking current data about available properties often use them. This information is expensive, however, so only a few community mapping efforts use this resource.

*Original data: Surveys.* Many GIS projects augment public and administrative data with information that community organizations collect themselves. Such original data collection is the basis of many asset mapping programs in which community groups and residents map local assets and resources. Data may be collected about assets such as social networks, health, recreation facilities, volunteer opportunities, trees and green space, murals, and community gathering sites. They can be gathered by volunteers, including youths, students, and residents. For original data collection to be most useful, data collectors must know why they are collecting the information and how it will be used.

### STEP 4: CREATE MAPS USING GIS

Most GIS mapping projects require a significant technology investment. There are five components of GIS:

*Hardware*. Hardware is the physical computer on which GIS operates. GIS software runs on a wide range of hardware types, from centralized computer servers to desktop computers. You do not have to buy a special kind of computer to run GIS. Because GIS requires a very large amount of memory, however, it is often a good idea to dedicate a computer to the project.

*Software*. GIS software provides the functions and tools needed to store, analyze, and display geographic information. See *http://www.geoplan.ufl.edu/software.html* for a comprehensive review of GIS software packages.

*Data*. Data are the most important ingredients of GIS projects. GIS transforms tabular data bases into layered geographic information or maps.

*People*. GIS technology is of limited value without the involvement of people who have the capacity to manage it and develop plans for applying it to real-world problems.

*Methods*. A successful GIS project operates according to a well-designed working collaborative and implementation plan.

As noted, mapping community data requires not only investments in hardware and software but also staff support. For most community groups, developing the in-house technological capacity is too expensive. Therefore, many community organizations develop partnerships with technology or mapping intermediaries, such as universities, to maintain GIS technology.

Because community mapping projects often use computers and the Internet, low-income and low-wealth communities may need to strengthen their technology infrastructure. Even though community groups are not expected to build and maintain GIS applications, they must have the technological capacity to be informed partners and users of these systems. Building organizational and community capacity to use technology is a challenging endeavor.

### STEP 5: USE MAPS TO PROMOTE COMMUNITY BUILDING AND NEIGHBORHOOD REVITALIZATION

The ultimate purpose of community mapping is to improve programs, policy advocacy, and research. Effective community groups will use GIS outputs and maps as a foundation for campaigns to promote community building and equitable development. In this step of the mapping process, community organizations transform data and spatial analysis into action.

### Resources

Craig, W. J., T. M. Harris, and D. Weiner, eds. 2002. *Community Participation and Geographic Information Systems*. London: Taylor and Francis.

Gravlee, C. C. 2002. "Mobile Computer-Assisted Personal Interviewing with Handheld Computers: The Entryware System 3.0." *Field Methods* 14, no. 3: 322–36.

Kirschenbaum, J., and L. Russ. 2002. *Community Mapping: Using Geographic Data for Neighborhood Revitalization*. Oakland, Calif.: PolicyLink.

## References

U.S. Geological Survey. 2003. "Geographic Information Systems." http://erg.usgs.gov/isb/pubs/gis_poster/.

# Appendix 7

# Criteria for Creating Triggers or Codes

*Editor's note:* As discussed in chapters 2 and 12, Brazilian adult educator Paulo Freire's education for critical consciousness has become an important approach in community organizing around the world, particularly with low-income and less educated groups. As in other popular education methods, one step in the Freirian approach involves the development of triggers or codes, which are based on themes that emerge in group discussion and are presented back to the group to facilitate deeper dialogue about root causes, other consequences of the issue or problem, and action plans to bring about change. Here, Freirian scholar and educator Nina Wallerstein presents her own tips for the selection and development of triggers that can facilitate this process in either classroom or community settings.

To help facilitate groups in developing triggers or codes, the following steps may be helpful.

1. Identify the issue that you want to address. This issue should be a problem that people can relate to on an emotional and social level. It should be an issue that will trigger full participation in the discussion. In choosing an issue, think about the following criteria:

    a.  It should be familiar to your class or community participants and should represent a problem that people care about and want to solve;

    b.  It should include both a personal and a socio-cultural dimension, so that discussion can lead to both personal and social actions to change the situation; and

Reprinted by permission of the author.

    c.   It should not present an overwhelming problem, but should enable participants during the discussion to strategize short- or long-term actions for change.

2. Identify the physical form that will best portray this issue: a socio-drama, written role-play, song, slide or series of slides, video segment, or picture. Good visual triggers contain people so that discussion participants can imagine what the people in the picture might be feeling. Juxtaposition of images also works to present the multiple sides of an issue.

3. Role-plays or socio-dramas can be easily developed with the following steps:
       a.   Brainstorm a list of possible feelings or reactions to the issue.
       b.   Decide on each character who will represent the different feelings or reactions. (It is best to have a minimum of three characters with three points of view. With two characters, the problem can become too polarized for people to identify solutions.)
       c.   Create the scripts for each character. This script can be either written out verbatim or sketched out as an outline.
       d.   Remember not to write a solution into the script, but only present the problem. The action strategies should come out of the group discussion following the role-play or socio-drama.
       e.   Keep it short. Each role-play or socio-drama should last no more than 5 or 10 minutes.

# Appendix 8      A Checklist for Action

The following checklist will become so routine that these questions will frame your perspective of any setting for action. Your need to answer these questions will guide everything you do, and your ability to answer them will powerfully increase the likelihood of your success.

- From whom do we want to get a response?
- What responses do we want to get?
- What action or series of actions has the best chance of producing that response?
- Are the members of our organization able and willing to take these actions?
- How do the actions we decide to take lead to the needed development of our organization?
- How do our actions produce immediate gains in a way that helps us achieve our long-term goals?
- Is everything we are doing relevant to the outcomes we want to produce?
- How will we assess the effectiveness of our chosen approach to help refine the next steps we should take?
- What are we doing to keep this interesting?

BARBARA ISRAEL
AMY A. SCHULZ
EDITH PARKER
ADAM BECKER

Scale for Measuring
Perceptions of Control at the
Individual, Organizational,
Neighborhood, and
Beyond-the-Neighborhood
*Appendix 9* Levels

*Note from Barbara Israel:* My colleagues at the University of Michigan and I initially developed the Perceived Control Scale with respondents from Detroit, Michigan, who are primarily of African American or European American descent (Israel et al. 1994, Schulz et al. 1995). The Revised Perceived Control Scale presented here is a revision of this earlier scale and has been tested with African American women living on the east side of Detroit as part of a longitudinal, community-based, participatory research project known as the Eastside Village Health Worker Partnership (Becker et al. 2002, Schulz et al. 1998, Schulz et al. 2003).

The scale assesses individual perceptions of control or influence at four levels of analysis—individual, organizational, neighborhood, and beyond the neighborhood. In accordance with our conceptualization of empowerment across all four levels, the intent of the items at the individual level is to assess perceptions of individual influence over decisions that affect the individual's life in general. At the organizational and neighborhood levels, the intent is to assess both perceptions of individual influence within an organizational and neighborhood context and the perceived influence of the organization and neighborhood. Items measuring perceived control beyond the neighborhood level are intended to assess the perceptions of influence of the neighborhood in broader areas, such as the city, state, and national levels (Becker et al. 2002). Questions measuring perceived con-

Reprinted by permission of the authors.

trol at the organizational level pertain to the organization that respondents identify as being most important to them.

The scale provides a partial measure of empowerment, examining individual perceptions of control or influence at multiple levels. It does not, however, measure the development of conscientization, or critical consciousness (see chapters 2 and 12), nor does it assess the broader social, political, economic, and cultural contexts that affect empowerment. The scale is further limited in that it does not measure actual control or obtain a collective assessment, at the organizational, neighborhood, or beyond the neighborhood levels of perceived or actual control. For these reasons, we strongly suggest that this survey instrument be used in combination with qualitative approaches such as focus groups, community observations, and in-depth semistructured interviews. Finally, concepts of neighborhood, community, control, and empowerment may differ across cultures and regions; and these differences should be taken into account when the scale is adapted to other areas or population groups.

Despite these limitations, the perceived control indices presented here have considerable potential use for health educators and other social change professionals engaged in empowerment interventions. See Israel et al. (1994) and Becker et al. (2002) for a more detailed look at the instrument's conceptual grounding and development, its strengths and limitations, and its applications in the field.

### Revised Perceived Control Scale Items: Multiple Levels of Empowerment Indices

For the first nine items, the interviewer asked the participants: "For each of the following, please tell me whether you agree strongly, agree somewhat, disagree somewhat, or disagree strongly."

1. I can influence decisions that affect my life.
2. I am satisfied with the amount of influence I have over decisions that affect my life.
3. I can influence decisions that affect my neighborhood.
4. I am satisfied with the amount of influence I have over decisions that affect my neighborhood.
5. By working together with others in my neighborhood, I can influence decisions that affect my neighborhood.
6. My neighborhood has influence over things that affect my life.
7. By working together, people in my neighborhood can influence decisions that affect the neighborhood.
8. People in this neighborhood have connections to people who can influence what happens outside the neighborhood.
9. People in my neighborhood work together to influence decisions at the city, state or national level.

Participants were asked a number of general questions about organizational membership. For the last five items of the Revised Perceived Control Scale, the interviewer asked the participants: "Thinking about the organization that you identified as most important to you, would you say that you agree strongly, agree somewhat, disagree somewhat, or disagree strongly with the following statements?"

10. I can influence the decisions that this organization makes.
11. This organization has influence over decisions that affect my life.
12. This organization is effective in achieving its goals.
13. This organization can influence decisions that affect the neighborhood or community.
14. I am satisfied with the amount of influence I have over decisions that this organization makes.

### Indices

- Perceived control at the individual level includes items 1 and 2 above (alpha=.61).
- Perceived control at the organizational level includes items 10 through 14 above (alpha=.67).
- Perceived control at the neighborhood level includes items 3 through 7 above (alpha=.77).
- Perceived control beyond the neighborhood level includes items 8 and 9 above (alpha=.64).
- Perceived control at multiple levels includes all 14 items above (alpha=.77).

(The alpha coefficients presented here were generated from the longitudinal survey questionnaire administered as part of the Eastside Village Health Worker Partnership [Becker et al. 2002]).

### References

Becker, A. B., B. A. Israel, A. J. Schulz, E. A. Parker, and L. Klem. 2002. "Predictors of Perceived Control among African American Women in Detroit: Exploring Empowerment as a Multi-Level Construct." *Health Education and Behavior* 29, no. 6: 699–715.

Israel, B. A., B. N. Checkoway, A. J. Schulz, and M. A. Zimmerman. 1994. "Health Education and Community Empowerment: Conceptualizing and Measuring Perceptions of Individual, Organizational, and Community Control." *Health Education Quarterly* 21, no. 2: 149–70.

Schulz, A. J., B. A. Israel, E. A. Parker, M. Lockett, Y. Hill, and R. Wills. 2003. "Engaging Women in Community-Based Participatory Research for Health: The East Side Village Health Worker Partnership." In *Community-Based Participatory Research for Health*, edited by M. Minkler and N. Wallerstein, 293–315. San Francisco: Jossey-Bass.

Schulz, A., B. A. Israel, M. Zimmerman, and B. Checkoway. 1995. "Empowerment As a Multi-Level Construct: Perceived Control at the Individual, Organizational and Community Levels." *Health Education Research* 10, no. 3: 309–27.

Schulz, A. J., E. A. Parker, B. A. Israel, A. B. Becker, B. Maciak, and R. Hollis. 1998. "Conducting a Participatory Community-Based Survey: Collecting and Interpreting Data for a Community Health Intervention on Detroit's East Side." *Journal of Public Health Management and Practice* 4, no. 2: 10–24.

# Appendix 10

# Ten Principles for Effective Advocacy Campaigns

1. Communicate values. Effective advocacy communication is predicated upon the strong, clear assertion of basic values, moral authority, and leadership.

2. American political discourse is fundamentally oppositional. People are more comfortable being against something than for something.

3. Most issues are decided by winning over the undecided. Typically, the percentage on one side of an issue is offset by a roughly equivalent percentage on the other side. It is the undecided or conflicted percentage left in the middle that determines the outcome.

4. More than anything else, Americans want to be on the winning side. The dominant factor influencing the undecided to choose one side or another is the perception that they're joining the winning side. So for advocacy campaigns, acting like a winner—projecting confidence, asserting the moral high ground, aggressively confronting the opposition—is a prerequisite to winning.

5. Make enemies, not friends. Identify the opposition, and attack their motives. Point your finger at them, and name names.

6. American mass culture is fundamentally alienating and disempowering. Most Americans don't feel they can make a difference or that they count, and they feel unqualified or unprepared to make important decisions about complex social questions. The key is to educate, empower, and motivate your target audiences.

Reprinted from a handout distributed by the Public Media Center, by permission of the author.

7. Successful advocacy and social marketing campaigns, which generally have limited budgets, mainly utilize communications strategies based on social diffusion through opinion leaders and not on mass media. Effective social policy movements develop through the creation of substantive messages which empower, challenge, and target a few key audiences that, in turn, influence larger constituencies.

8. Responsible extremism sets the agenda. To move the media, you must communicate as responsible extremists, not as reasonable moderates.

9. Social consensus isn't permanent and must continually be asserted and defended. Social advocacy is an ongoing process that doesn't end with the passage of a law or resolution of a specific problem.

10. In the same way that biological diversity is essential to planetary survival, strategic diversity is critical to successful social movements. Multiple, independent advocacy campaigns on a single issue should be encouraged, while centralized monocultural efforts should be avoided.

# Appendix 11

# Ten Commandments of Community-Based Research

1. Thou shalt not define, design, nor commit community research without consulting the community!

2. As ye value outcomes, so shall ye value processes!

3. When faced with a choice between community objectives and the satisfaction of intellectual curiosity, thou shalt hold community objectives to be the higher good!

4. Thou shalt not covet the community's data!

5. Thou shalt not commit analysis of community data without community input!

6. Thou shalt not bear false witness to, or concerning members of the community!

7. Thou shalt not release community research findings before the community is consulted (premature exposition)!

8. Thou shalt train and hire community people to perform community research functions!

9. Thou shalt not violate confidentiality!

10. Thou shalt freely confess thyself to be biased and thine hypotheses and methodologies to be likewise!

Reprinted by permission of the author.

# About the Contributors

ADAM BECKER, Ph.D., is an assistant professor in the Department of Community Health Sciences at Tulane University. His current projects include a participatory investigation with high school students to explore and address root causes of violence, a participatory evaluation emphasizing youth leadership development as an HIV prevention strategy among young African American men who have sex with men, and a grounded theory study of internal and external factors in the development of community-based organizational capacity.

ANGELA GLOVER BLACKWELL is founder and president of PolicyLink, a national nonprofit organization dedicated to advancing a new generation of policies that achieve economic and social equity guided by the wisdom, voice, and experience of local constituencies. Ms. Blackwell previously served as senior vice president of the Rockefeller Foundation, where she directed the foundation's domestic and cultural divisions and developed programs centered on issues of leadership, inclusion, race, and policy. She also founded the innovative Urban Strategies Council in Oakland, California, and worked as a partner with Public Advocates, a nationally known public interest law firm. Ms. Blackwell is co-author of *Searching for the Uncommon Common Ground: New Dimensions on Race in America* (Norton 2002). She received her undergraduate degree from Howard University and her law degree from the University of California, Berkeley.

LYNN BLANCHARD is a research assistant professor in the Department of Pediatrics at the University of North Carolina School of Medicine. She holds a joint appointment as a lecturer in health behavior and health education at the School of Public Health, where she received her master's and doctorate degrees in public health. A former doctoral fellow at the Bush Institute for Child and Family Health Policy, her current research interests include evaluation of the efficacy of peer support for parents of young children with special needs, community attitudes toward HIV vaccine trials, and parent-professional partnerships.

CHERIE R. BROWN is founder and executive director of the National Coalition Building Institute in Washington, D.C., a leadership training organiziation that trains community leaders, government officials, and campus administrators. She received a master's degree of education in counseling and consulting psychology from Harvard

University and for twenty years has been doing training in prejudice reduction and coalition building in the United States, Canada, Europe, and the Middle East. Her publications and videos include *The Art of Coalition Building: A Guide for Community Leaders* (American Jewish Committee 1984) and *Working It Out: Blacks and Jews on the College Campus* (National Coalition Building Institute 1985).

LELAND BROWN, M.P.H., is founder and director of the Global Bridges Group, a minority-owned business whose mission is to enhance collaboration, promote dialogue, and increase understanding among diverse communities, cultures, and institutions. He currently works with the California Center for Public Dispute Resolution on issues including land use, air quality, and environmental concerns. Mr. Brown teaches a graduate course on conflict resolution at John F. Kennedy University. He received his master's degree in health policy and planning from the School of Public Health, University of California, Berkeley.

FRANCES D. BUTTERFOSS is professor and head of the Health Promotion and Disease Prevention Section at the Center for Pediatric Research in Norfolk, Virginia, a joint program of the Children's Hospital of the King's Daughters and Eastern Virginia Medical School. She received her Ph.D. from the Norman School of Public Health at the University of South Carolina at Columbia. Butterfoss coordinates local child health and statewide immunization coalitions and provides technical assistance and training for health coalitions nationwide. Her research focuses on evaluating the effectiveness of community coalitions for health promotion.

CHRISTINA GOETTE CARPENTER is the Youth POWER coordinator in the community health education section of the San Francisco Department of Public Health. She received her B.A. in sociology from the University of California, Berkeley, and her M.P.H. from the Department of Health Sciences at San Jose State University.

RAYMOND A. COLMENAR is a senior associate at PolicyLink in Oakland, California. Previously, he was a program officer in the Rockefeller Foundation's Equal Opportunity Division, where he developed and implemented various employment and community building initiatives. He also is the former director of the South of Market Problem Solving Council in San Francisco and a former policy analyst for the city and county's department of human services, where he analyzed welfare and other social policies. Mr. Colmenar has a master of public policy degree from the Goldman School of Public Policy at the University of California, Berkeley, and a bachelor of arts degree in Management Science from the University of California, San Diego. He serves on the board of LISTEN, Inc., a national youth leadership intermediary, and is an advisor to the Aspen Institute's Roundtable on Comprehensive Community Initiatives' Race and Community Revitalization Project.

CHRIS M. COOMBE is a Ph.D. candidate in health behavior and health education in the School of Public Health at the University of Michigan and a National Institute of Mental Health fellow at the Institute for Social Research. She holds a master's degree in public health from the School of Public Health, University of California, Berkeley. With more than twenty-five years of community experience,

Coombe focuses on community-based participatory research and the effects of social inequalities on health.

GALEN EL-ASKARI, M.P.H., is a partner in Walton El-Askari and Associates, which provides consultation services in the areas of health education, community organizing and community development, designing and planning programs, administration, and evaluation. Her primary experience, skills, and interests lie in developing and evaluating programs that build the capacities of communities and agencies to leverage resources to influence local policies and institutions to improve the quality of life for children and families.

EUGENIA ENG is professor of health behavior and health education and director of the M.P.H. degree program and the Community Health Scholars Postdoctoral Program in the School of Public Health at the University of North Carolina at Chapel Hill. With funding from the National Institutes of Health and private foundations, she has developed and tested a lay health advisor model to address socially stigmatizing health problems such as pesticide poisoning, breast cancer, and sexually transmitted diseases. Eng has helped practitioners and researchers around the world design and conduct the action-oriented community diagnosis, a community assessment procedure that combines the principles of community organizing with those of the social ecological framework for health promotion.

ROBERT FISHER is professor in the School of Social Work and director of urban and community studies at the University of Connecticut. He received his Ph.D. in urban and social history from New York University and his B.A. in history from Rutgers University. He is the author of *Let the People Decide: Neighborhood Organizing in America* (Twayne 1994) and co-editor of *Mobilizing the Community: Local Politics in the Era of the Global City* (Sage 1993).

NICHOLAS FREUDENBERG is a distinguished professor and director of urban public health at Hunter College, City University of New York. He was a founding member of the New York City Coalition to End Lead Poisoning and participated in its activities throughout the 1980s. For the past twenty-five years, he has worked with communities in New York City on a variety of public health and policy issues, including asthma, environmental hazards, HIV, and substance abuse.

ROBERT M. GOODMAN, Ph.D., M.P.H., M.A., is the director of the multidisciplinary masters of public health program and professor at the Graduate School of Public Health at the University of Pittsburgh. Formerly, he was Usdin Family Professor in Community Health Sciences at the Tulane University School of Public Health and Tropical Medicine. He directed the Center for Community Research at the Wake Forest University School of Medicine and was a faculty member at the University of North Carolina and the University of South Carolina schools of public health. Dr. Goodman has written extensively on issues concerning community health development, community capacity, community coalitions, evaluation methods, organizational development, and the institutionalization of health programs. He has been the principal investigator and evaluator on projects for the Centers for

Disease Control, the National Cancer Institute, the Centers for Substance Abuse Prevention, the Children's Defense Fund, and several state health departments.

HERBERT CHAO GUNTHER has been president and chief executive officer of Public Media Center, the nation's leading nonprofit strategic marketing, advocacy, and communications agency, since its founding in 1974. The agency builds partnerships with nonprofit organizations and philanthropic foundations to develop campaigns that raise public awareness of health, social, environmental, and other issues, including population, gender equity, health care access, AIDS education, media fairness, corporate responsibility, social justice, and human and civil rights. All agency initiatives and programs reflect a fundamental institutional commitment to strengthening democratic values and civil society.

LORRAINE M. GUTIERREZ is a professor with a joint appointment in the School of Social Work and the Department of Psychology at the University of Michigan, Ann Arbor. She also directs the Edward Ginsberg Center for Community Service and Learning. Gutierrez received her Ph.D. in social work and psychology at the University of Michigan. Her research focuses on multicultural issues in communities and organizations. Current projects include community-based research on technology access for Latino communities, identification of multicultural issues in community practice, and methods for multicultural social work education. Gutierrez has published on topics such as empowerment practice and women of color.

TREVOR HANCOCK is a public health physician and health promotion consultant based in Victoria, British Columbia. Much of his work in the past twenty years has been in the area of healthy cities and communities, an approach he helped to pioneer. In the early 1980s he assisted in designing the first community health survey and health status report for the city of Toronto. As an adviser to the World Health Organization in Europe, he helped organize the first technical workshop on healthy city indicators in Barcelona in 1987 and has maintained his interest in the subject ever since. In 1999 he co-authored with Ronald Labonte and Rick Edwards a major review for Health Canada of population health indicators at the community level.

SONJA HERBERT conducts media advocacy trainings and strategic consultations with the Berkeley Media Studies Group, a project of the Public Health Institute. She received her master's degree in public health from the University of California, Berkeley. Her background includes federal health policy advocacy with the Sexuality Information and Education Council of the United States, and she has chaired the board of directors of the National Women's Health Network. Committed to harnessing the power of the Internet for social change, Sonja leads workshops on community organizing on line and teaches web design to teenagers in a community-based digital divide program.

MARK S. HOMAN, M.S.W, has been a full-time faculty member in the Social Services Department of Pima Community College since 1978 and currently serves as department chair. He also is an adjunct faculty member in the Department of Sociology and Social Work at Northern Arizona University and in the Graduate School of Social Work at Arizona State University. A strong advocate of community empowerment, he has worked for twenty-five years with diverse populations in urban, rural, and reservation communities on a broad range of issues, including neighborhood stabilization and empowerment, hunger, reproductive rights, children with special health needs, family planning, and community development programs. He is the author of *Promoting Community Change: Making it Happen in the Real World* (Wadsworth 2003) and *Rules of the Game: Lessons from the Field of Community Change* (Wadsworth 1998).

BARBARA ISRAEL, Dr.P.H., M.P.H., is a professor in the Department of Health Behavior and Health Education at the University of Michigan School of Public Health and is deputy editor of the journal *Health Education and Behavior*. She received her doctorate in public health from the University of North Carolina at Chapel Hill. Dr. Israel has published widely in the areas of community-based participatory research, community empowerment, evaluation, stress and health, and social networks. She has extensive experience conducting community-based participatory research in collaboration with partners in diverse ethnic communities.

DANIEL KASS is a research scientist with the Environmental and Occupational Disease Epidemiology Unit of the New York City Department of Health and Mental Hygiene, where he conducts research on housing and health. He holds a master's degree from the School of Public Health at the University of California, Los Angeles, and is completing a doctorate in public policy at New York University.

JOSH KIRSCHENBAUM coordinates PolicyLink's Community Building in the Digital Age initiative, an effort to understand how information technology can be used as a neighborhood revitalization tool. Previously, he was at the University of California, Berkeley, where he directed a defense conversion research program and managed partnerships between the university and the city of Oakland. He holds a B.A. from Brown University and a master's degree in city and regional planning from the University of California, Berkeley.

SUSAN KLITZMAN is an associate professor in and director of the Urban Public Health Program at Hunter College, City University of New York. During the late 1990s, she managed the Childhood Lead Poisoning Prevention Program at the New York City Department of Health. Currently, she is a member of the New York City Board of Health.

JOHN P. KRETZMANN is co-director of the Asset-Based Community Development Institute at Northwestern University's Institute for Policy Research. A former community developer and organizer, he writes on community building themes and is co-author of *Building Communities from the Inside Out: A Path toward Finding and Mobilizing a Community's Assets* (ACTA 1997), one of the field's most cited works.

RONALD LABONTE has worked in community health promotion for more than twenty-five years in settings ranging from local government to community groups to labor unions to United Nations agencies. He is currently director of the Saskatchewan

Population Health and Evaluation Research Unit, professor of community health and epidemiology at the University of Saskatchewan, and professor of kinesiology and health studies at the University of Regina. He received his Ph.D. from the University of Toronto.

LAUREN LARIN is a research assistant to Dr. Marc Pilisuk at the Saybrook Graduate School and Research Center in San Francisco and a graduate of the Peace and Conflict Studies Program at the University of California, Berkeley.

EDITH A. LEWIS is an associate professor in the School of Social Work at the University of Michigan, Ann Arbor. She received her master's degree in social work from the University of Minnesota and her Ph.D. in social welfare from the University of Wisconsin–Madison, where she also held an appointment as lecturer. Her current research interests include women's empowerment, community organizing with people of color, and the incorporation of African American structures and traditional strengths into group work and other intervention approaches.

JOANN McALLISTER, Ph.D., has been involved with criminal justice and community organizations in the development and evaluation of batterer intervention and domestic violence prevention programs since 1993. Currently, she evaluates prevention and intervention programs for youth and adults; conducts research on batterer intervention and criminal justice responses to domestic violence; and trains court probation, social, and medical service personnel to screen and intervene with domestic violence offenders. She is the co-author of Doing Democracy (New Society Press), a guide to social movement theory and practice, and an adjunct faculty member at Saybrook Graduate School and Research Center in San Francisco.

MARIAN McDONALD is associate director for minority and women's health for the National Center for Infectious Diseases at the Centers for Disease Control and Prevention in Atlanta. Active in minority health and women's health for three decades, she was formerly a health education professor at Tulane University's School of Public Health and Tropical Medicine, where she taught courses on community organization and race, gender, and ethnicity in health promotion. A poet and lifelong cultural worker, her poetry has appeared in numerous publications in the Americas.

JOHN L. McKNIGHT is director of the community studies program at the Institute for Policy Research at Northwestern University, where he is a professor in both the School of Speech and the School of Education and Social Policy. He has worked with communities across the United States and Canada and is author of *The Careless Society: Community and Its Counterfeits* and co-author of the workbook *Building Community from the Inside Out*.

MEREDITH MINKLER, Dr.P.H., is professor of health and social behavior and director of the Dr.P.H. Program at the School of Public Health, University of California, Berkeley. She has more than twenty-five years of experience in working with underserved communities on community-identified issues through community building, community organizing, and community-based participatory research. Her current research interests include local efforts to foster community-based participatory research among diverse groups and document the impact of participatory research on public policy. Dr. Minkler is co-author or editor of six books and more than one hundred articles and book chapters about community-based participatory research, community health education, health promotion, community building, and gerontology, including *Forgotten Caregivers: Grandmothers Raising Children of the Crack Cocaine Epidemic* (with Kathleen M. Roe; Sage 1993), *Critical Perspectives on Aging* (with Carroll L. Estes; Baywood 1998), and *Community Based Participatory Research for Health* (with Nina Wallerstein; Jossey-Bass 2003).

EDITH PARKER, Dr.P.H., M.P.H., is an associate professor in the Department of Health Behavior and Health Education at the University of Michigan School of Public Health. She received her master's and doctoral degrees from the University of North Carolina School of Public Health. Her work focuses on the development, implementation, and evaluation of community-based participatory public health interventions. She is currently involved with the Community Action against Asthma project, the Eastside Village Health Worker Project, and the Detroit Community–Academic Urban Research Center, all located in Detroit.

CHERI PIES is currently the director of family, maternal, and child health programs for Contra Costa Health Services in the Public Health Division and a clinical associate professor at the School of Public Health, University of California, Berkeley. She received her master's degree in social work from Boston University and her master's and doctoral degrees in public health from the School of Public Health at the University of California, Berkeley. Dr. Pies has served as a consultant in AIDS prevention and education, women's health issues, family planning and reproductive technologies, the development and evaluation of community-based programs, and participatory action research activities. Her research interests include reproductive ethics, lesbian and gay health care concerns, and the use of qualitative methodologies in public health research.

MARC PILISUK is professor emeritus at the University of California, Davis and Berkeley, and professor at the Saybrook Graduate School and Research Center in San Francisco. He received his doctorate in clinical and social psychology from the University of Michigan. Dr. Pilisuk combines research and activism in the areas of conflict resolution, social support, health and caring, and environmental and social justice. His most recent co-authored books include *The Healing Web: Social Networks and Human Survival* (University Press of New England 1986).

KATHLEEN M. ROE is professor and chair of the Department of Health Sciences, San Jose State University, and director of the Center for Community Health Studies. She received master's and doctoral degrees from the School of Public Health at the University of California, Berkeley, where she also served as lecturer. Roe is a consultant to health education programs on the local and national levels and to state and local health departments. Her research interests include qualitative methodologies, contemporary women's history, children's perceptions of AIDS, grandparent caregiving, and program evaluation. Recent publications include the co-authored book *Grandmothers As Caregivers: Raising Children of the Crack Cocaine Epidemic* (Sage 1993).

KEVIN ROE, M.P.H., is the community organizer for Magnet, a gay men's health and community center in San Francisco's Castro District. For the past seven years, as part of the Community Health Studies Group, he has served as one of the evaluators for San Francisco's HIV prevention community planning process. He is the HIV/AIDS trainer for the Institute for Community Health Outreach's state community health outreach worker certification program and has worked on the Project Inform National HIV Treatment Hotline since 1995. He received his master's degree in public health from San Jose State University in 2003.

BETH ROSENTHAL is a consultant, researcher, and trainer in organizational, community, and collaboration development for nonprofits, government agencies, and foundations. Based in New York City, she received her M.S. from Columbia University. Her consulting firm, Collaboration and Change, builds capacity for advocacy, strategic partnerships, community organizing, and leadership development. Ms. Rosenthal is on the faculty of New York University's Wagner School of Public Service. Her publications include the workbook *Strategic Partnerships: How to Create and Maintain Interorganizational Collaborations and Coalitions* (Education Center for Community Organizing, Hunter College School of Social Work 1994).

JACK ROTHMAN is professor emeritus of social welfare in the School of Public Policy and Social Research at the University of California, Los Angeles. He received his doctorate from Columbia University and taught for many years at the University of Michigan in the School of Social Work. Rothman's areas of research are community organizing, social planning research use, and intervention research. His latest publications are *Intervention Research: Design and Development for Human Service* and *Practice with Highly Vulnerable Clients: Case Management and Community-Based Service*.

LISA RUSS is the associate director of the Movement Strategy Center, where she provides support to youth empowerment organizations and coordinates a network of consultants who work with social justice groups. Previously, she worked in several neighborhood organizations in San Francisco, where she struggled to use GIS mapping to track neighborhood change during the dot-com boom, an experience that convinced her there must be a better way and inspired her to co-author the article reprinted in this book.

VICTORIA SANCHEZ, Dr.P.H., is an associate research scientist with the Pacific Institute for Research and Evaluation in Chapel Hill, North Carolina. She completed her doctorate at the School of Public Health at the University of North Carolina and her master's degree at the School of Public Health of the University of California, Berkeley. She has held numerous positions in community-based organizations and health departments, including program coordinator for the Adolescent Social Action Program dissemination grant in northern New Mexico.

JENNIFER SARCHÉ is currently leading the community education team in the HIV Research Section of the San Francisco Department of Public Health. She is a past program director for Building Bridges for Peace, an organization that builds communication and leadership skills among young women from the United States, Israel, and Palestine. Ms. Sarché holds a master's degree in public health from the University of California, Berkeley.

AMY A. SCHULZ is a research associate professor in the Department of Health Behavior and Health Education at the University of Michigan School of Public Health. Her current research focuses on social factors that contribute to health, with a particular focus on health disparities and urban communities. Her work emphasizes a community-based participatory approach, linking research with community-level interventions to address social conditions linked to health. She received her doctorate in sociology in 1994 and her master's degree in public health in 1981, both from the University of Michigan.

CINDY BERENSTEIN SIBLEY is as a part-time lecturer at California State's Hayward University and a counselor at an elementary school in Menlo Park. She has a B.A. in psychology from San Diego State University, an M.P.H. in community health education from San Jose State University, and an M.S. in educational psychology from Hayward University.

SUSAN STALL is an associate professor of sociology and women's studies at Northeastern Illinois University, Chicago. She is a community sociologist and activist who focuses on women's organizing, community building, and leadership development in both rural and urban settings. As an activist, she worked with residents in public housing to form the citywide advocacy organization, Chicago Housing Authority Residents Taking Action. She is co-author of *The Dignity of Resistance: Women Residents' Activism in Chicago Public Housing* (Cambridge University Press 2004).

LEE STAPLES is a clinical professor at Boston University School of Social Work, where he teaches community organizing and macro social work practice. He received his Ph.D. in sociology and social work from Boston University. Since the late 1960s, he has been engaged in numerous social change efforts as organizer, supervisor, staff director, trainer, consultant, coach, and educator. His work has included welfare rights, housing, child care, mental health consumers, labor, neighborhood, and public health organizing. Dr. Staples has done extensive training and consulting with nongovernment organizations in the Balkans and currently is involved in a variety of community organizing efforts, including immigrant rights, affordable housing, environmental justice, and mental patients' rights.

RANDY STOECKER is a professor of sociology at the University of Toledo. He has been doing community-based research since the mid-1980s, when a community activist made him agree to contribute something to the community in exchange for granting an interview. He works mostly with community organizing and development groups and with community Internet efforts, which includes managing the COMM-ORG web site and list serve (http://comm-org.utoledo.edu). He also publishes regularly on community-based research, community organizing and development, and community Internet.

MILDRED THOMPSON leads PolicyLink research documenting the value of community involvement in strengthening health delivery systems. She has participated in research and advocacy efforts focused on reducing health disparities and has co-authored academic journal articles and reports aimed at advancing effective strategies and promoting positive policy change. Previously, she served for ten years as an executive administrator with Alameda County Public Health Department. Ms. Thompson has an M.S.W. from New York University as well as a nursing degree and has taught at San Francisco State University and Mills College. She serves on several boards and commissions, including Alameda County's Children and Families Commission; Partnership for Public's Health; Girls, Inc; the African American Wellness Project; and the Zellerbach Family Foundation. She is a Robert Wood Johnson Urban Health Initiative fellow.

LILY VELARDE is the University of New Mexico's master's of public health practicum director and a founder of the Adolescent Social Action Program at the School of Medicine, University of New Mexico. She is active in Hispanic youth leadership programs and was a recent past president of the New Mexico Public Health Association. Velarde holds a master's degree in public administration and a Ph.D. from the University of New Mexico.

LAWRENCE WALLACK is professor in the School of Community Health and dean of the College of Urban and Public Affairs at Portland State University. He also is professor emeritus at the School of Public Health of the University of California, Berkeley, and a senior fellow at the Rockridge Group in Oakland, California. Dr. Wallack is primary author of *New for a Change* (Sage 1999) and *Media Advocacy and Public Health: Power for Prevention* (Sage 1993) as well as co-editor of *Mass Communication and Public Health: Complexities and Conflicts* (Sage 1990). He received his master's and doctoral degrees from the School of Public Health of the University of California, Berkeley, and has been a consultant for the World Health Organization and numerous other community, philanthropic, and government organizations.

NINA WALLERSTEIN is a professor in the Department of Family and Community Medicine and founder and director of the master's in public health program at the University of New Mexico. She received her doctoral and master's degrees in community health education at the School of Public Health of the University of California, Berkeley. For more than twenty-five years, she has been involved in empowerment, popular education, and participatory research with youth, women, tribes, and community building efforts. She is co-editor of *Community Based Participatory Research for Health* (Jossey-Bass 2003), co-author of *Participatory Evaluation Workbook for Community Initiatives: New Mexico Healthier Communities* (University of New Mexico and New Mexico Partnership for Healthier Communities 1997), and author of three adult education books and more than seventy-five articles and book chapters on participatory intervention research, adolescent health promotion, empowerment theory, and popular health education. Her current research interests focus on understanding and assessing the role of social capital and community capacity in tribal communities.

CHERYL L. WALTER, Ph.D., works for the California Institute on Human Services at Sonoma State University, where she is currently the lead evaluator for a federal grant to improve the special education system in California. In 2000, she completed her doctorate at the School of Social Welfare at the University of California, Berkeley, where she also received her M.S.W. and her M.P.H. Formerly a consultant to the Alameda County Health Care Services Agency, Walter was principal author of the overall design of the county's MediCal managed care plan. She also served as a board member and development director of the Women's Cancer Resource Center in Berkeley and executive director of the Gay and Lesbian Resource Center in Santa Barbara, California.

SHERYL WALTON, M.P.H., is the director of community capacity building at the Public Health Division of Berkeley's Health and Human Services Department and a partner in Walton El-Askari and Associates. A community health educator, she specializes in supporting residents, parents, community groups, and agencies seeking to build on the assets and strengths of low-income, multicultural communities to improve health and quality of life. She offers consultation in areas such as community assessment, leadership development, media and policy advocacy, training and curriculum development, and participatory research and evaluation.

ABRAHAM WANDERSMAN is professor of psychology at the University of South Carolina, Columbia. He received his Ph.D. from Cornell University, with specialization in social psychology, environmental psychology, and social organization and change. Wandersman was interim co-director of the Institute for Families and Society at the University of South Carolina. His research interests include environmental issues and community responses, citizen participation in community organizations and coalitions, and interagency collaboration. His publications include the co-authored *Prevention Plus III* (U.S. Department of Health and Human Services 1989) and the co-edited *Empowerment Evaluation: Knowledge and Tools for Self-Assessment and Accountability* (Sage 1996).

CAROLINE C. WANG is assistant professor of health behavior and health education at the School of Public Health, University of Michigan. She has directed and consulted on photovoice projects in rural China, Ann Arbor, Flint, and the San Francisco Bay Area and is co-editor of *Visual Voices: 100 Photographs of Village China by the Women of Yunnan Province* (Yunnan People's Publishing House 1995) and editor of *Strength to Be: Community Visions and Voices* (2000).

# Index